Translational Medicine and Drug Discovery

This book, edited by two leaders known for driving innovation in the field, focuses on the new discipline of translational medicine as it pertains to drug discovery and development within the pharmaceutical and biotechnology industries. Translational medicine seeks to translate biological and molecular knowledge of disease and how drugs work into innovative strategies that reduce the cost and increase the speed of delivering new medicines for patients. This book describes these general strategies, biomarker development, imaging tools, translational human models, and examples of their application to real-life drug discovery and development. The latest thinking is presented by researchers from many of the world's leading pharmaceutical companies, including Pfizer, Merck, Eli Lilly, Abbott, and Novartis, as well as from academic institutions and public–private partnerships that support translational research. This book is essential for anyone interested in translational medicine from a variety of backgrounds (university institutes, medical schools, and pharmaceutical companies) in addition to drug development researchers and decision makers.

Bruce H. Littman, MD, is the founder of Translational Medicine Associates, LLC, and was the Vice President and Global Head of Translation Medicine at Pfizer, Inc., where he worked for 19 years, first in Experimental Medicine and then in Translational Medicine before starting his own company. He has published and presented extensively in the areas of early drug development, biomarker qualification, and personalized medicine. He was former cochair and is a current member of the Inflammation and Immunity Steering Committee of the Biomarker Consortium. Prior to his pharmaceutical career, Dr. Littman was a faculty member of Virginia Commonwealth University School of Medicine for 13 years. He is a Founding Fellow of the American College of Rheumatology, former President of the Virginia Society of Rheumatologists, and a Fellow of the American College of Physicians.

Rajesh Krishna, PhD, FCP, FAAPS, is an area lead director in product value enhancement at Merck Research Laboratories. Dr. Krishna is the editor of three books on new drug development. In addition to authoring some 120 articles and oral/poster presentations, Dr. Krishna has served as a section editor for the *Journal of Clinical Pharmacology*, associate editor for *BMC Clinical Pharmacology*, and an editorial board member for *BMC Medicine*. He is a Fellow of the American College of Clinical Pharmacology and the American Association of Pharmaceutical Scientists, where he was the 2010 Chair of the Clinical Pharmacology and Translational Research section. He is an affiliate member of the Institute of Translational Medicine and Therapeutics at the University of Pennsylvania and an adjunct assistant professor in clinical pharmacology at Thomas Jefferson University.

Translational Medicine

and Drug Discovery

EDITED BY **BRUCE H. LITTMAN**

Translational Medicine Associates, LLC

RAJESH KRISHNA

Merck Research Laboratories

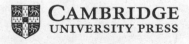

CAMBRIDGE
UNIVERSITY PRESS

32 Avenue of the Americas, New York NY 10013-2473, USA

Cambridge University Press is part of the University of Cambridge.

It furthers the University's mission by disseminating knowledge in the pursuit of education, learning and research at the highest international levels of excellence.

www.cambridge.org
Information on this title: www.cambridge.org/9781107435940

© Cambridge University Press 2011

First published 2011
First paperback edition 2014

A catalogue record for this publication is available from the British Library

Library of Congress Cataloguing in Publication data

Translational medicine and drug discovery / [edited by] Bruce H. Littman, Rajesh Krishna.
    p. ; cm.
Includes bibliographical references and index.
ISBN 978-0-521-88645-1 (hardback)
1. Drug development.   2. Molecular pharmacology.   I. Littman, Bruce H., 1944–
II. Krishna, Rajesh.   III. Title.
[DNLM: 1. Drug Discovery.   2. Translational Research – methods. QV 744]
RM301.25.T73   2011
615'.19–dc22   2010037116

ISBN 978-0-521-88645-1 Hardback
ISBN 978-1-107-43594-0 Paperback

Contents

Ole J. Bjerrum
    Department of Pharmacology and Pharmacotherapy
    Faculty of Pharmaceutical Sciences
    University of Copenhagen
    Denmark

Roberto A. Calle
    Cardiovascular, Metabolic, and Endocrine Diseases Research Unit
    Pfizer Pharmatherapeutics Research and Development
    Groton, CT

Jill Fiedler-Kelly
    Cognigen Corporation
    Williamsville, NY

Gregory Gaich
    Division of Endocrinology and Cardiovascular Discovery Research
        and Clinical Investigation
    Eli Lilly & Co.
    Indianapolis, IN

Thaddeus H. Grasela
    Cognigen Corporation
    Williamsville, NY

David B. Lee
    Deputy Director
    The Biomarkers Consortium
    Foundation for the National Institutes of Health
    Bethesda, MD

Hans H. Linden
    European Federation of Pharmaceutical Sciences
    EUFEPS Central Office
    Stockholm
    Sweden

Bruce H. Littman
    President
    Translational Medicine Associates, LLC
    Stonington, CT

Gerard J. Marek
    Abbott Laboratories
    Neuroscience Development
    Abbott Park, IL

John S. Millar
    Institute for Translational Medicine and Therapeutics
    Institute for Diabetes, Obesity, and Metabolism
    University of Pennsylvania
    Philadelphia, PA

David E. Moller
    Division of Endocrinology and Cardiovascular Discovery
        Research and Clinical Investigation
    Eli Lilly & Co.
    Indianapolis, IN

Adam J. Schwarz
    Lilly Research Laboratories
    Indianapolis, IN

Robert Slusser
    Rancho Palos Verdes, CA

Dominic G. Spinella
    Executive Director, Translational Medicine
    Pfizer, Inc.
    San Diego, CA

S. Aubrey Stoch
    Department of Clinical Pharmacology
    Merck Research Laboratories
    Rahway, NJ

Johannes T. Tauscher
Lilly Research Laboratories
Indianapolis, IN

Ann E. Taylor
Translational Medicine Diabetes and Metabolism
Novartis
Cambridge, MA

Mervyn Turner
Chief Strategy Officer
Merck & Co., Inc.
and
Senior Vice President of Emerging Markets
Merck Research Laboratories
Rahway, NJ

Elizabeth Gribble Walker
Director
Predictive Safety Testing Consortium Critical Path Institute
Tucson, AZ

David Wholley
Director
The Biomarkers Consortium
Foundation for the National Institutes of Health
Bethesda, MD

Drug discovery and development has evolved in an accelerated fashion during the latter half of the 20th century and the first decade of the 21st century from the serendipity of folk medicine and herbal remedies to a more refined observational and hypothesis-driven biological approach and finally to the present-day translational approach that relies on an understanding of disease and human biology at a molecular level. Advances in information, molecular and biomarker technologies, and quantitative systems pharmacology have further enabled this rapid evolution. Along with these important advances and changes, however, has come an unsustainable attrition rate that has increased the cost of discovering and developing new drugs and threatens the future of the pharmaceutical industry as we have known it. The combination of modern, science-driven translational drug discovery and development and unsustainable attrition rates has created a new reality that has had its greatest impact on the earliest stages of drug development. This reality is mandating changes in strategies, technologies, and disciplines in an effort to improve confidence and the success rate of new drug targets, mechanisms, and molecules. Ultimately, these changes are designed to affect the endgame: improved productivity in terms of new drug approvals for unmet medical needs at a sustainable cost from the modern drug discovery engine.

One of the most significant changes embraced by the pharmaceutical and biotech industry is the creation and evolution of the discipline of translational medicine. We hypothesize that the successful implementation of translational medicine strategies will herald an era in which, from the initial decision to pursue a specific drug target forward, the line of sight is on proof of concept and not just the nomination of a drug development candidate. The effective use of biomarkers will enable development decisions regarding early drug candidates based on human drug target validation for the disease, pharmacodynamics, proof of mechanism, and proof of concept for the drug target and molecule. Specifically, biomarkers can be leveraged to define what constitutes adequate target engagement and as decision-making tools to confirm three hypotheses regarding the target: (1) The relationship of target modulation to the biological changes that will result in a desirable effect in a disease population; (2) the ability of the compound to hit and modulate the target hard enough and long enough at a well-tolerated dose to test the concept; and (3) the level of efficacy and safety resulting from target modulation that is likely to be medically and commercially acceptable.

This book describes how the discipline of translational medicine has evolved to meet these drug development challenges and highlights current translational strategies and drug development paradigms across a diverse spectrum of therapeutic areas. Within Section I, experts define biomarkers and discuss the principles of the translational medicine discipline, describe the challenges and opportunities in translational paradigms unique to each disease area, and propose thoughtful solutions. Section II describes how biomarkers should be qualified to support the drug development process and how government and industry have responded to the needs and high costs of developing the tools and technologies required to develop new drugs efficiently and speed their delivery to patients. Finally, in Section III, we take a glimpse into the trends and changes needed for further success in the 21st century. An effort has been made in this volume to be transparent regarding cultural and management circumstances that must be dealt with and how companies should balance risk and drug development investments to be able to maximize the value from these translational medicine paradigms.

We expect that this volume will benefit drug discoverers and developers alike. Scientists in academia, regulatory institutions, and pharmaceutical industry laboratories, as well as those working on all aspects (chemistry, biology, physiology, pathophysiology, pharmacology, therapeutics) of translational discovery and clinical research, will find the book useful. Ultimately, we feel that it can serve as a useful training and educational tool for anyone interested in early drug development.

Bruce H. Littman, Stonington, CT
Rajesh Krishna, Rahway, NJ

**Translational Medicine
and Drug Discovery**

Translational Medicine: History, Principles, and Application in Drug Development

Translational Medicine: Definition, History, and Strategies

Bruce H. Littman

What is translational medicine? This discipline, although defined differently by various groups in academia, regulatory institutions, and industry, shares the fundamental vision of translational medicine, which is to efficiently and effectively translate basic scientific findings relevant to human disease into knowledge that benefits patients. Pfizer was one of the first pharmaceutical companies to embrace experimental medicine and translational medicine as a recognized discipline within the sphere of early drug development, and this author was intimately involved in the evolution of this discipline since its inception at this company. This chapter therefore describes the significance, role, and practice of translational medicine in drug development from a Pfizer perspective, although the concepts are considered to be widely applicable to drug development at any academic, public, or private institution. At Pfizer, translational medicine was defined as "the *integrated application* of innovative pharmacology tools, biomarkers, clinical methods, clinical technologies, and study designs to improve confidence in human drug targets and increase confidence in drug candidates, understand the therapeutic index in humans, enhance cost-effective decision making in exploratory development, and increase success in Phase 2 leading to a sustainable pipeline of new products." Because this book focuses on drug development, this will be the definition for the purposes of this chapter.

In the late 1980s and early 1990s, pharmaceutical companies were rapidly adopting a drug discovery strategy that depended on selecting drug targets based on what was known about key pathways important in disease expression, enzymes that catalyzed rate-limiting steps along the pathway, or cellular receptors that were ligated by important relevant mediators. After these targets were selected, chemical libraries were screened for leads that modulated the activity of these pathways. These chemical leads were optimized into new chemical entities (NCEs) and progressed into in vitro and in vivo biological testing to confirm their druglike properties. This drug discovery strategy and its associated activities were quite different from earlier methods that directly screened NCEs or naturally occurring

Fig. 1.1a
The remit of
translational medicine
during drug
development.

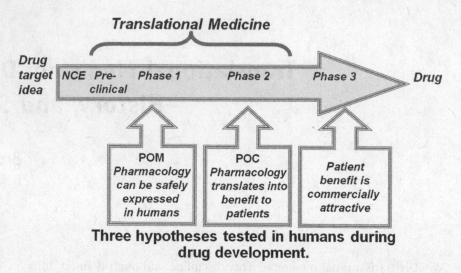

Three hypotheses tested in humans during drug development.

substances for efficacy in animal disease models. It was thought that knowing the drug's target and mechanism of action and having a scientific rationale for efficacy and safety from the beginning would increase the success rate for drug discovery. The new approach resulted in fuller pipelines that stretched resources, and companies needed to develop a strategy for identifying the compounds with the greatest probability of developmental success ("winners") and those less likely to be successful ("losers") as early as possible. To execute this new strategy, pharmaceutical companies formed "experimental medicine" organizations, the primary mission of which was to demonstrate that a drug was safe and active on its target in humans (defined as proof of mechanism or POM) and to determine whether this expression of pharmacology translated into meaningful efficacy in patients (defined as proof of concept or POC). Within the pharmaceutical industry, it was these groups of clinician–scientists that developed and refined their translational skills and evolved into translational medicine groups. Their role often involved the translation of biomarkers from the laboratory into the clinic using transparent criteria for qualification and validation for a specific decision-making purpose such as POM and POC (Figure 1.1a).

Compared with experimental medicine, however, translational medicine groups began to work further upstream in the drug discovery and development process. Experimental medicine groups generally did not have any responsibility for drug projects prior to identification of the drug candidate or, in some cases, prior to the first in human (FIH) studies. Translational medicine groups, in contrast, became involved in all early phases of drug discovery from target identification forward. They often conducted studies in patient populations to increase confidence in drug targets or test the translatability of biomarkers from preclinical models to humans in parallel with the early stages of drug discovery in the laboratory. The frequent failure of animal models to predict efficacy in humans led to a more cost-effective and efficient strategy to get drug candidates to humans earlier to aid target selection and optimize candidate selection because humans were recognized as the "ultimate model

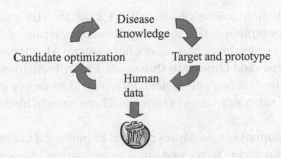

Disease knowledge

Candidate optimization

Target and prototype

Human data

Fig. 1.1b
Translational medicine now brings human experiments into the drug discovery process earlier so that they contribute much more to target selection and candidate optimization.

organism" (Figure 1.1b).[1] This strategy was supported by the U.S. Food and Drug Administration (FDA) in the United States through the exploratory investigational new drug (IND) mechanism and subsequently in the European Union (EU) through the exploratory Clinical Trials Application (CTA) mechanism.[2]

This chapter will focus on the role of translational medicine groups in the pharmaceutical industry, how their work supports the aforementioned decision-making strategies, and how these strategies may undergo subsequent change as we embark on an era of personalized medicine.

1.1. Biomarkers in Drug Development: A Common Understanding

In 2003 at Pfizer, different groups and individuals focusing on different stages and disciplines of drug development, including discovery, toxicology, biomarker development, clinical research, translational medicine, and drug metabolism, had different understandings of what biomarkers were, how they could be used, and how they were validated or qualified. To move translational research objectives forward and achieve universal buy-in for the use of biomarkers for development decisions, it was important to develop a common lexicon. Leaders of these various disciplines not only wanted to accomplish this for Pfizer, but they also wanted to do this for the drug development community as a whole. The following definitions were agreed on and used in many internal and external communications and presentations.

Biomarker: A characteristic that is measured and evaluated as an indicator of normal biologic processes, pathogenic processes, or pharmacological responses to a therapeutic intervention (consistent with the National Institutes of Health [NIH] Workshop definition).[3]

Diagnostic: A biomarker that has clinical applicability for patient management (e.g., in diagnosis, in identification of a subpopulation of patients who would benefit most from a drug or suffer adverse events from a drug, to aid dose selection).

Surrogate end point: A biomarker accepted by regulatory agencies as a substitute for a standard clinical endpoint for drug approval (e.g., human immunodeficiency virus [HIV] load for HIV antiviral, low-density lipoprotein [LDL] lowering for cardiovascular events, blood pressure lowering for hypertension, hemoglobin $A1_C$ for diabetes).[4]

Biomarker Types and Linkage to Outcome: Every biomarker could be defined based on two parameters: its type and its degree of linkage to efficacy or safety outcomes in humans. Three types of biomarkers were defined:

Target Biomarker: Measures physical or biological interactions with the molecular target (e.g., positron emission tomography [PET] ligand demonstration of receptor occupancy, measurement of enzyme inhibition, measure of receptor blockade).

Mechanism Biomarker: Measures a biological effect presumed to be downstream of the target. For example, the biomarker may be physiological (e.g., blood flow), biochemical (e.g., change in downstream substrate turnover), behavioral (reaction time), genetic (e.g., change in gene expression), or proteomic (e.g., change in protein profile in tissues or biofluids).

Outcome Biomarker: Substitutes for a clinical outcome measure that is independent of the mechanism or target of a compound or predicts an outcome of a disease or toxicity following treatment.

Linkage to Outcomes: This second dimension for describing a biomarker refers to its linkage to human efficacy or safety outcomes. The linkage is labeled low, medium, or high based on the following definitions:

Low = There is no consistent information on the linkage of biomarker change to efficacy or safety outcomes in humans. Linkage to outcomes in animal models may exist.

Medium = Biomarker differences are associated with efficacy or safety outcome data in humans but have not been reproducibly demonstrated in clinical studies.

High = Biomarker differences have been reproducibly demonstrated to be correlated with disease efficacy or safety outcomes in two or more longitudinal studies in humans.

Examples of how biomarkers were classified using this system are provided in Figure 1.2.

Fig. 1.2
Examples of biomarker classification by type and linkage to outcome.

Type

	Low	Medium	High
Target	NK-1 receptor occupancy (PET) for an NK1 antagonist	Prothrombin time for a thrombin, Factor Xa or TFVIIa inhibitor	D2 receptor occupancy for anti-psychotics
Mechanism	Cell infiltration after MIP1α skin challenge for a CCR1 antagonist	uTIINE for MMP inhibitor for osteoarthritis progression	MIC for efficacy of antibiotics
Outcome	Reduced rate of loss of cartilage volume by MRI in OA progression	QTc prolongation for risk of fatal arrhythmia	Viral load in HIV Transaminase elevation for hepatoxicity

Linkage to Human Efficacy/Safety

The process of achieving acceptance of the validity of biomarker data for decision making also required a common understanding of the definition and requirements for validation or qualification, including the following:

Validation: Characterization of the biomarker that confirms its fitness for a specific purpose. The degree of rigor required varies with the purpose but always requires organizational agreement. This has more recently been termed "qualification."

Technical Validation: The process of selecting all technical attributes required to demonstrate fitness for the purpose, setting appropriate performance requirements for each attribute, and evaluating the biomarker against these requirements. Examples of some of the elements of the technical evaluation process that may be required are demonstrations of selectivity and specificity, accuracy, precision, responsiveness to pharmacology or disease, and robustness of all necessary procedures and assay steps under conditions similar to those that will be encountered in use (e.g., in a clinical methods study, storage, stability, and matrix effects are considered).

Note: The term "clinical validation" is not recommended because it is included in the linkage to outcome dimension of this biomarker classification. Full clinical validation such as may be required to achieve surrogate endpoint status can be viewed as meeting the criteria for high linkage to outcome, but for many purposes this degree of validation is not required.

Biomarker Translation: The activities needed to ensure that the biomarker (assay and underlying biology) is valid between preclinical species, between preclinical species and humans, or both.

Refer to Chapter 8 for additional information on the process of biomarker qualification.

The roles of biomarkers in drug development relate to their ability to be translated to humans from preclinical models to define criteria for POM, to measure pharmacodynamic (PD) activity in animals and humans for purposes of dose selection and pharmacokinetic (PK) – PD modeling and simulation, to substitute for efficacy and safety clinical endpoints in defining POC, to select appropriate populations of subjects for a clinical trial, and to predict clinical outcomes. These uses will be discussed later in this chapter.

1.2. Pharmacology: Testing the Target (POM)

If preclinical data on compounds and predictions of efficacious doses in humans were 100% accurate, new compounds could simply undergo

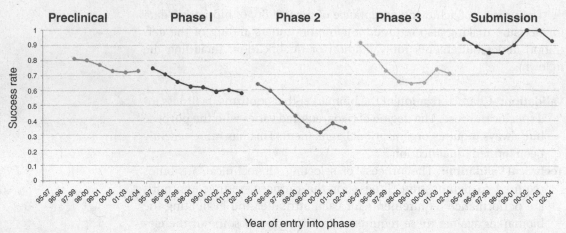

Fig. 1.3
Drug candidate survival by phase for drug candidates entering each phase from 1994 to 2004 and assessment of each candidate's status after 3 years. For example, for the 1994–1996 time window, drug candidates were monitored until the end of 1999; for the 1995–1997 time window, drug candidates were monitored until the end of 2000. For candidates entering Phase 2 during the period from 1995 to 2002, survival went from 64% to 32%. (Data courtesy of CMR International, a Thomson Reuters Business.)

Phase 1 testing for pharmacokinetics and safety (on completion of toxicological testing) and then be evaluated in appropriately powered Phase 2 trials with a high probability of success. Across the industry, however, success rates in Phase 2 decisions have decreased to half their level in the early 1990s (Figure 1.3).[5] The most common reason for failure in Phase 2 in the 1990s was lack of efficacy, and the failure rate for unprecedented mechanisms (i.e., new mechanisms) is considerably higher than the industry average.[6] Why is this the case, and how did the industry respond?

There are many areas of uncertainty regarding the translation of preclinical pharmacology data to humans. The simplistic strategy of accepting the validity of predicted efficacious doses or drug exposure and performing large Phase 2 trials after they are achieved could be the fastest route to Phase 3, but it leaves many unanswered questions when it is not successful. What do you do next if the drug fails to achieve an efficacy signal? Is the molecular target still valid? Has the mechanism been fully tested? Has the target been fully engaged? Do we just need a more potent NCE or one with better (higher or longer) exposure? In fact, this was the situation in which many companies found themselves during the late 1990s as failure rates in Phase 2 doubled (Figure 1.3). These questions cannot rationally be answered unless we know whether the drug actually expressed its intended pharmacology as a result of modulating the drug target.

Translational medicine groups addressed this issue by developing clinical experimental methods and biomarkers that could be used to evaluate the pharmacological activity of drug candidates in Phase 1 studies, usually in the FIH or first multiple-dose Phase 1 study. These methods and biomarkers are translated from preclinical animal or in-vitro studies to humans to confirm that a compound is active on its target and expresses its mechanism of action. As defined earlier in this chapter, these may be target biomarkers if they directly measure drug–target interactions (e.g., receptor occupancy using a PET ligand) or mechanism biomarkers if they measure downstream consequences of target modulation. Criteria for moving forward into Phase 2 are based on the translation of preclinical results and

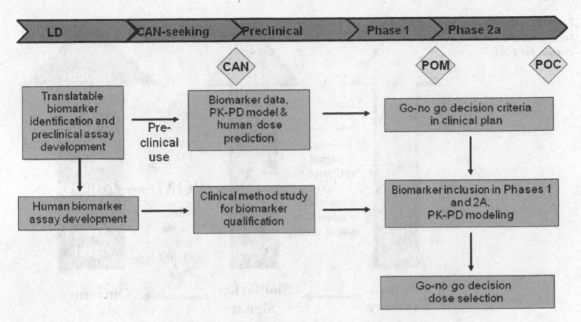

Fig. 1.4 Biomarker translation for decision making: candidate selection (CAN), POM, and POC (as presented by the author at BioIT, Boston, MA, 2006).

defined as POM. This process is illustrated in Figure 1.4. In general, the POM biomarker criteria are based on a similar biomarker signal in animals that resulted in downstream outcomes in disease models. Although efficacy in preclinical disease models often does not translate into efficacy in the human disease, efficacy in the animal disease model is a result of the compound's pharmacology and is a downstream outcome. Because most companies would not be advancing the drug candidate if it did not have efficacy in an animal disease model, using the model to help define POM is both logical and acceptable. Figure 1.5 illustrates how POM criteria are translated to humans and describes the principles for creating these criteria. In all cases, the clinical methods, biomarkers, and "doability" in the setting of a clinical trial must be validated to a level at which all stakeholders agree to use the results for the POM decision.

The process of validation or qualification can be illustrated using the example of an ultraviolet light type B (UVB) skin irradiation challenge model for a p38 mitogen-activated protein (MAP) kinase inhibitor program for rheumatoid arthritis (RA) that was developed at Pfizer. The validation plan included the following steps:

■ Technically validate all biochemical assays using murine and human skin biopsies;
■ Evaluate these endpoints in hairless mice after exposure to UVB irradiation and determine the effect of the p38 inhibitor;
■ Confirm UVB effects on the same endpoints in human skin;
■ Evaluate reproducibility of UVB-induced changes in humans to determine sample size for a Phase 1 clinical study; and
■ Benchmark the changes seen with murine p38 inhibition in skin with the efficacy outcomes in a collagen-induced arthritis disease model.

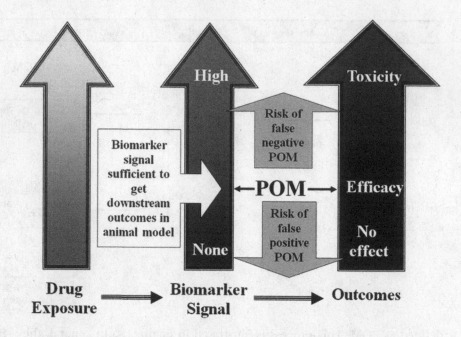

Figure 1.6 summarizes the outcome of these efforts. Here the downstream mechanism biomarkers are biochemical, and the model could be performed in healthy volunteers during the course of a Phase 1, single-dose trial. The drug candidate's level of inhibition of UVB-induced murine responses downstream of p38 MAP kinase at a dose and exposure that had efficacy in the collagen arthritis model is the level of inhibition needed for POM in humans using the same skin model. The same model could be used for compound differentiation or optimization either in the preclinical phase or in humans through modeling of drug exposure and pharmacodynamic response relationships (PK/PD modeling) and simulation.

As described earlier in the text, mechanism biomarkers do not necessarily have to be biochemical. For some mechanisms and indications, POM criteria may require confirmation of drug activity in a target population using a translated behavioral biomarker rather than a biochemical endpoint. For example, Figure 1.7 describes how POM was defined and achieved for an anorectic agent being developed for obesity. Here reduced

<u>Proof of Mechanism</u>
- ♦ **Every first Phase 2 trial must be a valid test of the drug target**
  - – **Understand the required level of pharmacological activity from preclinical work**
  - – **Translate to humans as go/no go decision criteria for proof of mechanism (POM)**
  - – **Prove the compound safely expresses adequate pharmacology in Phase 1 = POM**
  - – **Only start Phase 2 if POM is achieved**
- ♦ **Phase 2 result speaks to the validity of the drug target, enables data-driven program decisions, and predicts late-phase success**

Table 1.1. Examples of POM Using Biomarkers Translated from Preclinical Models

Inflammation/Immunology: Flow cytometry for changes in cell surface activation markers, intracellular biomarkers (cytokines, etc.); lymphocyte subpopulation changes; pathway-relevant gene expression changes (blood, tissue); endotoxin challenge models; skin challenge models; direct measurement of mediators in serum or urine; immunization models

Obesity programs: Food intake and energy balance

ADHD: Cognitive effects, functional imaging

Osteoporosis: Bone biomarkers

Psychotherapeutic programs: PET receptor occupancy

Oncology programs: Angiogenesis biomarkers (dce-MRI, vessel density), tyrosine kinase inhibition (target phosphorylation), metabolic response (FDG-PET)

Atherosclerosis: Lipids, inflammation biomarkers

POM decision criteria are derived from the biomarker change associated with desired downstream outcomes in animal models that are translated to humans for POM decisions.
dce-MRI: dynamic contrast-enhanced magnetic resonance imaging.
FDG-PET: Fluorodeoxyglucose positron emission tomography.

food consumption was validated as a mechanism biomarker and translated from a mouse model to humans. Other examples of POM for various types of projects are listed in Table 1.1.

What if POM is for a compound whose target is nonhuman and instead belongs to a pathogen? Antiviral agents and antibiotics usually target molecules that are coded for by the genome of the pathogen. Frequently, the preclinical work for antiviral agents includes the development of an

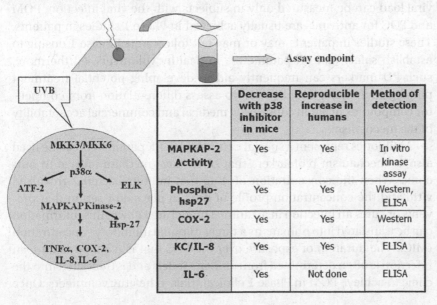

	Decrease with p38 inhibitor in mice	Reproducible increase in humans	Method of detection
MAPKAP-2 Activity	Yes	Yes	In vitro kinase assay
Phospho-hsp27	Yes	Yes	Western, ELISA
COX-2	Yes	Yes	Western
KC/IL-8	Yes	Yes	ELISA
IL-6	Yes	Not done	ELISA

Fig. 1.6
UVB skin challenge model for determining POM for a p38 MAP kinase inhibitor. A defined optimal dose of UVB radiation is applied to the skin at time of peak drug exposure, and at a predetermined optimal time point a biopsy is taken of the area and processed for biochemical assays. ELISA, enzyme-linked immunosorbent assay; COX-2, cyclooxygenase-2; KC, keratinocyte chemoattractant (murine equivalent of human IL-8, interleukin 8); ATF-2, activating transcription factor 2; ELK, extracellular signal-regulated kinases; MAPKAP, mitogen activated protein kinase-activated protein kinase 2; Hsp-27, heat shock protein 27; TNFα, tumor necrosis factor-α; MKK, mitogen-activated protein kinase kinase. (Courtesy of Dr. Alan Clucas, Pfizer Global Research and Development and as previously publicly presented.)

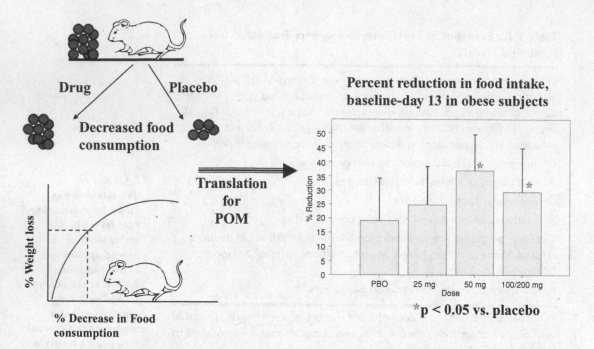

Fig. 1.7
Example of POM for an anorectic compound for obesity. In the animal model, mice spontaneously eat less food and lose weight when they are dosed with the compound compared with mice dosed with a placebo. The percent reduction in food consumption seen acutely that is associated with acceptable longer term weight loss is translated to the clinic as a behavioral biomarker for the purpose of a POM definition. (Previously publicly presented by Pfizer Global Research and Development.)

assay that measures viral replication and its inhibition by the candidate drug in vitro. It is important when this assay is developed that it also be qualified for use in vivo in human subjects. The measurement of viral load and its change after treatment are often used to define POM and, with medium or high linkage to outcome, may also be a case where an efficacy signal can be obtained to achieve POC at the same time. For both POM and POC, it is important to define the level of change in viral load or viral replication that has clinical significance. If this is not known in advance, then clinical methods studies are needed to create this linkage to outcome and qualify the biomarker for decision making. Because viral replication and viral load can be measured only in subjects with the viral infection, POM and POC for antivirals are usually achieved in Phase 1 studies in patients. These studies in patients may or may not follow initial Phase 1 dosing to establish safety and PK parameters in healthy volunteers. Furthermore, such PD markers can frequently aid in developing potential treatment paradigms that can then be used to assess differentiation from competitor compounds or aid in confirming medical and commercial acceptability of the mechanism.

Antibiotics represent a special case in which PK parameters can be used also as mechanism biomarkers that often have medium linkage to outcome. When the concentration of drug that inhibits bacterial growth in vitro and the concentration profile of drug in plasma or serum that prevents or cures an infection in an animal model are known, this information can be translated into humans as a target minimal inhibitory concentration (MIC). The duration of exposure over the MIC that is required to cure an infection is often determined from animal models and is translated into the clinic to achieve POM in Phase 1 clinical trials in healthy volunteers. Once the required duration of exposure over MIC is achieved at a well-tolerated dose in Phase 1 there is a high probability that POC will be positive in a patient population. For this reason, POM for antibiotics often becomes a signal to increase investment and triggers a large pivotal Phase 2 trial.

In all cases, if POM is achieved in Phase 1, it is concluded that the drug modulates its target sufficiently to test the efficacy of the drug mechanism in Phase 2. Requiring a positive POM first will clearly reduce Phase 2 attrition if the drug target is actually important for disease expression. A positive POM with failure to achieve an efficacy signal in Phase 2 (negative POC), however, still provides value for two reasons. First, it enables the company to discard that drug target for the disease indication, and the organization will not ask for another candidate with the same mechanism. Eliminating work on a mechanism that did not provide a positive POC allows companies to direct resources more rapidly to more successful projects. Second, a positive POM gives value to the compound because it demonstrates that the drug is active at a safe dose and could be tested in other indications or enter an "indication discovery" paradigm.

1.3. Study Design Considerations for POM

1.3.1. Population

Whenever possible, POM should be tested in the context of a traditional Phase 1 single- or multiple-dose study in healthy volunteers. This population will deliver the cleanest evaluation of safety, will not be taking other medications, and will not have other disease-related issues that could confound PK or PD endpoints. If the drug target and its associated downstream pharmacology is not expressed appropriately in a healthy volunteer population, and if it is not possible to use a clinical model in healthy volunteers that stimulates the expression of the drug's target (like the UVB skin model described earlier in text), however, it will be necessary to select a disease population that does allow for the measurable expression of the drug's mechanism. Often this population is a subset of the overall disease population known to have abnormal expression of the pathway that is to be inhibited or stimulated by the candidate drug. Regardless of the nature of the population selected, the study design involving such a patient stratification or enrichment approach should allow for an evaluation of the PD activity of the candidate drug over a wide range of doses such that the full range of PD expression can be elicited. Last, if POM and POC can be achieved in the same Phase 1 study, provided a target population is used, the study design may become a hybrid in which some goals, such as safety and PK (and sometimes PD) properties, are characterized in a healthy population, and then a target population is selected for evaluation of (pharmacodynamics and) efficacy. For example, an antiviral HIV drug may be evaluated in a Phase 1 study with a single-dose first stage in healthy volunteers followed by a multiple-dose second stage in HIV-positive subjects. This design allows for a clean evaluation of single-dose pharmacokinetics and safety that aids dose selection to achieve targeted exposures in the second stage with evaluation of effects on viral load and lymphocyte subpopulations for POM and POC.

1.3.2. Risk

When considering study design for a POM study, two areas of risk need to be considered and mitigated. The first relates to safety of the mechanism. If the pharmacology of the drug results in significantly increased safety risk, the population selected must derive some benefit to justify the risk. For example, immunosuppressive drugs may be safely given to healthy volunteers in a single-dose Phase 1 study, but a multiple-dose Phase 1 study often requires a population that could benefit from immunosuppression because there is a risk of opportunistic infection in subjects receiving even short-term immunosuppression. Likewise, cancer drugs often have a narrow therapeutic index and are usually tested in cancer patients first. Theoretically, if an oncology drug has a mechanism that is safe and measurable in healthy subjects, it can be studied in healthy volunteers first. Because healthy volunteer studies are small and can be done quickly, a follow-on study using safe and active doses can be conducted next in which all cancer patients receive an active dose and POC will require less time overall. For a drug with a nontoxic and nonmutagenic mechanism, one can argue that this course is also the best to follow from a risk–benefit perspective for the cancer patients in the study. In the traditional dose escalation cohort design, the initial cohorts receive doses that are usually not sufficiently pharmacologically active to produce tumor responses. These patients pay an opportunity cost because they may also be eligible for other studies that offer some potential efficacy.

The second area of risk to consider is whether the POM decision can be made using the study design without a significant risk of a false-positive or -negative result. Understanding the variability around the measurements (effect size) and selecting a sufficient number of subjects who will receive pharmacologically active doses to ensure the appropriate power helps to reduce the risk of false positive or negative results. It is better to err on the side of a false-positive decision because then the drug will go on to a POC study for final evaluation, whereas a false-negative decision results in terminating a drug candidate that actually should have gone on to a POC study.

1.3.3. Feasibility

When considering POM study design, feasibility in a clinical trial setting is extremely important. A common misconception is to design a scientifically rigorous study that has the perfect comparator controls and study population but is not doable in a reasonable period of time in the real world. For example, suppose the "molecularly correct" population when considering the biochemical pathway targeted by the drug represents 50% of the overall disease population and the evaluation of the drug mechanism requires that the population not be treated with some other class of drugs commonly used in the disease (60% of patients). If it is assumed that 40% of the disease population will not use that type of drug and 50% of those have the right molecular characteristics, only 20% of the disease population is potentially eligible for the study. Other typical exclusion criteria will frequently bring that number down further making the study recruitment a significant challenge. Thus, study feasibility often requires some compromises in study design or a study design that becomes more rigorous in selecting the optimal population only for the appropriate pharmacologically active doses after safety and PK data are obtained in a broader population.

1.3.4. Endpoints

POM usually requires biomarker endpoints that confirm the interaction and activity of a new drug on its molecular target, downstream pathways, or both as described earlier in the text. This requirement translates into a study design in which several factors must be taken into consideration. These factors include not only those discussed earlier, such as the appropriate population and effect size for confirming changes in the endpoint, but also such factors as the optimal time after dosing for measuring change in the endpoints, sample collection requirements, and so forth. These factors should have been optimized as part of the biomarker translation and qualification process. The POM study design should mimic the conditions used during that qualification. This is no time to insert unproven sample collection techniques or assay modifications when one assumes that the changes are not significant. Sometimes the POM or POC decision criteria are not based on the required degree of biomarker change in a group that received the same safe dose but rather on observing a significant dose response in the endpoint and may use PK–PD modeling methods (see Section 1.3.5). POM endpoints should preferably be measured over a range of drug doses anyway, and, under these circumstances, the POM decision may be based on observing a slope for the dose response that is significantly different from zero and the required degree of change is modeled and found to be within the well-tolerated dose range. Compared with a POM study in which each dose group must be large enough to test for a significant and acceptable degree of postdose change in the biomarker, the size of the population required for this type of dose-response analysis is often smaller and delivers more information about response over the entire dose range.

1.3.5. PK–PD and PD–PD Models

Regardless of the POM definition, the measurement of biomarker end-points over the full range of exposures allows for the development of PK–PD models that can be applied to other significant questions using simulations. In some cases in which PK is not available, feasible, or applicable, disease or PD–PD modeling can be performed. The dose-response endpoint for POM discussed earlier in the text may be viewed as one form of PK–PD model, but results of early studies often also raise new issues that can be addressed through PK–PD models, especially when dose is not a good surrogate for exposure. For example, suppose a drug caused electrocardiogram changes with Q-T prolongation at high exposures. One could combine the PK–PD model for the desired pharmacology using the POM biomarkers with a model for Q-T prolongation and decide if there is a large enough therapeutic window to continue. The same concept applies to any safety issue. Sometimes PK–PD models with POM biomarkers can be used to benchmark a new drug against a marketed drug with a similar mechanism if the requirement for POM is superiority with respect to therapeutic index, dosing frequency, or safety differentiation. In these cases, the model would require at least an equivalent degree of mechanistic activity while demonstrating the required differentiation features. Suffice it to say that PK–PD modeling lends itself nicely to any quantitative biomarker signal used for POM and often results in reduced sample sizes and greater certainty around the POM decision itself. Figure 1.8 describes the results of a PK–PD model from a single-dose study conducted by Pfizer under an exploratory IND (Expl-IND) in which a lipid-lowering compound with a novel mechanism failed to meet criteria for POM based on superiority to atorvastatin (Lipitor).

Fig. 1.8
Use of PK–PD model and a lipid biomarker to examine superiority of a novel lipid-lowering agent compared with atorvastatin. In this case, the new drug did not show lipid changes (*solid curve representing the standard error range*) superior to atorvastatin within an acceptable (safe and well-tolerated) dose range (*right of the vertical line*). A decision to terminate the compound was made after a single-dose study conducted under an Expl-IND.

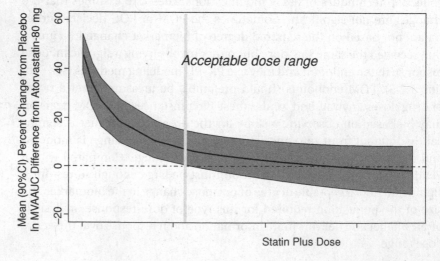

1.4. Confirming the Hypothesis That a Drug Target (Mechanism of Action) Will Be Efficacious (POC)

POC has been defined differently by many companies. For some it means that the drug project is likely to succeed all the way to the market. For the purposes of this chapter and from the viewpoint of translational medicine groups, it is defined as confirmation that the drug target and mechanism of action of the compound will provide an efficacy signal at a safe and well-tolerated dose (Figure 1.1a). In other words, it is POC for the drug target using a compound that may still have significant issues that require larger studies to identify and resolve. POC must provide sufficient evidence to invest further in the drug project and often triggers more detailed planning and resources for larger Phase 2B or 3 trials. When designing a clinical program to reach the POC decision point, translational medicine groups recognize the historically high attrition rates in Phase 2 and design these programs to be as rapid, cost-effective, and efficient as possible. Programs are designed to identify the losers quickly and to conserve resources by focusing on the efficacy question and by leaving other important commercial and medical questions to be answered later. In other words, they identify the most favorable situation for seeing an efficacy signal such that, if it is not seen not seen, it is highly unlikely that efficacy will occur in larger studies. Several principles are used when developing a POC strategy and designing a POC clinical study.

1.5. Study Design Considerations for POC

1.5.1. Population

The first step is to identify the disease phenotype and patient population that are "molecularly correct" for the drug mechanism. Here there are three principles to consider. The first principle is that every chronic disease has multiple genetic and environmental causes, but the drug candidate usually has just one molecular target or mechanism of action. Drug activity will modulate pathways downstream of the drug target. Within a patient population, the importance of that pathway for disease expression varies directly with the degree of abnormal pathway activity. Some patients with the disease will have abnormal pathway activity based on their genetic background and environmental factors. For other patients this pathway is less abnormal, and other molecular and environmental factors are more important for their disease expression. The second principle is that the magnitude of the clinical response to a drug that targets a specific pathway will be proportional to the degree of abnormal pathway expression. This

Fig. 1.9
Three distributions of pathway expression for different drug targets demonstrating sizes of disease subpopulations with good clinical responses to drugs targeting each pathway (*shaded areas*). From Webb CP, Thompson JF, & Littman BH (2009). Redefining Disease and Pharmaceutical Targets Through Molecular Definitions and Personalized Medicine. In: *Biomarkers in Drug Development: A Handbook of Practice, Application, and Strategy*, edited by Bleavins MR, Rahbari R, Jurima-Romet M, and Carini C. John Wiley and Sons, Inc., Hoboken, NJ (2010).

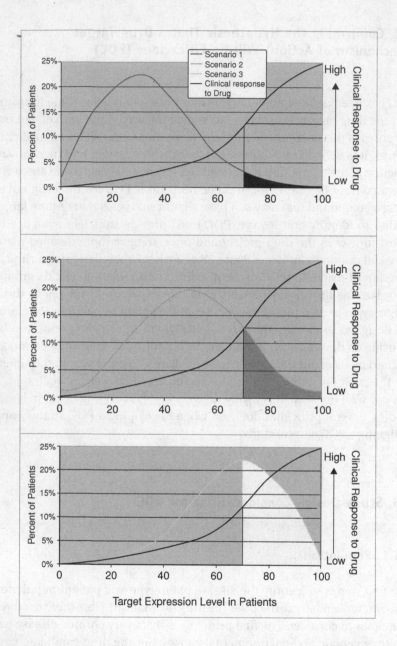

means that an efficacy signal will be easier to generate in this population. These two principles are illustrated in Figure 1.9 and are similar to those considered for personalized medicines.[7] The third principle is that the population selected must be one that will uniformly achieve drug exposure levels and duration of drug exposure that ensure that the drug's mechanism is active as defined previously for POM. Thus, if the absorption, distribution, metabolism, and elimination (ADME) characteristics of the drug would lead to highly variable drug exposure, subjects should also be selected to provide for adequate exposure in all subjects. For example, if the drug is a CYP2D6 substrate, and if high exposure is known to be associated with significant adverse events, subjects should be prescreened to select those that will metabolize the drug similarly (to exclude poor metabolizers). This prescreening reduces variability, allowing for inclusion of high doses that would have led to adverse events in poor metabolizers, and allows the study to include a wide dose range to fully test efficacy of the mechanism. Selecting the optimal patient population for a POC clinical study should use these three principles and validated biomarkers to identify the correct subjects. Thus, the organization accepts the notions that (1) if an efficacy signal is not seen in this optimal population it is unlikely to be seen at all and (2) a negative POC will kill the drug and its mechanism for that indication.

1.5.2. Efficacy Endpoints

The second step in designing the POC study is to select a primary efficacy endpoint that has low variability (to allow small sample size) and will be responsive relatively quickly. Because POC studies are conducted early in development, they are usually not supported by long-term toxicology studies, and drug exposure may be limited to 4 weeks or less (assuming only 4-week toxicology studies were completed). In some cases, if short-term efficacy endpoints are not acceptable, the organization must accept larger up-front investments to support longer POC trials. For example, a drug for obesity that requires a trial for weight loss (as opposed to some metabolic or food consumption endpoint) may require longer than 4 weeks of exposure. Often, conventional clinical endpoints will suffice, but sometimes biomarkers with medium or high linkage to clinical outcome are selected. For example, metabolic responses in fluorodeoxyglucose (FDG)-PET studies in cancer patients have been shown in longitudinal studies in breast and lung cancer patients to correlate with clinical outcomes later.[8] The FDG-PET response is therefore a mechanism biomarker that has high linkage to clinical outcome. Here an early metabolic response using FDG-PET quantitative imaging may be used in a POC study because there is evidence that it will probably predict longer term clinical outcomes.

The study population can also be selected to reduce variability of the efficacy (biomarker) endpoint. For example, in rheumatoid arthritis (RA) patients the clinical response to a disease-modifying antirheumatic drug (DMARD) is associated with reduction in C-reactive protein (CRP).[9] The production of CRP is primarily driven by interleukin-6 (IL-6).[10] The –174 G to C single nucleotide polymorphism (SNP) in the promoter region of the IL-6 gene determines the amount of IL-6 produced as a result of IL-1 or lipopolysaccharide (LPS or endotoxin) stimulation.[11] The C allele results in a lower IL-6 response, and cells homozygous for the C allele do not increase IL-6 production in response to these stimuli in vitro.[11] Thus, when selecting RA patients for a study that uses CRP or IL-6 as a biomarker with high linkage to efficacy outcomes, variability of the endpoint can be reduced by ensuring that all subjects have at least one copy of the G allele. Because the

C allele frequency is reported to be 0.4, approximately 16% of the population will be homozygous C/C, leaving 84% eligible for the study.[11] If a new DMARD candidate does not reduce CRP fairly quickly, it is unlikely to have efficacy.

1.5.3. Dose Selection

Often companies and clinician-scientists are inclined to simplify POC studies and reduce cost by studying just one dose, frequently the maximum tolerated dose, and comparing efficacy at this dose to placebo. They choose to defer an understanding of the dose response in patients to larger Phase 2 studies if an efficacy signal is confirmed in the POC study. Clearly this option may be preferred in some cases, and classic, more deterministic statistical measures of efficacy (mean change on placebo vs. mean change on active drug) can be used for the primary efficacy endpoint. POC, however, may also be defined as observing a significant dose response for the efficacy signal in a smaller study where the slope of the dose response is statistically different from zero. With this design, one assumes that unusual dose-response curves are not likely (e.g., U-shaped dose response). This assumption is safe if it is based on POM study PK–PD data that demonstrate a typical E_{max}-shaped dose-response curve for the drug's pharmacology. The doses selected for the POC study can also be based on the POM study PK–PD data to ensure that they fall within the optimal, relatively linear range of pharmacological activity.

1.5.4. Cost, Speed, and Risk

Finally, the study design must reflect the organization's tolerance for risk, cost, and speed. If the result of the POC trial will determine whether the organization builds a new plant and invests heavily in a Phase 2B/3 clinical program for a compound that is expected to generate huge revenues, the POC study result must have a low likelihood of delivering a false-positive or -negative result. In this case, the POC study may end up looking like a relatively large Phase 2B trial. In contrast, if the POC study will result in a more typical Phase 2B study investment, the organization can tolerate a false-positive result but would not like to end up with a false-negative result that kills the compound and the mechanism for the indication. If there are safety issues that require 4 weeks of dosing to become apparent, then a 4-week study is best even if efficacy can be observed in much shorter studies. If some aspects of safety and efficacy require larger numbers of subjects to evaluate, and if there is a desire to reduce costs, one may consider using adaptive designs for the study that require certain initial results prior to stopping the study, recruiting additional subjects to particular dose groups, or adding new dose groups to the study. Importantly, the study design must reflect the organization's tolerance for cost, speed, and risk,

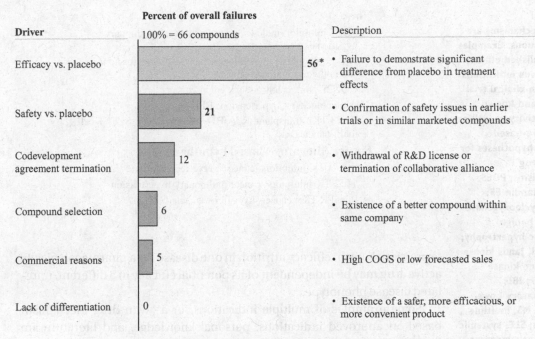

Percent of overall failures

Driver	100% = 66 compounds	Description
Efficacy vs. placebo	56*	• Failure to demonstrate significant difference from placebo in treatment effects
Safety vs. placebo	21	• Confirmation of safety issues in earlier trials or in similar marketed compounds
Codevelopment agreement termination	12	• Withdrawal of R&D license or termination of collaborative alliance
Compound selection	6	• Existence of a better compound within same company
Commercial reasons	5	• High COGS or low forecasted sales
Lack of differentiation	0	• Existence of a safer, more efficacious, or more convenient product

* Only 1 indication RIP out of 37 indication RIPs by efficacy vs. placebo had an established MOA

Fig. 1.10
Lack of efficacy is the usual root cause of Phase 2 failure. This analysis of the root cause of attrition done at Pfizer was based on 66 failed compounds, where 65 had an unprecedented mechanism of action. COGS, cost of goods.

and there must be the willingness to accept more innovative study designs in this phase of development and acceptance of the outcome, especially if it involves termination.

1.5.5. Multiple Indications (Serial or Parallel)

After a novel drug with an unprecedented mechanism of action achieves POM, the choice of indication for the POC study may or may not be simple. Often a drug target is selected with a primary indication in mind, and the clinical plan for the compound is clear about the indication of choice for the POC study. As noted earlier in text, however, the Phase 2 success rate across the pharmaceutical industry is on the order of 30% to 35% and is lower for unprecedented mechanisms.[5,6] Analyses of the root cause of Phase 2 attrition by Pfizer (Figure 1.10) and Kola and Landis both point to lack of efficacy as the most common cause.[6] Often, however, the molecular pathways modulated by the drug's mechanism are known to be important for disease expression in more than one indication. The following four points underpin the logic of a parallel indication approach. First, mechanisms are conserved and used by different organ systems for different purposes. Second, different diseases often have the same abnormally expressed targets and pathways, but the importance of the pathway for disease expression may be different. Third, Phase 2 attrition for efficacy may be due to a previously unsuspected minor role of the target for disease

Fig. 1.11
Drug mechanisms are promiscuous. Examples of established efficacy for various indications based on clinical trial results and known drug activity as well as literature-based efficacy hypotheses for other drug mechanisms. PDE5, prostaglandin E5; COX2, cyclooxygenase 2; BPH, benign prostatic hypertrophy; JAK3 TKi, Janus kinase 3 tyrosine kinase inhibitor; IBD, inflammatory bowel disease; MS, multiple sclerosis; SLE, systemic lupus erythematosus; EGFR TK, epidermal growth factor receptor tyrosine kinase; TIE2 TKi, inhibitor of receptor tyrosine kinase for angiopoietin; PDGFR TKi, platelet-derived growth factor receptor tyrosine kinase inhibitor.

- **Now:**
  - PDE5 inhibitor: male erectile dysfunction, pulmonary hypertension
  - NK-1 antagonists: hyperalgesic pain (RA), depression, chemotherapy induced emesis
  - COX2i: pain, colon polyps, colon cancer
  - Alpha blockers: hypertension, BPH
  - JAK3 TKi: transplant, RA, IBD, psoriasis, MS, SLE, T-cell malignancies, etc.
- **Future (literature-based hypotheses)?**
  - EGFR TK inhibitors: cancer, nerve regeneration
  - TIE2 TK inhibitors: cancer, pulmonary hypertension
  - PDGFR TKi: cancer, liver fibrosis, scleroderma

expression. Fourth, efficacy attrition in one disease for a pharmacologically active drug may be independent of its potential efficacy in a different, unrelated disease phenotype.

Some examples of multiple indications for a given drug mechanism based on approved indications, personal knowledge, and literature are listed in Figure 1.11. To maximize the chance of getting a product from a drug that has achieved POM, the organization should consider performing multiple POC studies in parallel if each can be tested quickly and at low cost in a "molecularly correct" population using traditional endpoints or outcome biomarkers looking for a big signal. In contrast, if one indication really drives the value of the compound, a serial approach that is dependent on a positive POC for the primary indication first may be the most acceptable strategy.

What are the predicted results in terms of Phase 3 starts if multiple indications are tested in parallel? Based on the data described in Figure 1.10, where the 66 Phase 2 failures represent 80% of the total number of Phase 2 starts (this assumes 20% success in Phase 2 for compounds with unprecedented mechanisms), the probability that any one indication might have a positive efficacy signal is approximately 32.1%, and the compound safety failure rate is approximately 25.5%. Other assumptions include that the efficacy results for each indication are stochastically independent (i.e., the outcome of one has no impact on the outcome of the other), that attrition due to safety runs across all indications irrespective of how many are tested, and that the efficacy outcomes and safety outcomes are independent of each other. Given these assumptions, the probability of getting one Phase 3 start can be calculated for any specific number of indications tested (Figure 1.12). For example, the probability of getting one Phase 3 start if four indications are tested is 0.6. The cost-effectiveness of this strategy depends on the use of biomarkers and study designs that are looking for big efficacy signals with small numbers of subjects selected to be the best possible responders to the drug's mechanism.

1.6. Human Indications Screening

Another approach that addresses the Phase 2 attrition issue and is related to parallel evaluation of indications is based on the idea of first reducing a portion of the risk of failure due to lack of efficacy. This strategy is called human indications screening and should be done early in development through the use of mechanism biomarkers and biomarkers with medium or high linkage to outcome in the context of resource-sparing Expl-INDs or CTAs. Such an approach can greatly increase the confidence that a novel drug target will result in a successful efficacy outcome and is especially valuable when animal disease models do not exist or are not predictive of eventual efficacy in humans. The clinical plan for this approach involves two stages that may be combined in a single protocol, particularly if the mechanism biomarker for POM also has medium or high linkage to outcome. As depicted in Figure 1.13a, the clinical goals include the following:

Stage 1: Achieve POM: Pharmacology expressed in humans at a safe dose.

Stage 2: Look for an efficacy signal using informative target populations where efficacy can be evaluated. When the mechanism is "promiscuous," consider parallel evaluation of different target populations to screen for efficacy signals. Thus, efficacy can be evaluated with target or mechanism biomarkers that have medium or high linkage to outcome (e.g., CRP decrease in RA, food consumption decrease for obesity, glucose decrease for diabetes, cognitive effect for attention-deficit/hyperactivity disorder [ADHD], bone biomarkers for osteoporosis, FDG-PET response in cancer) or with standard endpoints if their variability (effect size) is acceptable (e.g., forced expiratory volume in 1 second [FEV1] for asthma, Visual Analogue Scale [VAS] pain scale, viral load in HIV).

Fig. 1.12
The probability of getting one Phase 3 start when testing multiple indications.

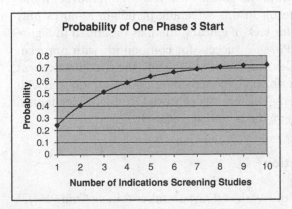

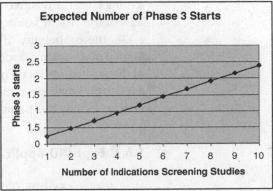

Fig. 1.13
Human indication screening. Parallel efficacy screening paradigm is illustrated. 13A: importance of confirming POM before testing multiple indications for an efficacy signal. 13B: The logic of performing a parallel screening evaluation of multiple indications to maximize the likelihood of achieving at least one POC and subsequent Phase 3 start for compounds that have proven their pharmacological activity (positive POM). This logic is based on the known Phase 2 failure rate and percentage of times failure is due to lack of efficacy. NCE, new chemical entity.

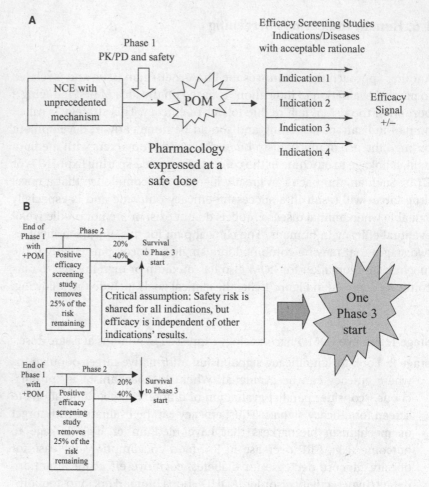

Because this is a screening tool, the statistical approach is adjusted to look for a clear (large) efficacy signal and for "flat liners" and is not powered to look for small differences. Studies are therefore small and within the size and cost range of a traditional Phase 1 program. The goal is to accelerate compound or drug target development for positive indications knowing that much of the efficacy risk has been removed. If one assumes that a positive result in this screening paradigm removes only 25% of the risk of failure for lack of efficacy, then, as described in Figure 1.13b, the probability of Phase 2 success for compounds with unprecedented mechanisms doubles from 20% to 40%. Thus, the cost effectiveness of this strategy relies on performing the screening studies rapidly and with a relatively small investment. The recently approved Expl-IND mechanism enables exactly this paradigm if it is used aggressively.[2]

1.6.1. Expl-IND Application

How does the Expl-IND route work and save resources? In its *Guidance for Industry, Investigators, and Reviewers,*[2] the FDA states that the "exploratory

IND study is intended to describe a clinical trial that occurs very early in Phase 1, involves very limited human exposure, and has no therapeutic intent... "Such exploratory IND studies are conducted prior to the traditional dose escalation, safety, and tolerance studies that ordinarily initiate a clinical drug development program. The duration of dosing in an exploratory IND study is expected to be limited (e.g., 7 days)." Examples of the purposes of Expl-IND studies that are mentioned include (1) "Gain an understanding of the relationship between a specific mechanism of action and the treatment of a disease"; (2) "Provide important information on pharmacokinetics, including, for example, biodistribution of a candidate drug"; (3) "Select the most promising lead product from a group of candidates designed to interact with a particular therapeutic target in humans"; and (4) "Explore a product's biodistribution characteristics using various imaging technologies". The preclinical resources supporting an Expl-IND study are significantly less than those needed for a standard IND.

Guidance on dosing states that "the starting dose is anticipated to be no greater than 1/50 of the no observed adverse event level (NOAEL) from the 2-week toxicology study in the sensitive species on an mg/m^2 basis. The maximum clinical dose would be the lowest of the following: $\frac{1}{4}$ of the 2-week NOAEL; $\frac{1}{2}$ of the AUC at the NOAEL in the 2-week rodent study, or the AUC in the dog at the rat NOAEL, whichever is lower; or the dose that produces a pharmacological response or at which target modulation is observed in the clinical trial." This last stated limit to dose escalation is critical.

Probably the most important piece of translational research when using the Expl-IND route to confirm an efficacy signal for a novel drug mechanism is to define the pharmacologically active dose and understand its relationship to the highest dose that will be allowed based on animal safety studies. This strategy requires that the pharmacologically active dose be less than or equal to 25% of the 2-week rat safety study NOAEL or one-half of its rat area under the curve (AUC). A translatable mechanism biomarker can be used to define pharmacological activity in rats and humans for this purpose. A biomarker signal at some level is defined as "pharmacological activity," and dose escalation must stop when this signal is observed in the clinical trial. Because the goal is to look for a downstream efficacy signal resulting from this pharmacology in humans, it is essential to define the level of that biomarker signal based on its association with downstream outcomes in an animal model. To ensure that it is a true test of the mechanism in patients, POM must be built into the study as part of the dose escalation design, and the pharmacologically active dose must be defined accordingly and safely reached. The Phase 1 study generally has an initial stage that is a cohort dose escalation single- and multiple-dose design up to the highest allowed dose (defined by the pharmacologically active dose in the protocol), and then a final cohort of molecularly correct patients (as described earlier in the text) may receive this dose for a maximum of 7 days. Although therapeutic intent is not allowed, the potential for efficacy may be evaluated in every cohort if the mechanism biomarker has medium or high linkage to outcome and if the population is appropriate, but if a different population is required, or an outcome biomarker requires special conditions or resources, or both, then this final stage of the study may require a change of site to meet subject selection and biomarker qualification requirements for measuring an efficacy signal. Because a drug candidate with this type of efficacy confirmation carries a higher risk of future failure than do compounds that achieve traditional POC as described earlier in the text, success using this paradigm may be labeled proof of viability (POV) for the drug target.

1.6.2. Low Cost Attrition and Portfolio Economics

One of the main benefits of the indication-screening strategy is to eliminate bad compounds, drug targets, mechanisms, and indications as quickly as possible and at a low resource cost. If it is assumed that a company has finite resources for drug development and a portfolio of drug projects at various stages of development, a successful translational medicine group will enable that company to make scientifically driven decisions about the termination or progression of these projects at an early stage and thus greatly increase its productivity. One way of looking at the benefits of indication screening is to consider the cost to resolve risk for a drug project to achieve its POC milestone. In this way one can compare the relative costs to achieve a similar degree of risk reduction. This type of analysis is illustrated in Figure 1.14 using typical development costs for necessary activities and people in full-time equivalents (FTEs). Here one can see that it costs approximately $18 million to reach a positive or negative POV in an indication-screening paradigm using an Expl-IND for a novel drug mechanism with an associated efficacy signal. Because most novel

Fig. 1.14
Risk resolved to achieving POC vs. resource costs for two strategies: Indications Screening under an Expl-IND compared with a typical resource sparing Phase I and 2A approach. POV is reached when an indications screening study delivers a positive efficacy signal. FTE, full-time equivalent.

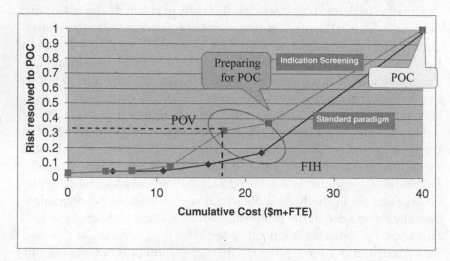

drug mechanisms typically fail, this cost is rather low compared with the $40-million cost to achieve a positive or negative POC decision with the more conventional paradigm. If 80% deliver negative POV results (approximated from Phase 2 survival data for candidates with unprecedented mechanisms), the cumulative cost to get one positive POC including the costs following POV is approximately $102 million for the indication-screening approach and approximately $200 million for the conventional approach; thus, the indication-screening paradigm is about half the cost of the latter. The risk resolved by a positive POV will vary by project. Figure 1.14 assumes that it will be approximately 30%, which is a realistic number for many projects.

At this point it is also important to consider the size of the early drug development portfolio and organizational structure. With a large early portfolio a company will benefit from this indication-screening strategy and will be more likely to adopt it because it wants to put its resources behind the winners and discard the losers as soon as possible (knowing that it will have a reasonable number of winners left). If the portfolio is small, however, the organization may not embrace this strategy, fearing to a greater extent the possibility of a false-negative decision. The impact of a false-negative decision on the viability of a company with a small portfolio is much greater. Even a company with an overall large early candidate portfolio may act like a small company with a much smaller early candidate portfolio if it has divided up that portfolio into independent units (frequently by therapeutic area) and each unit ends up with just a few early candidates. From the point of view of the acceptance of data-driven decisions based on an indication-screening strategy, it is much better to maintain as large an early development portfolio as possible and ensure that one body has governance over the entire early portfolio.

1.7. Commercial Profile and Translational Medicine

1.7.1. Impact on Survival

Commercial requirements for new products often drive the goals of drug projects in the pharmaceutical industry. Translational biomarkers and the strategies used to make development decisions for novel compounds can also be used to determine whether compounds meet goals that were created based on requirements for commercial success. A good example was cited earlier in the text and is illustrated in Figure 1.8. Here a new lipid-lowering mechanism and competing candidates were evaluated in relation to Lipitor. Superiority to Lipitor (Pfizer) was a requirement for commercial success. In this example, PK–PD modeling using a mechanism biomarker enabled rapid decisions on continued development. The high commercial requirements led to the attrition of these compounds (as is often the case), but here the cost was low.

Commercial requirements can have other broad positive and negative effects on translational medicine, drug discovery, and drug development efforts. If a company is only looking for "blockbusters," the universe of drug targets and indications they pursue is greatly restricted. In addition, these blockbuster commercial requirements often include high efficacy and safety hurdles to justify pricing goals. If there are no validated biomarkers that can be used to address these requirements efficiently early in development, only a small part of the risk of failure may be addressed by translational medicine activities and strategies. High commercially driven goals are most often evaluated in large comparative studies, which can lead to the discontinuation of projects late in development when it is expensive to do so. Another problem exists for unprecedented drug mechanisms. If there are no existing products with that mechanism, it is extremely difficult to predict the clinical profile and potential commercial attractiveness. For example, neurokinin-1 (NK1) receptor antagonists were found by Merck to have activity as antidepressants.[12] Pfizer, Merck, and others performed studies in patients with depression and compared the efficacy of NK1 receptor antagonists with that of serotonin reuptake inhibitors (SSRIs). The researchers found that the NK1 antagonists did not offer superior efficacy or safety and thus were not commercially attractive in competition with generic SSRIs. As a result, no NK-1 antagonists advanced to registration for depression, and most died expensively in Phase 2 or Phase 3.[12]

These requirements for commercial blockbusters may also prevent researchers from building on new science and new unproven areas of medical need. A recent *Business Week* interview with the CEO of Novartis, Dr. Daniel L. Vasella, focused on this issue.[13] At Novartis, a shift in strategy to more of a medical-need and science-driven focus, rather than a commercial focus, has resulted in a 40% increase in the number of drug candidates and a 60% improvement in drug candidate survival to late-phase development over the last 3 years. Dr. Vasella believes that good drugs will become commercial successes even if their initial indication is dictated by the importance of the mechanism for a relatively small patient group with high medical need. At Novartis, the success of imatinib (Gleevec) has reinforced this view. Gleevec started as an extremely effective drug for a targeted indication (Philadelphia chromosome positive chronic myeloid leukemia) with a few thousand new patients per year and grew to now include six other high-medical-need indications with revenues of $3.7 billion in 2008. Its effectiveness also justified a high price.

Vasella's strategy for Novartis is similar to the translational medicine strategy for making POM and POC decisions for novel drugs using a molecularly correct patient subpopulation. He believes that "focusing early on narrowly defined groups of patients will lead to more targeted and effective therapies with fewer side effects" and that this profile will also lead to faster and less expensive drug development programs with a high survival rate to regulatory approval. Of course Novartis does hope that the Gleevec model will become the rule and that commercial success will come from broadening the indication(s) later. If a company has this philosophy, it will support its translational medicine group by hiring first-class clinician-scientists, investing in translatable biomarker discovery and development for POM and POC decisions, and fostering a culture in which the criteria for further investment are based on the translation of preclinical results to humans and human data, not just potential commercial rewards.

1.7.2. Impact on Decision Making

Clearly, all things being equal, development decisions can and should be made in part based on commercial projections because all drug companies need to make a positive return of investment for their shareholders. Also, medical need can drive commercial value, and when decisions are aligned with both it is not difficult to make that decision. Regardless of how decision criteria are decided, translational medicine groups flourish when organizations make development decisions based on previously agreed criteria aligned with good scientific logic. Sometimes, however, commercial interests lead a company to hope that early negative data will be balanced or overcome by later positive findings and to decide to take more investment risk. Taking greater risk is often also justified by the desire to bring forward an important new drug sooner – especially if it benefits patients and meets an unmet medical need. During this author's time at Pfizer, the company generally followed good science and made appropriate development decisions. Sometimes, however, a previously agreed portfolio management strategy was changed when it was time to make hard, risky decisions. Under these conditions the work of translational medicine groups may become irrelevant, and their morale suffers. Here are three such anecdotes based on experiences at Pfizer. The first one involves a 5-lipoxygenase (5-LO) inhibitor approach for asthma and chronic obstructive pulmonary disease (COPD). Pfizer had several candidates and wanted to pick the best one to compete with Ziluton, Abbott's 5-LO inhibitor. That drug established precedence for the mechanism in asthma, but it was not an ideal drug because it had a short half-life, was dosed four times a day, and had only modest efficacy. Pfizer's candidates had better pharmacokinetics, but the best of them still produced nausea and vomiting at predicted efficacious doses. A Phase 1 comparative PK–PD study against Ziluton was performed using a mechanism biomarker, urinary leukotriene 4 (LTE4) level, to measure PD activity. The maximum tolerated dose of the best Pfizer compound had less 5-LO inhibition than did Ziluton. When the data were presented, the development team chose to push forward anyway with their planned large and expensive Phase 2 trials in asthma and COPD. This course was endorsed by the portfolio management group. Of course, both studies failed to demonstrate efficacy, and the compound was killed approximately

1 year and $5 million later. This outcome was predictable, but an organization hungry for a commercial success was willing to take more risk.

A second example involves CP-690,550, Pfizer's Janus kinase 3 (JAK3) inhibitor. This immunosuppressive mechanism is potent, and the compound was and still is being developed for patients with solid organ transplants and for RA.[14] A 14-day, multidose, Phase 1 study was conducted in psoriasis patients, and it was clear from both biomarker and clinical data that even the lowest doses tested had some immunosuppressant activity whereas high doses had some off-target adverse events. Toxicology studies showed that very high exposures of CP-690,550, like those of all potent immunosuppressant drugs, led to opportunistic infections and lymphomas. Thus, the key to successful development was finding the right dose and regimen. The Phase 1 data suggested the need to test low doses on the order of 1 mg to 5 mg once or twice a day, but low-dose tablets were not yet available. The team wanted to start the first Phase 2, 6-week RA study using the available tablet sizes rather than wait 6 months for smaller tablets. They were hoping that they would still demonstrate a dose response for efficacy, a clearly less effective dose, and an acceptable safety profile for a dose in Phase 3. There was never any doubt that this potent immunosuppressive mechanism would be efficacious in RA, but the optimal dose going forward was the main issue. The development team and the portfolio management group, anxious to start Phase 2, decided to take a chance to see if they could still demonstrate an acceptable dose response. A year later, the study did demonstrate excellent efficacy in RA, but the dose response for the primary clinical endpoint was flat across all three doses tested at the 6-week time point, although a dose response was apparent for some secondary endpoints.[14] Lower dose tablets were then used for a second RA dose-ranging study to find a less effective dose and clearly establish the basis for the Phase 3 dose.[15] Although the team performed its research tasks flawlessly, it probably would have been able to start Phase 3 earlier had the first Phase 2 trial been deferred until smaller strength tablets became available.

The third example involves Pfizer's cholesterol ester transfer protein (CETP) inhibitor program. Torcetrapib was the lead compound, and it exhibited potent CETP inhibition with elevation of high-density lipoprotein (HDL) cholesterol. HDL was a useful mechanism biomarker, with medium linkage to cardiovascular outcomes, but CETP mass and activity (target biomarker) were also measured. High HDL is associated with a lower risk of cardiovascular events, but it was and is still unknown whether elevating HDL through CETP inhibition would also have this favorable outcome. In Phase 1 studies, high doses of torcetrapib led to a reduction in LDL cholesterol and large increases in HDL.[16] These changes, however, were associated with increased blood pressure, and, with these findings, the development strategy put great emphasis on finding backup compounds that did not increase blood pressure and could be used to replace torcetrapib. Compounds were found that had similar or better CETP inhibition without blood pressure changes in animal models and in humans; meanwhile, torcetrapib was advancing rapidly in Phase 2.[17] It was also decided to develop torcetrapib in a combination with Lipitor to lower LDL and improve its clinical profile at the lower doses that were thought not to significantly elevate blood pressure but still significantly increase HDL. The dose of torcetrapib was modeled against blood pressure and lipid data, and, although there was a clear risk for a small increase in blood pressure, it was hoped that the efficacy would still be great enough to reduce cardiovascular events. There was agreement by experts inside and outside Pfizer that the benefit of HDL elevation and LDL lowering would likely outweigh any negative effects of a small blood pressure increase. In addition, Pfizer was reacting to investors who wanted Pfizer to develop torcetrapib in time to make up for the loss of revenue from the patent expiration of Lipitor. Instead of accepting a 1- to 2-year delay and switching to one of the backup compounds, Pfizer advanced torcetrapib and put the backup compounds that did not raise blood pressure on hold after Phase 1 studies to wait for outcomes data on torcetrapib. The rest is history. Cardiovascular events and blood pressure were higher on the torcetrapib–Lipitor combination than on Lipitor alone, and development was stopped.[18,19] Hundreds of millions of dollars were spent, and we may never know whether the result would have been different with one of the backup compounds that did not elevate blood pressure. The hypothesis that CETP inhibition would result in reduced cardiovascular risk and atherosclerotic plaque regression is still untested. Was the unfavorable result due to a failed hypothesis that raising HDL by CETP inhibition would have the same beneficial effects seen in people with high HDL levels? Was the elevated blood pressure responsible for the unfavorable outcomes? Recent data suggest that an off-target mechanism is responsible for elevation of blood pressure.[20] Whatever the reason, it is clear that the development of other CETP inhibitors will now have a huge safety hurdle to overcome (see Chapter 3, Section 3.9).

These three examples clearly show the impact and influence of organizational culture and specifically what can happen when a company takes on greater risk by making development decisions that give more weight to commercial goals than to the potential significance of existing scientific data. This also can lead to an environment in which the work of translational medicine groups is viewed as "nice-to-have" but not essential when in reality it is clearly the most essential part of early human drug development.

1.7.3. Translational Medicine and the Personalized Medicine Option

If early decisions are made based on mechanistic activity, and an efficacy signal in a molecularly correct disease subpopulation is identified by appropriate biomarkers, why not continue with targeted drug development to seek approval and labeling for that same narrow subpopulation? In fact, this approach could be less expensive and more rapid with a higher success rate to regulatory approval than one that attempts to broaden the indication to the entire disease population. Alternatively, development for the broad disease population could proceed in parallel but be obtained later with some of the costs being paid by revenues from the drug after approval for the subpopulation. Novartis has taken this approach for an anti-IL-1 antibody (Ilaris) by first developing it for Muckle–Wells syndrome and using this molecularly correct population to show safety and efficacy and enable more rapid development for other indications.[21] Ilaris has now been approved for this indication, and development for broader indications is expected to follow. In addition, Regeneron has obtained approval for its IL-1 trap using this same approach.[22] This strategy has the advantage of being able to obtain real-life safety information outside of the confines of a clinical trial. Any potential safety issues could be approached prospectively in the broader program. If universal health care and electronic medical records become a reality in the United States, it may be possible to obtain almost real-time safety monitoring for newly marketed drugs, which would further enable this type of strategy and might even speed drug approvals in general.

If it is decided to pursue development in a disease subpopulation identified by a biomarker, there will be additional qualification hurdles for the biomarker assay because it will have to be approved as a diagnostic device and used in the Phase 3 program. Such companion diagnostics are becoming more common, and this development path is not particularly difficult with a robust assay. Thus, the efforts of translational medicine groups to make development decisions using a molecularly correct population can also offer the option for the company to pursue a personalized medicine product.

1.8. Conclusion

This chapter has summarized the methods, strategies, hurdles, and consequences of supporting the translational medicine discipline within a pharmaceutical company. Because this has become more commonplace across the industry, over the next 5 to 10 years we will see if these investments pay off in terms of drug development productivity.

1.9. References

1. Littman BH, & Williams SA. (2005). Opinion: The ultimate model organism: Progress in experimental medicine. Nature Rev. Drug Discovery. 4, 631–638.

2. Guidance for industry, investigators, and reviewers. Exploratory IND studies. January 2006. Available at www.FDA.gov and http://www.fda.gov/downloads/Drugs/GuidanceComplianceRegulatoryInformation/Guidances/UCM078933.pdf

3. Biomarker Definitions Working Group. (2001). Biomarkers and surrogate endpoints: Preferred definitions and conceptual framework. Clin. Pharmacol. Ther. 69, 89–95.

4. Lathia CD, Amakye D, Dai W, Girman C, Madani S, Mayne J, et al. (2009). The value, qualification, and regulatory use of surrogate end points in drug development. Clin. Pharmacol. Ther. 86, 32–43.

5. Data courtesy of CMR International, and derived from CMR International 2009 Pharmaceutical R&D Factbook, CMR International, a Thomson Reuters Business (2009).

6. Kola I, & Landis J. (2004). Opinion: Can the pharmaceutical industry reduce attrition rates? Nature Rev. Drug Discovery. 3, 711–715.

7. Webb CP, Thompson JF, & Littman BH. (2010). Redefining disease and pharmaceutical targets through molecular definitions and personalized medicine (pp. 593–623). In: Biomarkers in Drug Development: A Handbook of Practice, Application, and Strategy, edited by Bleavins MR, Rahbari R, Jurima-Romet M, & Carini C. Hoboken, NJ: John Wiley & Sons, Inc.

8. Juweid ME, & Cheson BD. (2006). Positron-Emission tomography and assessment of cancer therapy. N. Engl. J. Med. 354, 496–507.

9. Aletaha D, & Smolen JS. (2002). The rheumatoid arthritis patient in the clinic: Comparing more than 1,300 consecutive DMARD courses. Rheumatology. 41, 1367–1374.

10. Li, S-P, & Goldman ND. (1996). Regulation of human C-reactive protein gene expression by two synergistic IL-6 responsive elements. Biochemistry. 35, 9060–9068.

11. Fishman D, Faulds G, Jeffery R, Mohamed-Ali V, Yudkin JS, Humphries S, et al. (1998). The effect of novel polymorphisms in the interleukin-6 (IL-6) gene on IL-6 transcription and plasma IL-6 levels, and an association with systemic-onset juvenile chronic arthritis. J. Clin. Invest. 102, 1369–1376.

12. Friedman L. (2002). NK-1 antagonists: The next generation of depression therapy? Curr. Psychiatry. 1, 60–61.

13. Capell K. Novartis: Radically remaking its drug business. CEO Dan Vasella's growth mantra for Novartis is to follow the science, not financials. Business Week, June 11, 2009.

14. Kremer JM, Bloom BJ, Breedveld FC, Coombs JH, Fletcher MP, Gruben D, et al. (2009). The safety and efficacy of a JAK inhibitor in patients with active rheumatoid arthritis. Results of a double-blind, placebo-controlled phase IIa trial of three dosage levels of CP-690,550 versus placebo. Arthritis Rheum. 60, 1895–1905.

15. Fleischmann RM, Genovese MC, Gruben D, Kanik KS, Wallenstein GV, Wilkinson B, et al. (2009). Safety and efficacy after 24 week (wk) dosing of the oral JAK inhibitor CP-690,550 (CP) as monotherapy in patients (pts) with active rheumatoid arthritis (RA). Arthritis Rheum. 60(Suppl 10), 1924.

16. Clark RW, Sutfin TA, Ruggeri RB, Willauer AT, Sugarman ED, Magnus-Aryitey G, et al. (2004). Raising high-density lipoprotein in humans through inhibition of cholesteryl ester transfer protein: An initial multidose study of torcetrapib. Arterioscler. Thromb. Vasc. Biology. 24, 490–497.

17. LaMattina J. Slides 3–5, Pfizer presentation to investors, November 30, 2006. Available at: http://media.pfizer.com/files/investors/presentations/LaMattina_Intro_112906_part2.pdf.

18. Nissen SE, Tardif J-C, Nicholls SJ, Revkin JH, Shear CL, Duggan WT, et al. (2007). Effect of torcetrapib on the progression of coronary atherosclerosis. N. Engl. J. Med. 356, 1304–1316.

19. Barter PJ, Caulfield M, Eriksson M, Grundy SM, Kastelein JJP, Komajda M, et al. (2007). Effects of torcetrapib in patients at high risk for coronary events. N. Engl. J. Med. 357, 2109–2122.

20. Forrest MJ, Bloomfield D, Briscoe RJ, Brown PN, Cumiskey AM, Ehrhart J, et al. (2008). Torcetrapib-induced blood pressure elevation is independent of CETP inhibition and is accompanied by increased circulating levels of aldosterone. Br. J. Pharmacol. 154, 1465–1473.

21. Lachmann HJ, Kone-Paut I, Kuemmerle-Deschner JB, Leslie KS, Hachulla E, Quartier P, et al. (2009). Use of canakinumab in the cryopyrin-associated periodic syndrome. N. Engl. J. Med. 360, 2416–2425.

22. Hoffman HM, Throne ML, Amar NJ, Sebai M, Kivitz AJ, Kavanaugh A, et al. (2008). Efficacy and safety of rilonacept (interleukin-1 Trap) in patients with cryopyrin-associated periodic syndromes: Results from two sequential placebo-controlled studies. Arthritis Rheum. 58, 2443–2452.

Translational Medicine and Its Impact on Diabetes Drug Development

Roberto A. Calle and Ann E. Taylor

2.1. Introduction

Type 2 diabetes is one of the largest medical burdens in the United States. At present it is estimated that 23.6 million people in the United States have diabetes (7.8% of the population) of which 5.7 million remain undiagnosed.[1] Of this total, approximately 95% have type 2 diabetes. In addition to insulin, eight different drug classes are available for the treatment of type 2 diabetes. In spite of all these drugs being available, many of them generic, only 49.8% of patients reach the American Diabetes Association–recommended targets for glucose control.[2] Moreover, many patients require the addition of a second therapy to maintain glucose control. Thirty-six percent require a second therapy with a mean time to failure from start of initial therapy of 1.51 years. Thus, many patients require multiple medications and often eventual insulin replacement.[3] Furthermore, many of the existing drugs have characteristics and potential adverse effects that make them less than ideal.[4]

Macrovascular and microvascular complications continue to take a heavy toll on patients with diabetes. An estimated 57.9% of people with type 2 diabetes have one or more complications. As a nation, the United States spends $57.1 billion a year in health care related to diabetes and its complications.[5] With an estimated 57 million people now having prediabetes, this metabolic pandemic can only be expected to grow unless serious steps are taken at the public health and drug development levels. Therefore, the need for better drugs for type 2 diabetes is now stronger than ever. (See Table 2.1.) A sound translational medicine approach is one of the approaches in which we can accelerate and improve our probabilities of success in developing new drugs and perhaps also develop biomarkers to determine which drugs best serve the needs of which patients, enabling a personalized medicine strategy for this disease.

Table 2.1. Summary of the Benefits, Adverse Effects, and Potential Concerns of Diabetic Drugs[a]

	Long-Term Data	Other Benefits	HbA$_{1c}$ Decrease	Route	Hypoglycemia Risk	Body Weight Change	GI Effects	Other Potential Concerns
SUs (1946)	Proven efficacy/ safety	Low cost	0.8%–2.0%	Oral	Yes	Gain	No	CV events?
Biguanides (metformin) (1957)	Proven efficacy/ safety	Low cost	1.0%–1.5%	Oral	No	None or possible loss	Yes	Lactic acidosis (very rare)
α-Glucosidase inhibitors (1995)	Limited data	CV benefits?	0.5%–0.8%	Oral	No	No	Yes	Unknown
Glinides (1997)	Limited data	Rapid acting	0.8%–1.5%	Oral	Low	Gain	No	Unknown
TZDs (1997)	Improve β-cell function	Lipid profile (pioglitazone)	0.8%–1.0%	Oral	No	Gain	No	Edema, heart failure, bone fracture
GLP-1 agonists (2005)	Unknown	Potential for improved β-cell mass?	0.6%–1.0%	Injection	No	Loss	Yes	Risk of pancreatitis
Amylin analogues (2005)	Unknown		~0.6%	Injection	No	Loss	Yes	Unknown
DPP-4i (2006)	Unknown		0.5%–0.9%	Oral	No	Neutral	Yes	Potential risk of pancreatitis

GI, gastrointestinal; SUs, sulfonylureas; CV, cardiovascular; TZDs, thiazolidinediones.
[a] Modified with permission from (4).

2.2. Primary Challenges

2.2.1. Efficacy

2.2.1.1. Glucose Lowering

Demonstration of a beneficial effect on glucose lowering is the primary goal for new antidiabetic agents. To get to that point there is a hierarchy of questions that need to be answered:

1. Does the compound modulate the target with the desired magnitude predicted to provide efficacy at a safe and well-tolerated dose (proof of mechanism)?
2. Does the compound's modulation of the target result in a reduction in circulating blood glucose (proof of concept), and how does the magnitude of effect compare to that of extant therapies?
3. What other clinical benefits can this compound provide beyond improved glycemic control?

The sooner these questions can be answered, the earlier a decision can be made regarding the viability of a compound as a new antidiabetic agent. In general, to support a decision to proceed to Phase 3 development, a Phase 2 study is needed to provide safety, tolerability, and glucose-lowering efficacy data. In the current environment of multiple available drugs, it is expected that a new candidate drug in early development will show evidence of a potential for better glucose-lowering efficacy than existing therapies have, a clinical benefit in addition to glucose lowering, or both. HbA1c is highly valued as the endpoint of these Phase 2 studies as it is a validated surrogate endpoint accepted by regulatory agencies for approval of antidiabetic agents and is also the gold standard for judging glucose control in diabetic patients. Therefore, a successful proof-of-concept study with this endpoint significantly reduces the risks of a full development investment. Unfortunately, a thorough assessment of HbA1c change requires at least a 12-week study to account for its dependence on red blood cell turnover and a relatively large sample size to account for its variability. As an example, typically, a dose-ranging study with placebo and 4 doses would require a sample size of approximately 75 subjects per group (375 subjects) for a power of 80% ($\alpha = 0.05\%$) to detect a change of 0.6% HbA1c units. The time and money required to execute such a study call for a relatively high level of confidence in success to commit those resources. The complexity increases if the goal is to show efficacy superiority over an existing therapy or other benefits such as better tolerability. Clearly, efficient prosecution of a portfolio of mechanisms and compounds calls for decisions to be made as to which ones deserve further advancement at earlier stages than an HbA1c-anchored proof-of-concept study.

In general, one key characteristic sought in all new antidiabetic agents is that the glucose-lowering effect be inherently glucose-dependent (i.e., with intrinsic limitation in the degree of glucose lowering as the glucose levels approach normoglycemia). A corollary of this desire for glucose dependence, from the point of view of drug development, is that the typical use of healthy volunteers with normal glucose levels in standard Phase 1 studies limits the ability to test glucose lowering directly early on. Short-term studies with nonglycemic target–related biomarkers are a necessary strategy to increase confidence in the safety and efficacy projections for novel compounds. To enable early decision making, it is important to consider which nondiabetic populations could be considered for study early on, what the duration of those studies should be and what endpoints are most likely to yield useful and predictive information. In addition to target-related biomarkers, it is possible to include glycemic endpoints other than HbA1c as dictated by the mechanism and the study population.

The selection of the population for Phase 1, its minimum duration, and its endpoints will also be influenced by the depth of knowledge of the mechanism and whether it has enabled identification of target-specific biomarkers that can provide a proof of mechanism, that is, a confirmation that the compound tested is modulating the intended target in the manner and magnitude desired. Development of target or mechanistic biomarkers that change acutely or in short-term studies and that do not depend on an early efficacy signal for glucose lowering are tremendously enabling, for they permit the compound to be tested in a single dose or a very short-term multiple dose study in healthy volunteers. Target or mechanistic biomarkers can be incorporated into the standard Phase 1 studies that one would carry out in healthy volunteers as part of a development program, allowing proof of the activity of the molecule early in development. One recent example of this strategy's being successfully applied is the development of dipeptidyl peptidase-IV inhibitors (DPP-4i) for the treatment of type 2 diabetes. DPP-4i were developed with great speed largely thanks to the identification of biomarkers that enabled early clinical evaluation of the compounds and their likelihood of success (see Case Study #1).

If no specific target biomarker is available, the selection of the population, the minimum duration of the studies, and the endpoints to be measured are largely influenced by what might be called the *systemic mechanism* of the candidate drug, which refers to the physiologic means by which modulation of the putative diabetes target is hypothesized to influence glucose balance and thus lead to lower circulating glucose levels. Examples of systemic mechanisms available to clinicians include insulin secretion by insulin secretagogues (e.g., sulfonylureas), improved hepatic or peripheral insulin sensitivity (e.g., peroxisome proliferator-activated receptor-γ [PPAR-γ] agonists), and inhibition, delay, or both of nutrient absorption (e.g., α-glucosidase inhibitors).

If the systemic mechanism is thought to be one that changes and achieves a steady state rapidly, such as acute insulin secretion or delay of nutrient absorption, a single-dose study or short-term study of 7 to 14 days may be sufficient to demonstrate the impact on a glycemic endpoint.[6,7] If the systemic mechanism is projected to require a longer duration to be fully implemented (such as some insulin sensitizers), the use of a glycemic endpoint may require longer studies, probably with a minimum of 3 to 8 weeks.[8,9] It is quite possible that mechanisms that induce insulin sensitization in a shorter period of time could be developed. However, as of now, the only example of insulin sensitizers we have are the PPAR-γ agonists (thiazolidinediones), which, as modulators of nuclear receptors regulating protein expression, take a longer time to express their full activity. Until examples of faster-acting insulin sensitizers become available and the uncertainty around the time to detect an efficacy signal with an insulin sensitizer is reduced, the most sensible strategy to reduce false negatives is to approach those mechanisms with longer duration studies.

In choosing a population for early development studies in which pharmacodynamic (PD) measures beyond a target biomarker could be obtained, two options become apparent:

1. Use of nondiabetic populations with abnormal metabolism (e.g., insulin resistance, impaired glucose tolerance) in which closely related endpoints could be measured; or
2. Early entry into the type 2 diabetes population.

The identification of subjects with impaired glucose tolerance can be enhanced by starting with a high-risk population such as persons who are overweight. If the target is an insulin secretagogue, the response of subjects with impaired glucose tolerance can be assessed relatively simply using oral glucose tolerance tests (OGTTs), which provide early information on both glucose and insulin responses.[10] The recruitment of subjects with type 2 diabetes can be more difficult (and complicated by variable concomitant medications). The amount of information gathered by going directly to patients with type 2 diabetes is invaluable, however, as relatively straightforward measures of glucose can start validating the target. If the target being pursued is one with scarce information and no target biomarker, this option may be the most expeditious. In this case, if glucose reduction is not demonstrated, a target biomarker is especially useful to clarify whether the failure was due to inadequate pharmacokinetics (PK), suboptimal tissue distribution, inadequate duration of therapy, or a failure of the target hypothesis. These questions cannot be answered without a target biomarker to confirm target engagement.

Regarding the endpoint to be measured, the researcher can choose from among several static or dynamic tests.

Static: fasting plasma glucose, mean glucose from continuous glucose monitoring or from multiple daily glucose measures, fructosamine, 5-α-glucitol, HbA1c, proinsulin

Dynamic: glucose area under the curve (Glu AUC) in response to a glucose or meal challenge, insulin area under the curve (Ins AUC), glucose infusion rate (GIR) (Table 2.2)

Each of the tests has its advantages and disadvantages, and the best choice depends on the systemic mechanism by which the drug is expected to improve glycemia and the population chosen for the early studies. The advantage of many of these static measures is that they are proximal (e.g., fasting plasma glucose, fructosamine) to the approvable endpoint. In addition, they are easily translatable as they are in clinical use for monitoring diabetes control. The use of fasting plasma or mean glucose levels can be a relatively simple approach for early development amenable to implementation in short 1- to 2-week studies and is particularly suitable for insulin secretagogue agents expected to induce glucose lowering fairly acutely. The disadvantages are that detection of changes in fasting glucose level requires studying subjects with type 2 diabetes and that glucose variability is fairly large, thus requiring a larger sample size. The use of fructosamine has the advantage of acting as an integrated measure of glucose control over the prior 2 to 3 weeks and does not require fasting for an accurate measurement. It is well accepted that directionally it will match glucose and HbA1c, although the degree of correlation with HbA1c on magnitude of effect is less clear, as shown by the contradicting data available in the literature.[11,12] The use of 5-α-glucitol in either plasma or urine might be appropriate in cases in which the mechanism of action is expected to largely affect postprandial glucose.[13]

Measures like C-peptide and proinsulin, although not translatable to direct clinical care endpoints, have been used as specific markers of pancreatic β-cell function. Preservation of stimulated C-peptide response, for example, has been associated with better outcomes in patients with type 1 diabetes.[14,15] In type 2 diabetes and prediabetes, higher ratios of proinsulin to insulin have been correlated in several studies with deteriorating β-cell function[16–18]; conversely, lowering of relative hyperproinsulinemia as fasting proinsulin, proinsulin/insulin, or proinsulin/C-peptide ratio has been interpreted as evidence of improved β-cell health.[19,20]

One of the best ways to interrogate an autoregulated system, like glucose control, is to introduce a perturbation into the system. This approach is used extensively as a clinical research tool, but it also has utility as a means of assessing the effects of a candidate drug in clinical development. In the development of antidiabetic agents, the use of dynamic endpoints depends precisely on perturbing the system with an intervention that acutely raises glucose and then observing the system's response to that intervention. The intervention can vary from a relatively simple procedure like an OGTT or mixed-meal tolerance test (MMTT) to the more complex, like an intravenous glucose tolerance test (IVGTT) or a hyperglycemic clamp. Monitoring the response in terms of glucose, insulin, and C-peptide not only can determine whether the compound being tested affects the magnitude of the glucose excursion (Glu AUC), which will usually be the primary endpoint but, through the judicious use of modeling, data from the various GTTs can also shed light on whether the effect is mediated by enhancing the insulin secretory response or by improvements in insulin sensitivity.[21] The details of how to implement and interpret these approaches are beyond the scope of our discussion but are more extensively described in several chapters of an excellent textbook edited by Michael Roden: *Clinical Diabetes Research: Methods and Techniques*.[22] The reader is referred to these reviews for additional details.

2.2.1.1.1. Additional Benefits Beyond Glucose Lowering

2.2.1.1.1.1. Weight Loss

Epidemiologic studies have clearly shown the association of obesity and insulin resistance with the risk for development of type 2 diabetes.[23–26] Clinically, it is well documented that weight loss leads to improved glucose control in patients with diabetes.[27] The beneficial impact of weight loss was recently exemplified by the 1-year data from The Look Ahead Trial study showing that diabetic patients in the intensive lifestyle modification group achieved decreases in weight of 8.6% and that this result was associated with greater improvements in mean HbA1c compared with the control group, while at the same time showing a statistically significant reduction in the use of antidiabetic medication.[28] Therefore, drugs that contribute to weight loss would be useful in the treatment of type 2 diabetes.

As a large number of patients with type 2 diabetes are also overweight or obese, it is possible to select a population for a Phase 2 study that can asssess efficacy for both weight loss and HbA1c lowering. Not only do the two conditions often coexist, but the endpoints can be assessed in a study of similar duration and sample size. A clinical trial powered to detect a decrease in HbA1c of 0.6% units, as described at the beginning of this chapter, has ample power to detect a clinically relevant weight loss signal.

If the sole effect of the drug is to cause weight loss, the U.S. Food and Drug Administration (FDA) has been reticent in granting an indication for type 2 diabetes. The most recent draft FDA guidance for the development of drugs for diabetes, however, signifies that this approach has changed.[29] Now, compounds may be accepted for an indication of glucose lowering if the weight loss results in robust glucose-lowering efficacy in obese diabetic patients and safety can be established for both lean and obese

Table 2.2. Tests with Dynamic Endpoints

Dynamic Test	Standard Intervention	Efficacy Endpoint: ↓ in Glucose Excursion AUC	Insulin Secretion Assessment	Insulin Sensitivity Assessment	Technical Complexity[a]
OGTT	75 g of glucose administered orally	Yes	Early insulin release (Glu AUC_{0-30})	Insulin sensitivity index; feasible with modeling	++
MMTT	7 kcal/kg of liquid meal (e.g., Ensure Plus) administered orally	Yes	Early insulin release (Glu AUC_{0-30})	Insulin sensitivity index; feasible with modeling	++
IVGTT	0.3 g/kg body weight glucose i.v. bolus	Yes	1st phase / acute insulin release (AIR_{0-10}); 2nd phase feasible with extended sampling	Feasible; made more accurate with i.v. insulin modification	+++
Hyperglycemic clamp	Variable i.v. glucose infusion[b]	No	Characterizes 1st and 2nd phases of insulin secretion	Feasible	++++
Hyperinsulinemic euglycemic clamp	Insulin infusion followed by variable glucose infusion to maintain euglycemia	No	No (infusing insulin)	Yes, gold standard	+++++

[a] Compared with complexity of single static measures, such as fasting plasma glucose = +.
[b] Rate adjusted to reach and maintain a predetermined plasma glucose level.

Each of these tests, except the hyperinsulinemic euglycemic clamps, can also be used to look at C-peptide and proinsulin secretion. AIR, acute insulin response to glucose.

diabetic patients. It should be noted that experience from several weight loss drugs, including sibutramine, orlistat, and rimonabant, suggest that, in general, obese diabetic patients do not lose as much weight as do nondiabetic patients.[30,31] For the mechanisms that have been studied, on average the diabetic patients lost approximately 60% of what the nondiabetic patients lost. The different populations have mostly been studied in separate studies, however, and so it is possible that other differences in baseline characteristics (weight, age, concomitant medications) have contributed to the different successes in weight loss.

Aside from the potential for weight loss alone to directly improve glucose control in type 2 diabetes, an antidiabetic mechanism that directly affects both weight and glucose control may provide an added benefit. In that situation, it may be advantageous to understand what portion of the benefit is derived from weight loss and what is weight-loss independent. In each case, being able to model the relationship of weight loss in type 2 diabetes and its effect on HbA1c is necessary. Mining the available literature for this relationship is possible. An example of the work done at Pfizer to model the relationship between weight loss and HbA1c lowering is illustrated in Case Study #2.

2.2.1.1.1.2. Cardiovascular Benefit

The main cause of morbidity and mortality in type 2 diabetes is cardiovascular disease.[32] The standard of care for reduction of cardiovascular risk calls for focusing on the use of multiple agents that can control lipids, glucose, and blood pressure as well as lifestyle modification to achieve the best possible control of known risk factors.[33] Nevertheless, an antidiabetic agent that delivers additional cardiovascular benefit would be a useful addition to the armamentarium against diabetes and its complications. At the very minimum, an antidiabetic agent must be neutral in its effect on cardiovascular risk (see Section 2.2.2). In many cases, the biomarkers that may be assessed to predict benefits on cardiovascular risk are the same ones that would be measured to characterize cardiovascular safety issues. The biomarkers with the best validation data in this area are lipids. As a large portion of diabetic patients harbor a dyslipidemia as a comorbidity, the opportunity to look for trends of beneficial effects in lipids is not beyond the reach of Phase 2 studies.[34,35] At the same time, inflammatory markers can also be monitored. C-reactive protein (CRP) is the best validated inflammatory marker for cardiovascular risk.[36–38]

2.2.1.1.1.3. β-Cell Preservation

The primary defect in the pathophysiology of type 2 diabetes has been debated for a long time. It is clear that the majority of patients who develop clinical type 2 diabetes have insulin resistance as a contributory factor.[39] Ultimately, however, it is the failure of the β cell to compensate for this increase in insulin requirements that leads to the clinical manifestation of hyperglycemia and its associated complications.[40–42] A drug that protects patients from further deterioration or even reverses the loss of functional β-cell mass would be a disease-modifying therapy. This type of disease-modifying antidiabetic (DMAD) agent would completely change the landscape of treatment for type 2 diabetes. Demonstration of this type of benefit is a significant challenge in translational medicine for type 2 diabetes.

Data from the United Kingdom Prospective Diabetes Study (UKPDS) indicate that β-cell function deteriorates at a rate of approximately 4% per year.[43] Therefore, demonstration of the benefit of such DMADs would require long-term studies to show that β-cell function is preserved or improved over a period of years. The design of these studies presents complex challenges as can be gleaned from the review of the ADOPT (A Diabetes Outcome Progression Trial) and the 1-year exenatide studies. From a clinical point of view, the potential benefit to the patient can be measured as the cumulative incidence of monotherapy failure after a fixed period of observation or as time to treatment failure. This approach was taken in the ADOPT study, which showed a lower incidence of monotherapy treatment failure with a thiazolidinedione as compared with metformin or a sulfonylurea after 5 years of therapy.[44] To address the issue of the mechanism of this effect, the investigators measured insulin sensitivity and β-cell function using the Homeostasis Model Assessment (HOMA-%S and HOMA-%B, respectively)[45] and confirmed a lower rate of β-cell function decline with a thiazolidinedione compared with metformin or a sulfonylurea. Unfortunately, the use of static fasting measures like HOMA-%B and HOMA-%S, which rely on fasting glucose and insulin, does not give the full mechanistic picture. The delayed β-cell deterioration could be an indirect effect of off-loading the β cell through peripheral insulin sensitization without a direct effect on the β cell, and this type of interplay is difficult to estimate by modeling. For a better understanding of this interaction, endpoints that correct the measurement of the insulin secretory response for differences in insulin sensitivity, like a disposition index (DI), are necessary*[46,47] In addition, understanding if the natural history of the disease has really been altered requires measuring β-cell function after a washout period off of the drug to demonstrate durability of the improvement on β-cell function. Such was the approach taken in a 1-year exenatide study (compared with insulin glargine) in which β-cell function was measured at the onset of therapy, during therapy, and after a 4-week washout period.[48] β-cell function was measured in this study using dynamic measurements that included a hyperglycemic clamp and arginine stimulation test to assess both first- and second-phase insulin release and a euglycemic hyperinsulinemic clamp to measure insulin sensitivity. This mechanistic

---

* DI: To obtain valid cross-sectional comparisons of β-cell function, the impact of β-cell compensation for insulin resistance must be taken into account. The DI was proposed by Bergman and colleagues [Bergman RN, Phillips LS, & Cobelli C. (1981). Physiologic evaluation of factors controlling glucose tolerance in man: Measurement of insulin sensitivity and beta-cell glucose sensitivity from the response to intravenous glucose. J. Clin. Invest. 68(6), 1456–1467] to account for these differences, and it was described as the product of insulin sensitivity and insulin secretion.

assessment is more robust but also clearly much more complex, thus requiring a more limited sample size. Even though significant improvements in insulin secretion were shown with exenatide as compared with insulin therapy, these beneficial effects were not maintained after the 4-week washout period. Thus, the clinical results with glucagon-like peptide-1 (GLP-1) agonists have not yet confirmed the preclinical suggestion that they can be disease modifying.

A true DMAD agent acting on the β cell should be able to

■ Improve or maintain β-cell function as measured by enhanced secretory response to insulin secretagogues;
■ Demonstrate durability of the improvement in β-cell function after washout of drug; and
■ Delay or prevent monotherapy failure as compared with other drugs.

By these criteria, none of the extant therapies has demonstrated a valid disease-modifying effect on type 2 diabetes.

One additional challenge in the development of a DMAD that preserves the β cell is how to demonstrate early that the proposed mechanism has the potential to eventually provide preservation of β-cell function that may lead to the types of outcome benefits discussed earlier in text. These early signals are important, particularly when we consider that some drugs that may eventually have the long-term benefit of β-cell preservation could have relatively modest improvements in glycemic control early on. Thus, gathering data early in the development process to support that a particular mechanism is improving β-cell functional health may make the difference between continuing a new compound into further development versus discontinuing it for lack of competitive efficacy. Measures like stimulated insulin, C-peptide response, and proinsulin, although not translatable to direct clinical care endpoints, have been used as specific markers of pancreatic β-cell function. For example, preservation of stimulated C-peptide response has been associated with better outcomes in patients with type 1 diabetes.[15] In type 2 diabetes and prediabetes, higher ratios of proinsulin to insulin have been correlated in several studies with deteriorating β-cell function[16–18]; conversely, the lowering of relative hyperproinsulinemia as fasting proinsulin, proinsulin/insulin, or proinsulin/C-peptide ratio has been interpreted as evidence of improved β-cell health.[19,20] Others have taken the approach of demonstrating restoration of the first phase of insulin secretion in subjects with type 2 diabetes, which is characteristically lost as β-cell function deteriorates.[49] This restoration of the first phase of insulin secretion has been argued to be evidence of improved β-cell health. None of these measures, however, has been validated to specifically predict preservation of β-cell function in a longitudinal study or to predict reduction in secondary failure of oral antidiabetic agents. The mechanisms with better data in this regard are the peroxisome proliferator-activated receptor-γ (PPAR-γ) agonists, for there are data with this class of drugs showing improvements in β-cell function and at least one study showing greater durability of glucose control compared with other mechanisms.[20,44,50] Because PPAR-γ agonists also cause (and are primarily thought to act through) insulin sensitization, however, ultimately one cannot separate the β cell and the insulin sensitization effects and their respective roles in the durability of response. As a result, the question of validation of these markers of β-cell health remains unanswered.

One additional hurdle is that current methods to assess β-cell function focus on insulin secretion responses, which might be confounded by direct insulin secretion mechanisms. Furthermore, acute insulin secretion can be confounded by glucolipotoxicity as well as by the duration of fasting that may allow more insulin granules to accumulate to be released. In the long term, increased insulin secretion may not be beneficial to the health of the β cell if the excess protein synthesis causes an unfolded protein response or endoplasmic reticulum stress.

Finally, the issue of how to determine whether this effect is mediated through an improvement in β-cell function, through an increase in β-cell mass, or both, is not one that we can address with present technology. Ultimately, it will be functional β-cell mass that counts. Approaches that have been proposed to measure β-cell mass and that may have potential for translation into humans include (1) the use of β-cell function assays as surrogates for β-cell mass, (2) angiographic and perfusion techniques to visualize changes in blood flow near islets due to functional activation or change in β-cell mass, (3) magnetic resonance imaging, and (4) labeling for tracer imaging with positron emission tomography (PET).[51–54] Technically, the approach that to date has shown the greatest feasibility as well as some level of validation in humans is the approach with functional assays (e.g., arginine stimulation test, IVGTT, hyperglycemic clamp), which, through studies in patients who have received pancreatic islet or pancreatic organ transplants, have shown a correlation with clinical outcomes.[54] Ideally, however, one would want to assess mass and function through independent measures. Although a matter of intense research, this is a goal that still remains elusive.

2.2.2. Safety

2.2.2.1. Cardiovascular

Antidiabetic agents are chronic therapy drugs; thus, long-term safety is of paramount importance. Specifically, knowing that the primary causes of morbidity in patients with diabetes are macrovascular complications and atherosclerosis, it is key to ensure that the drugs that are brought to the market, at the very least, have a neutral effect on cardiovascular risk. The need for cardiovascular safety is underscored by the recent FDA guidance requiring drug companies submitting New Drug Applications for antidiabetic agents to provide premarketing data demonstrating lack of cardiovascular harm.[55] The gold standard for cardiovascular risk assessment is an outcomes study. The incidence of cardiovascular events, even in a high-risk population such as patients with diabetes, requires large cohorts of patients followed by several years before the benefit can be demonstrated.[56] Typically, the results from large studies also use composite endpoints of different kinds of cardiovascular events, including myocardial infarctions, heart failure, and sudden death.

To assess the impact of a new diabetic therapy on cardiovascular risk in Phase 1 and 2 studies before making the investment in outcomes studies therefore requires the measurement of multiple risk factors for different cardiovascular mechanisms. Typical endpoints that are monitored in almost all early studies include blood pressure and lipids, for atherosclerosis risk, as well as ECG monitoring for arrhythmia and sudden death risk. Additional biomarkers that may be assessed, depending on the mechanism of action of the new compound and known safety risks of the class, also include inflammatory markers such as CRP and interleukin-6 (IL-6).[36–38,57,58] Studies of endothelial function, such as flow-mediated dilation (FMD), have been shown to be predictive of cardiovascular risk in some populations.[59,60] As a result, it has been suggested that these studies may serve as screenings for drug-related cardiovascular hazard. There is in fact some evidence that, in specific cases, drug-induced abnormalities in FMD may correlate with increased risk of cardiovascular complications (e.g., abacavir), although this evidence is still controversial.[61] The hurdles for accurate and reproducible measurements of endothelial function with FMD are large, however, and can lead to widely different results on the basis of technical differences.[62] Thus, although the measurement of FMD might be useful in specific cases, it cannot be recommended at present as a general screening strategy, and caution should be taken in interpreting FMD data as predictive of drug-related harm or lack thereof.

Unfortunately, no biomarker or measure of integrated cardiovascular risk exists that can serve as a general screening for compound or mechanism-related cardiovascular harm in early drug development. As long as this biomarker gap remains, the strategy for early assessment of cardiovascular risk for antidiabetic agents must be tailored to each proposed drug target. A careful assessment of the putative drug's mechanism of action and any potential links that it may have to pathways that may lead to increased cardiovascular risk can guide decisions of which endpoints must be monitored for safety.

2.2.2.2. Hypoglycemia

The Action to Control Cardiovascular Risk in Diabetes (ACCORD) and the Veterans Affairs Diabetes Trial (VADT) are two recent type 2 diabetes studies targeting intensive antidiabetic therapy to determine if tight glycemic control can reduce cardiovascular risk in diabetic patients. In the ACCORD study, the glycemic control portion was halted on recommendation of the data safety monitoring board due to a finding of increased rate of mortality in the intensive therapy arm as compared with the standard therapy arm.[63] Exploratory analysis of the mortality findings did not uncover an explanation, but, in both study arms, subjects with severe hypoglycemia had higher mortality than those without severe hypoglycemia.[64] Upon completion of the VADT, there was no decrease in its composite primary outcome of cardiovascular events and amputations for ischemia, but there was a non-statistically significant increase in cardiovascular deaths in the intensive therapy arm.[65] An exploratory analysis suggested that severe hypoglycemia within the prior 90 days was a strong predictor of the primary outcome and of cardiovascular death, although an association of severe hypoglycemia with all-cause mortality was apparent in the standard therapy arm only.[64] The results of these studies are a stark reminder that hypoglycemia remains a major hurdle for tight glycemic control and that its consequences can affect not only quality of life but also survival.

Thus, finding more efficacious antidiabetic drugs with minimal or no hypoglycemic risk is a priority. A focus on developing mechanisms that are glucose dependent, like the GLP-1 analogues and DPP-4i, can be expected to provide that safety. In looking for even more efficacious glucose-lowering agents, mechanisms are being explored that, like glucagon antagonists (which could block the liver's gluconeogenic response to hypoglycemia) and glucokinase agonists (which might block glucagon secretion from α cells), could hypothetically interfere with recovery from hypoglycemia. Particularly for mechanisms in which hypoglycemia is anticipated as a risk (e.g., full glucokinase agonists), it behooves the translational medicine clinician to capture hypoglycemia data with great care. For that purpose, and with the intention of facilitating comparisons across studies, it is advisable to use instruments that capture the adverse events of hypoglycemia following the conventions recommended by the American Diabetes Association (ADA) at the ADA workshop on hypoglycemia.[66] These recommendations establish accepted criteria for the definitions of the different severities of hypoglycemia and are mentioned as an acceptable classification in the FDA's draft guidance for industry on development of drugs for diabetes.[29]

For those mechanisms in which interference with counterregulatory mechanisms and hypoglycemia recovery is possible, it is important that this specific aspect be explored. For studying the potential changes in the responses of counterregulatory hormones and recovery from hypoglycemia, the use of a stepped hypoglycemic clamp is probably the most efficient and safe approach.[67] In this technique, an intravenous insulin infusion is used to increase circulating insulin levels, and a variable intravenous glucose infusion is used to manipulate the circulating glucose levels. This technique allows complete control and the potential for quick intervention for reversal of hypoglycemia if the subject is unable to self-regulate. At the same time, the adrenergic, glucocorticoid, and α-cell responses to hypoglycemia can be dissected, including definition of the thresholds for their activation, to confirm that they remain within the expected range and that the maximal response has not been blunted. Confirmation of a normal hormonal counterregulatory response would reduce the risk of unexpected profound and hard to reverse hypoglycemia with these mechanisms,[68] especially when tested in combination therapy with other mechanisms (e.g., insulin secretagogues, insulin) that may themselves induce hypoglycemia.

2.3. Case Studies

2.3.1. Case Study #1: Development of DPP-4i

The DPP-4i provide a new paradigm for the use of biomarkers in early drug development. DPP-4 is a key enzyme in the deactivation of the important gut hormone GLP-1, which mediates the improved clearance of glucose after oral rather than intravenous exposure. In this case, the direct measurement of circulating DPP-4 activity in the blood permitted a simple biomarker of response after a single dose of a new drug. Single doses of the DPP-4i vildagliptin were shown to have dose-dependent effects on DPP-4 activity as well as glucose-induced GLP-1 (Figure 2.1) and insulin and glucose responses (Figure 2.2) in Zucker fatty rats.[69]

These results allowed for modeling and prediction of the minimal suppression of DPP-4 activity that would be required for a clinically relevant impact on glucose levels. The suppression of DPP-4 activity in healthy volunteers could then be used as a surrogate to predict the efficacy of vildagliptin in patients with type 2 diabetes, thus significantly speeding up the early development of vildagliptin.

The first in-human studies in healthy volunteers were able to demonstrate inhibition of DPP-4 activity after a single dose. The amount and duration of DPP-4 activity inhibition after a single dose could be directly correlated with both the PK of drug exposure and the in vivo endpoint of increased active GLP-1 (Figure 2.3).[70] These first in-human, healthy volunteer, single-dose studies were able to accurately predict that a dose of 25 mg would be the approximate minimally effective dose for glucose lowering in diabetic patients, as was subsequently demonstrated.

Modeling could then be used to predict the exact intermediate dose of DPP-4i that would maximally affect glucose dynamics with once- or twice-a-day dosing. This approach allowed the early proof-of-concept trials to assess glucose lowering with a significantly simplified minimal number of appropriate dose groups.

Eventual Phase 2 and Phase 3 studies verified these predictions for optimal doses for glucose lowering. DPP-4i that were developed after the pioneers only needed to compare DPP-4 activity to be able to predict the

Fig. 2.1
The dose-response effect of vildagliptin when administered to Zucker fatty rats is shown for DPP-4 activity inhibition (A) and for glucose-dependent GLP-1 elevation (B). Reprinted with permission from Burkey et al., 2005 (69).

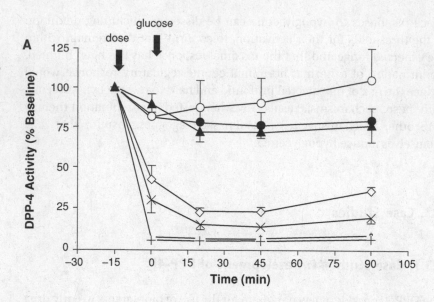

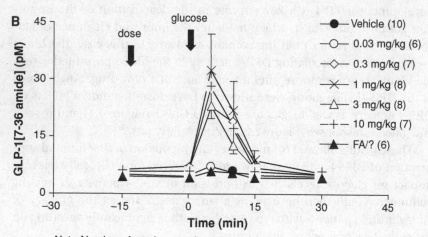

Note: Number of rats in parentheses.

long-term efficacy. Similarly, the strong PK–PD relationship after a single dose in healthy volunteers can be used to assess potential benefits of new formulations and of combination pills for special patient populations, including children.

2.3.2. Case Study #2: Development of 11-β-Hydroxysteroid Dehydrogenase Type 1 Inhibitors

The enzyme 11-β-hydroxysteroid dehydrogenase type 1 (11-b-HSD1) catalyzes the intracrine conversion of inactive cortisone to the active glucocorticoid cortisol in the liver. Because of its high level of expression in the liver relative to other tissues, inhibition of 11-b-HSD1 activity may reduce

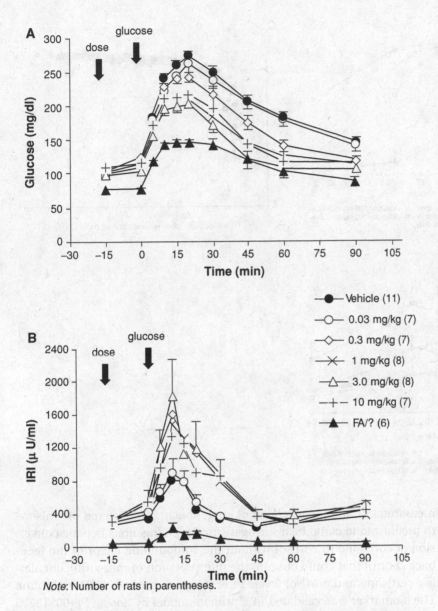

Fig. 2.2
The dose-response effect of vildagliptin when administered to Zucker fatty rats is shown for glucose excursion after an oral glucose challenge (A) and for glucose-dependent insulin secretion (B). Reprinted with permission from Burkey et al., 2005 (69).

Legend:
- Vehicle (11)
- 0.03 mg/kg (7)
- 0.3 mg/kg (7)
- 1 mg/kg (8)
- 3.0 mg/kg (8)
- 10 mg/kg (7)
- FA/? (6)

Note: Number of rats in parentheses.

glucocorticoid levels specifically in the liver and the splanchnic circulation.[71] The 11-b-HSD1 knockout mouse is protected from hyperglycemia associated with stress or obesity.[72,73] In addition, administration of a selective and potent 11-b-HSD1 inhibitor lowers body weight, insulin, fasting glucose, triglycerides, and cholesterol in diet-induced obese mice and lowers fasting glucose, insulin, glucagon, and triglycerides in murine diet-induced obesity and high fat/streptozotocin models of type 2 diabetes.[74]

PF-00915275 is a selective and potent 11-b-HSD1 inhibitor. Measurement of 11-b-HSD1 activity in the liver is not easily done. Therefore, to assess the effect of PF-00915275 on the target, it was proposed that a biomarker be developed based on the observation that the exogenous synthetic corticosteroid prednisone is a substrate for 11-b-HSD1 and thus that

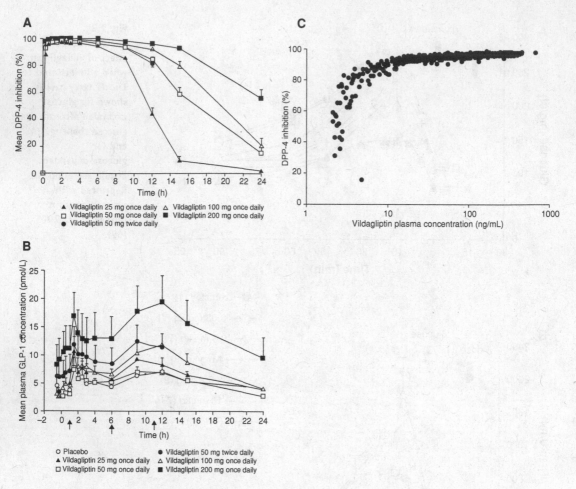

Fig. 2.3
Dose-response effect of vildagliptin after single-dose administration to healthy subjects on DPP-4 activity (A) and glucose-dependent GLP-I levels (B). Relationship between vildagliptin concentrations and DPP-4 inhibition, fitted to a simple Emax model (C). From Krishna R, Model-based evaluation of QTc interval risk: an increasing emphasis on early decision making J Clinical Pharmacol, 2009, 49: 1010-1. Reprinted by permission of Sage Publications.

measurement of the conversion of exogenously administered prednisone to prednisolone could be a surrogate for the endogenous hepatic conversion of cortisone to cortisol without the confounding factor of the feedback control that could obscure the interpretation of measuring circulating cortisone and cortisol levels in response to an 11-b-HSD1 inhibitor. The biomarker was validated in a primate model by dosing PF-00915275 to cynomolgus monkeys at doses from 0.1 to 3 mg/kg. As projected, dosing of PF-00915275 resulted in a dose-dependent decrease in the AUC of the prednisolone/prednisone ratio after an oral prednisone challenge of 10 mg/kg consistent with inhibition of 11-b-HSD1 activity (see Figure 2.4).[75]

Because the cynomolgus monkeys were normoglycemic, no insight into the level of inhibition needed to achieve glucose lowering could be obtained, although, judging by the levels of inhibition needed to see a statistically significant decrease in fasting insulin, one could hypothesize that inhibition of 11-b-HSD1 activity >57% was needed. To achieve additional confidence regarding projections of the magnitude of inhibition needed to see a clinical effect, researchers developed a novel

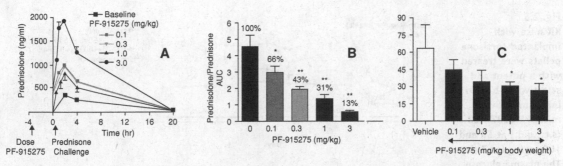

cortisone-induced diabetes mouse model to screen 11-b-HSD1 inhibitor compounds in vivo. KK mice have slightly elevated plasma glucose and insulin levels and are moderately insulin resistant. Subcutaneous implantation of a 21-day, slow-release pellet containing 35 mg of cortisone (C-35) caused these mice to become diabetic within 3 days of implantation. The cortisone pellet implantation resulted in a statistically significant increase in plasma glucose, insulin, triglycerides, and total cholesterol when compared with placebo pellet implanted controls. The newly diabetic mice were treated with a potent and selective 11-b-HSD1 inhibitor active in mice, PF-00877423 (s.c., q.d.) at 50 and 100 mg/kg for 7 days. The plasma glucose in mice treated with PF-00877423 at 100 mg/kg were significantly lower (>30% decrease) from Day 2 to Day 7 during the treatment period (see Figure 2.5). After compound withdrawal on Day 7, the glucose-lowering effect of PF-00877423 remained significant on Day 8 and then abated. Using plasma samples taken from a parallel group of KK mice treated with PF-00877423 at 50 mg/kg and 100 mg/kg (s.c., q.d.), PK parameters were defined for use in a PK/PD analysis of glucose changes using an indirect response/turnover model. The required glucose lowering of 30% was associated with minimal plasma levels of PF-0877423 at the time of PD steady state and were consistent with concentrations ~1.5-fold of EC_{50} determined in the rat FAO hepatoma cells (no mouse hepatoma cell lines were available for comparison). Because the PK/PD modeling estimated minimal concentrations that were consistent with EC_{50} values, all dose projections were based on maintenance of free EC_{50} levels (i.e., approximately 50% inhibition of 11-b-HSD1).

The ability of PF-00915275 to inhibit 11-b-HSD1 in humans was tested in a multiple-dose study in healthy volunteers.[76] On the basis of preclinical data, a criterion for proof of mechanism was set at 50% inhibition of 11-b-HSD1 activity. Doses between 0.3 and 15 mg q.d. were tested and found to be safe and well tolerated with a $t_{1/2}$ of approximately 30 hours. To assess inhibition of 11-b-HSD1, subjects received 10 mg of prednisone by mouth on the morning of Day 1 for baseline assessment, and on Day 11 at the same time they were dosed with PF-00915275. The mean ratio of prednisolone to prednisone AUC_{0-4} was measured as an index of 11-b-HSD1 inhibition. Figure 2.6 depicts the mean plasma concentration of prednisolone and the mean ratio of prednisolone to prednisone AUC_{0-4}.

Fig. 2.4 A, In vivo acute conversion of prednisone to prednisolone in cynomolgus monkeys upon receiving an acute prednisone challenge. B, AUC of prednisolone/prednisone ratio, which, as predicted, decreased with increasing doses of PF-00915275. C, Decrease in insulin fasting plasma insulin consistent with an insulin sensitization effect. From Bhat et al., 2008 (75). Reprinted with permission from The American Society for Pharmacology and Experimental Therapeutics.

Fig. 2.5
KK mice with implanted cortisone pellets were treated with a potent and selective 11-b-HSDI inhibitor active in mice, PF-00877423 (s.c., q.d.) at 50 and 100 mg/kg for 7 days. The plasma glucose levels in mice treated with PF-00877423 at 100 mg/kg were significantly lower (>30% decrease) from Day 2 to Day 7 during the treatment period and subsided after drug withdrawal. Unpublished observations printed with permission from Pfizer PharmaTherapeutics R&D.

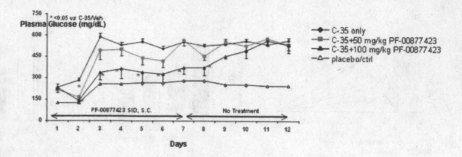

The maximum inhibition of prednisone to prednisolone conversion was 37% at the highest dose tested of 15 mg q.d. On the basis of these data, it was decided that PF-00915275 could not meet the criterion for proof of mechanism at the doses achievable in the clinic. Therefore, the compound was discontinued from further development.

2.3.3. Case Study #3: Effect of Weight Loss on HbA1c

Several mechanisms are considered to have potential for a weight loss effect in addition to an antidiabetic effect. Cannabinoid receptor subtype 1 (CB-1) antagonists and diacylglycerol acyltransferase 1 (DGAT1) inhibitors are typical examples of this category of mechanisms.[77,78] PF-001 is a compound acting on a mechanism also considered to have potential efficacy for weight loss and diabetes. PF-001 was tested at Pfizer for antidiabetic activity in a 12-week, proof-of-concept study in subjects with type 2 diabetes. The compound failed to achieve proof of concept, for the largest placebo-adjusted decrease in HbA1c at 12 weeks was 0.24% and there was no clear dose-response effect. The placebo effect was significant with a reduction of HbA1c in the placebo group of 0.61%. This study afforded an interesting opportunity to assess the effect of weight loss alone on HbA1c. A model was fitted for percent weight change from baseline versus time with placebo and drug effects.

- E_0 = placebo effect
- SLP = drug effect, %CFB/(ng/mL)
- k_1 = rate constant describing CFB effect
- k_2 = rate constant describing reversal of CFB effect

The structural equation was as follows:

$$CFB = \left\{ (E_0 + \eta_1) + (SLP + \eta_2)^* Css \right\}^* (1 - e^{-(k_1 + \eta 3)^* \, Time})$$
$$+ (k_2 + \eta_4)^* Time + \varepsilon_1$$

It was necessary to include a reversal effect in the equation due to directionality change in some individuals' data over time. Because a population approach was implemented for weight-loss assessment in which all subjects contributed data to the analysis, intersubject variability terms were

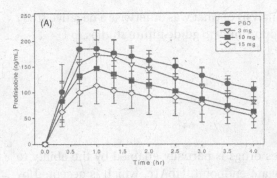 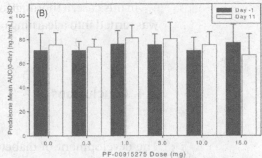

included in the structural model parameters, denoted as eta (η). Analysis of the data did not support any weight-loss activity beyond that afforded by the exercise and diet modification program that was part of the trial's design. For further analysis, the change from baseline for HbA1c was plotted versus percent weight loss, by dose and period. Because there was no appreciable difference between treatment arms, data were pooled and a simple linear regression was performed on HbA1c versus percent weight loss data (see Figure 2.7).

On the basis of this analysis, it would appear that decreases in weight are associated with decreases in HbA1c compared with baseline. Among the treatments studied, the placebo arm should provide the functional relationship between HbA1c change from baseline and percent weight loss not confounded by active compound: ~0.13% reduction in CFB HbA1c per 1% weight loss across all times in the study. When all of the data are incorporated (see Figure 2.7), the projection is that 10% weight loss translates to a decrease of 0.81% HbA1c change from baseline.

Fig. 2.6
Subjects were dosed with PF-00915275 with doses of 0.3 to 15 mg q.d. for 14 days. A, the mean plasma concentration of prednisolone; B, mean ratio of prednisolone to prednisone AUC_{0-4} for Day 11 versus baseline. The maximum inhibition of prednisone to prednisolone conversion was 37% at the highest dose tested of 15 mg q.d. From courtesy, 2008, (76). Reprinted with permission. Copyright 2008, The Endocrine Society.

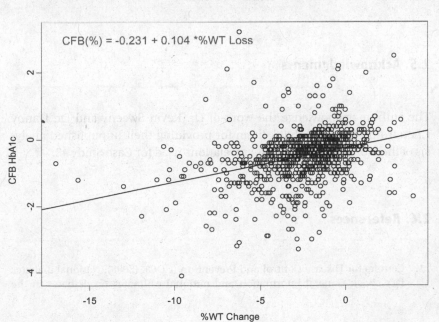

CFB(%) = -0.231 + 0.104 *%WT Loss

Fig. 2.7
Regression line for HbA1c change from baseline versus percent weight loss incorporating data from all doses. On the basis of the regression line for these data, a 10% weight loss translates to a decrease of 0.81% HbA1c change from baseline. Courtesy of Tim Rolph of Pfizer Pharmatherapeutics, CVMED Research Unit.

In this case, a thorough analysis of what was otherwise a negative study was turned into a learning opportunity to guide future studies.

2.4. Conclusions

The development of diabetes drugs is partially enabled by the ability to objectively measure a surrogate endpoint, HbA1c, which is accepted by regulatory agencies as the primary registrable endpoint. Furthermore, glucose measurements allow an estimation of the probability of a given drug candidate to meet sufficient HbA1c lowering to permit registration in studies lasting weeks or months. Nevertheless, the development of the next generation of antidiabetic agents is a challenging task that requires the identification of new targets that can deliver more than plain glucose lowering. The goals for this new generation of diabetes drugs include (1) effective glucose lowering without the burden of hypoglycemia, (2) reduction in micro- and macrovascular complications beyond that afforded by glycemic control alone, (3) true disease-modifying effects that prolong durability of glycemic control and significantly reduce the rate of secondary drug failure, and, finally, (4) all of these delivered by molecules with an impeccable safety profile. The last item is particularly important if we hope to implement these therapies early on, in the prediabetes stage, so that true primary prevention of type 2 diabetes is enabled rather than just treating patients when a large portion of the damage that leads to diabetic complications has already been done. Thus, demonstrating maximum clinical value for a mechanism, as well as safety, remains a serious challenge for persons involved in diabetes translational medicine.

2.5. Acknowledgments

The authors acknowledge the work of Dr. Kevin Sweeny and Dr. Danny Chen from Pfizer and thank them for providing their unpublished analysis of the HbA1c-to-weight loss correlations used for Case Study #3.

2.6. References

1. Centers for Disease Control and Prevention (CDC). (2008). National diabetes fact sheet: General information and national estimates on diabetes in the

United States, 2007. Atlanta, GA: U.S. Department of Health and Human Services, CDC.

2. Resnick HE, Foster GL, Bardsley J, & Ratner RE. (2006). Achievement of American Diabetes Association clinical practice recommendations among U.S. adults with diabetes, 1999–2002: The National Health and Nutrition Examination Survey. Diabetes Care. 29(3), 531–537.

3. Riedel AA, Heien H, Wogen J, & Plauschinat CA. (2007). Loss of glycemic control in patients with type 2 diabetes mellitus who were receiving initial metformin, sulfonylurea, or thiazolidinedione monotherapy. Pharmacotherapy. 27(8), 1102–1110.

4. Philippe J, & Raccah D. (2009). Treating type 2 diabetes: How safe are current therapeutic agents? Int. J. Clin. Practice. 63(2), 321–332.

5. American Association of Clinical Endocrinologists (AACE). (2007). State of diabetes complications in America: A comprehensive report Issued by the AACE. Available at: http://multivu.prnewswire.com/mnr/AACE/2007/docs/Diabetes_Complications_Report.pdf

6. Gonzalez-Ortiz M, Hernandez-Salazar E, & Martinez-Abundis E. (2005). Effect of the administration of a single dose of nateglinide on insulin secretion at two different concentrations of glucose in healthy individuals. J. Diabetes Complicat. 19(6), 356–360.

7. Hirose T, Mizuno R, & Yoshimoto T. (2002). The effects of nateglinide following oral glucose load in impaired glucose tolerance subjects: Rapid insulin stimulation by nateglinide in IGT subjects. Endocr. J. 49(6), 649–652.

8. Hammarstedt A, Sopasakis VR, Gogg S, Jansson PA, & Smith U. (2005). Improved insulin sensitivity and adipose tissue dysregulation after short-term treatment with pioglitazone in non-diabetic, insulin-resistant subjects. Diabetologia. 48(1), 96–104.

9. Rasouli N, Raue U, Miles LM, Lu T, Di Gregorio GB, Elbein SC, et al. (2005). Pioglitazone improves insulin sensitivity through reduction in muscle lipid and redistribution of lipid into adipose tissue. Am. J. Physiol. Endocrinol. Metab. 288(5), E930–E934.

10. Johanson EH, Jansson PA, Gustafson B, Sandqvist M, Taskinen MR, Smith U, et al. (2005). No acute effect of nateglinide on postprandial lipid and lipoprotein responses in subjects at risk for type 2 diabetes. Diabetes Metab. Res. Rev. 21(4), 376–381.

11. Dominiczak MH, Smith LA, McNaught J, & Paterson KR. (1998). Assessment of past glycemic control: Measure fructosamine, hemoglobin A1, or both? Diabetes Care. 11(4), 359–360.

12. Johnson RN, Metcalf PA, & Baker JR. (1983). Fructosamine: A new approach to the estimation of serum glycosylprotein. An index of diabetic control. Clin. Chim. Acta. 127(1), 87–95.

13. Dungan KM. (2008). 1,5-anhydroglucitol (GlycoMark) as a marker of short-term glycemic control and glycemic excursions. Expert Rev. Mol. Diagn. 8(1), 9–19.

14. Palmer JP, Fleming GA, Greenbaum CJ, Herold KC, Jansa LD, Kolb H, et al. (2004). C-peptide is the appropriate outcome measure for type 1 diabetes clinical trials to preserve beta-cell function. Diabetes. 53(1), 250–264.

15. Steffes MW, Sibley S, Jackson M, & Thomas W. (2003). Beta-cell function and the development of diabetes-related complications in the Diabetes Control and Complications Trial. Diabetes Care. 26(3), 832–836.

16. Inoue I, Takahashi K, Katayama S, Harada Y, Negishi K, Ishii J, et al. (1996). A higher proinsulin response to glucose loading predicts deteriorating fasting plasma glucose and worsening to diabetes in subjects with impaired glucose tolerance. Diabet. Med. 13(4), 330–336.

17. Larsson H, & Ahren B. (1999). Relative hyperproinsulinemia as a sign of islet dysfunction in women with impaired glucose tolerance. J. Clin. Endocrinol. Metab. 84(6), 2068–2074.

18. Pradhan AD, Manson JE, Meigs JB, Rifai N, Buring JE, Liu S, et al. (2003). Insulin, proinsulin, proinsulin:insulin ratio, and the risk of developing type 2 diabetes mellitus in women. Am. J. M. 114(6), 438–444.

19. Hanley AJ, Zinman B, Sheridan P, Yusuf S, Gerstein HC, & Diabetes Reduction Assessment with Ramipril and Rosiglitazone Medication (DREAM) Investigators. (2010). Effect of rosiglitazone and ramipril on beta-cell function in people with impaired glucose tolerance or impaired fasting glucose. Diabetes Care. 33(3), 608–613.

20. Smith SA, Porter LE, Biswas N, & Freed MI. (2004). Rosiglitazone, but not glyburide, reduces circulating proinsulin and the proinsulin:insulin ratio in type 2 diabetes. J. Clin. Endocrinol. Metab. 89(12), 6048–6053.

21. Cobelli C, Toffolo GM, Man CD, Campioni M, Denti P, Caumo A, et al. (2007). Assessment of beta-cell function in humans, simultaneously with insulin sensitivity and hepatic extraction, from intravenous and oral glucose tests. Am. J. Physiol. Endocrinol. Metab. 293(1), E1–E15.

22. Roden M. (2007). Clinical Diabetes Research: Methods and Techniques. First ed. West Sussex: John Wiley & Sons Ltd.

23. Chan JM, Rimm EB, Colditz GA, Stampfer MJ, & Willett WC. (1994). Obesity, fat distribution, and weight gain as risk factors for clinical diabetes in men. Diabetes Care. 17(9), 961–969.

24. Colditz GA, Willett WC, Rotnitzky A, & Manson JE. (1995). Weight gain as a risk factor for clinical diabetes mellitus in women. Ann. Intern. Med. 122(7), 481–486.

25. Ferrannini E, Natali A, Bell P, Cavallo-Perin P, Lalic N, & Mingrone G. (1997). Insulin resistance and hypersecretion in obesity. European Group for the Study of Insulin Resistance (EGIR). J. Clin. Invest. 100(5), 1166–1173.

26. Ford ES, Williamson DF, & Liu S. (1997). Weight change and diabetes incidence: Findings from a national cohort of US adults. Am. J. Epidemiol. 146(3), 214–222.

27. Anderson JW, Kendall CW, & Jenkins DJ. (2003). Importance of weight management in type 2 diabetes: Review with meta-analysis of clinical studies. J. Am. Coll. Nutr. 22(5), 331–339.

28. The Look AHEAD Research Group. (2007). Reduction in weight and cardiovascular disease risk factors in individuals with type 2 diabetes: One-year results of the Look AHEAD Trial. Diabetes Care. 30(6), 1374–1383.

29. U.S. Department of Health and Human Services, Division of Metabolism and Endocrinology Products, Food and Drug Administration, Center for Drug Evaluation and Research (CDER). (2008). Guidance for industry: Diabetes mellitus: Developing drugs and therapeutic biologics for treatment and prevention. Available at: http://www.fda.gov/downloads/Drugs/GuidanceCompliance RegulatoryInformation/Guidances/ucm071627.pdf

30. Franz MJ. (2007). The dilemma of weight loss in diabetes. Diabetes Spectr. 20(3), 133–136.

31. Lloret-Linares C, Greenfield JR, & Czernichow S. (2008). Effect of weight-reducing agents on glycaemic parameters and progression to type 2 diabetes: A review. Diabetic Med. 25(10), 1142–1150.

32. Morrish NJ, Wang SL, Stevens LK, Fuller JH, & Keen H. (2001). Mortality and causes of death in the WHO Multinational Study of Vascular Disease in Diabetes. Diabetologia. 44(Suppl 2), S14–S21.

33. American Diabetes Association. (2009). Standards of medical care in diabetes–2009. Diabetes Care. 32(Suppl 1), S13–S61.

34. Imperatore G, Cadwell BL, Geiss L, Saadinne JB, Williams DE, Ford ES, et al. (2004). Thirty-year trends in cardiovascular risk factor levels among US adults with diabetes: National Health and Nutrition Examination Surveys, 1971–2000. Am. J. Epidemiol. 160(6), 531–539.

35. Jacobs MJ, Kleisli T, Pio JR, Malik S, L'Italien GJ, Chen RS, et al. (2005). Prevalence and control of dyslipidemia among persons with diabetes in the United States. Diabetes Res. Clin. Pract. 70(3), 263–269.

36. Pai JK, Pischon T, Ma J, Manson JE, Hankinson SE, Joshipura K, et al. (2004). Inflammatory markers and the risk of coronary heart disease in men and women. N. Engl. J. Med. 351(25), 2599–2610.

37. Ridker PM, Cannon CP, Morrow D, Rifai N, Rose LM, McCabe CH, et al. (2005). C-reactive protein levels and outcomes after statin therapy. N. Engl. J. Med. 352(1), 20–28.

38. Ridker PM, Danielson E, Fonseca FA, Genest J, Gotto AM Jr, Kastelein JJ, et al. (2009). Reduction in C-reactive protein and LDL cholesterol and cardiovascular event rates after initiation of rosuvastatin: A prospective study of the JUPITER Trial. Lancet. 373(9670), 1175–1182.

39. Kahn SE. (2003). The relative contributions of insulin resistance and beta-cell dysfunction to the pathophysiology of type 2 diabetes. Diabetologia. 46(1), 3–19.

40. Festa A, Williams K, D'Agostino R Jr, Wagenknecht LE, & Haffner SM. (2006). The natural course of beta-cell function in nondiabetic and diabetic individuals: The Insulin Resistance Atherosclerosis Study. Diabetes. 55(4), 1114–1120.

41. Jensen CC, Cnop M, Hull RL, Fujimoto WY, Kahn SE, & the American Diabetes Association GENNID Study Group. (2002). Beta-cell function is a major contributor to oral glucose tolerance in high-risk relatives of four ethnic groups in the U.S. Diabetes. 51(7), 2170–2178.

42. Weyer C, Bogardus C, Mott DM, & Pratley LE. (1999). The natural history of insulin secretory dysfunction and insulin resistance in the pathogenesis of type 2 diabetes mellitus. J. Clin. Invest. 104(6), 787–794.

43. U.K. Prospective Diabetes Study Group. (1995). U.K. Prospective Diabetes Study 16. Overview of 6 years' therapy of type II diabetes: A progressive disease. Diabetes. 44(11), 1249–1258.

44. Kahn SE, Haffner SM, Heise MA, Herman WH, Holman RR, Jones NP, et al. (2006). Glycemic durability of rosiglitazone, metformin, or glyburide monotherapy. N. Engl. J. Med. 355(23), 2427–2443.

45. Matthews DR, Hosker JP, Rudenski AS, Naylor BA, Treacher DF, & Turner RC. (1985). Homeostasis model assessment: Insulin resistance and β-cell function from fasting plasma glucose and insulin concentrations in man. Diabetologia. 28(7), 412–419.

46. Ahren B, & Pacini G. (2004). Importance of quantifying insulin secretion in relation to insulin sensitivity to accurately assess beta cell function in clinical studies. Eur. J. Endocrinol. 150(2), 97–104.

47. Bergman RN. (2005). Minimal model: Perspective from 2005. Horm. Res. Paediatr. 64(Suppl 3), 8–15.

48. Bunck MC, Diamant M, Cornér A, Eliasson B, Malloy JL, Shaginian RM, et al. (2009). One-year treatment with exenatide improves beta-cell function, compared with insulin glargine, in metformin-treated type 2 diabetic patients. Diabetes Care. 32(5), 762–768.

49. Fehse F, Trautmann M, Holst JJ, Halseth AE, Nanayakkara N, Nielsen LL, et al. (2005). Exenatide augments first- and second-phase insulin secretion in response to intravenous glucose in subjects with type 2 diabetes. J. Clin. Endocrinol. Metab. 90(11), 5991–5997.

50. Gastaldelli A, Ferrannini E, Miyazaki Y, Matsuda M, Mari A, & DeFronzo RA. (2007). Thiazolidinediones improve beta-cell function in type 2 diabetic patients. Am. J. Physiol. Endocrinol. Metab. 292(3), E871–E883.

51. Freeby M, Goland R, Ichise M, Maffei A, Leibel R, & Harris P. (2008). VMAT2 quantitation by PET as a biomarker for beta-cell mass in health and disease. Diabetes Obes. Metab. 10(Suppl 4), 98–108.

52. Hirshberg B, Qiu M, Cali AM, Sherwin R, Constable T, Calle RA, et al. (2009). Pancreatic perfusion of healthy individuals and type 1 diabetic patients as assessed by magnetic resonance perfusion imaging. Diabetologia. 52(8), 1561–1565.

53. Medarova Z, & Moore A. (2009). MRI as a tool to monitor islet transplantation. Nat. Rev. Endocrinol. 5(8), 444–452.

54. Robertson RP. (2007). Estimation of beta-cell mass by metabolic tests. Diabetes. 56(10), 2420–2424.

55. U.S. Department of Health and Human Services, Division of Metabolism and Endocrinology Products, Food and Drug Administration, Center for Drug Evaluation and Research (CDER). (2008). Guidance for industry: Diabetes mellitus – evaluating cardiovascular risk in new antidiabetic therapies to treat type 2 diabetes. Available at: http://www.fda.gov/downloads/Drugs/GuidanceComplianceRegulatoryInformation/Guidances/ucm071627.pdf

56. Colhoun HM, Betteridge DJ, Durrington PN, Hitman GA, Neil HA, Livingstone SJ, et al. (2004). Primary prevention of cardiovascular disease with atorvastatin in type 2 diabetes in the Collaborative Atorvastatin Diabetes Study (CARDS): Multicentre randomised placebo-controlled trial. Lancet. 364(9435), 685–696.

57. Jenny NS, Tracy RP, Ogg MS, Luong LA, Kuller LH, Arnold AM, et al. (2002). In the elderly, interleukin-6 plasma levels and the -174G>C polymorphism are associated with the development of cardiovascular disease. Arterioscler. Thromb. Vasc. Biol. 22(12), 2066–2071.

58. Koenig W, Khuseyinova N, Baumert J, Thorand B, Loewel H, Chambless L, et al. (2006). Increased concentrations of C-reactive protein and IL-6 but not IL-18 are independently associated with incident coronary events in middle-aged men and women: Results from the MONICA/KORA Augsburg Case-Cohort Study, 1984–2002. Arterioscler. Thromb. Vasc. Biol. 26(12), 2745–2751.

59. Juonala M, Viikari JS, Laitinen T, Marniemi J, Helenius H, Rönnemma T, et al. (2004). Interrelations between brachial endothelial function and carotid intima-media thickness in young adults: The Cardiovascular Risk in Young Finns Study. Circulation. 110(18), 2918–2923.

60. Yeboah J, Crouse JR, Hsu F-C, Burke GL, & Herrington DM. (2007). Brachial flow-mediated dilation predicts incident cardiovascular events in older adults: The Cardiovascular Health Study. Circulation. 115(18), 2390–2397.

61. Hsue PY, Hunt PW, Wu Y, Schnell A, Ho JE, Hatano H, et al. (2009). Association of abacavir and impaired endothelial function in treated and suppressed HIV-infected patients. AIDS. 23(15), 2021–2027. 10.1097/QAD.0b013e32832e7140.

62. Bots ML, Westerink J, Rabelink TJ, & de Koning EJP. (2005). Assessment of flow-mediated vasodilatation (FMD) of the brachial artery: Effects of technical aspects of the FMD measurement on the FMD response. Eur. Heart J. 26(4), 363–368.

63. The Action to Control Cardiovascular Risk in Diabetes Study Group. (2008). Effects of intensive glucose lowering in type 2 diabetes. N. Engl. J. Med. 358(24), 2545–2559.

64. Skyler JS, Bergenstal R, Bonow RO, Buse J, Deedwania P, Gale EAM, et al. (2009). Intensive glycemic control and the prevention of cardiovascular events: Implications of the ACCORD, ADVANCE, and VA Diabetes Trials. Circulation. 32(1), 187–192.

65. Duckworth W, Abraira C, Moritz T, Reda D, Emanuele N, Reaven PD, et al. (2008). Glucose control and vascular complications in veterans with type 2 diabetes. N. Engl. J. Med. 360(2), 129–139.

66. American Diabetes Association Workgroup on Hypoglycemia. (2005). Defining and reporting hypoglycemia in diabetes: A report from the American Diabetes Association Workgroup on Hypoglycemia. Diabetes Care. 28(5), 1245–1249.

67. Evans ML, Pernet A, Lomas J, Jones J, & Amiel SA. (2000). Delay in onset of awareness of acute hypoglycemia and of restoration of cognitive performance during recovery. Diabetes Care. 23(7), 893–897.

68. Nauck MA, Heimesaat MM, Behle K, Holst JJ, Nauck MS, Ritzel R, et al. (2002). Effects of glucagon-like peptide 1 on counterregulatory hormone responses, cognitive functions, and insulin secretion during hyperinsulinemic, stepped hypoglycemic clamp experiments in healthy volunteers. J. Clin. Endocrinol. Metab. 87(3), 1239–1246.

69. Burkey BF, Li X, Bolognese L, Balkan B, Mone M, Russell M, et al. (2005). Acute and chronic effects of the incretin enhancer vildagliptin in insulin-resistant rats. J. Pharmacol. Exp. Ther. 315(2), 688–695.

70. Hu P, Yin Q, Deckert F, Jiang J, Liu D, Kjems L, et al. (2009). Pharmacokinetics and pharmacodynamics of vildagliptin in healthy Chinese volunteers. J. Clin. Pharmacol. 49(1), 39–49.

71. Basu R, Singh RJ, Basu A, Chittilapilly EG, Johnson CM, Toffolo G, et al. (2004). Splanchnic cortisol production occurs in humans: Evidence for conversion of cortisone to cortisol via the 11-beta hydroxysteroid dehydrogenase (11beta-hsd) type 1 pathway. Diabetes. 53(8), 2051–2059.

72. Morton NM, Holmes MC, Fiévet C, Staels B, Tailleux A, Mullins JJ, et al. (2001). Improved lipid and lipoprotein profile, hepatic insulin sensitivity, and glucose tolerance in 11-beta-hydroxysteroid dehydrogenase type 1 null mice. J. Biol. Chem. 276(44), 41293–41300.

73. Morton NM, Paterson JM, Masuzaki H, Holmes MC, Staels B, Fiévet C, et al. (2004). Novel adipose tissue-mediated resistance to diet-induced visceral obesity in 11-beta-hydroxysteroid dehydrogenase type 1-deficient mice. Diabetes. 53(4), 931–938.

74. Hermanowski-Vosatka A, Balkovec JM, Cheng K, Chen HY, Hernandez M, Koo GC, et al. (2005). 11beta-HSD1 inhibition ameliorates metabolic syndrome and prevents progression of atherosclerosis in mice. J. Exp. Med. 202(4), 517–527.

75. Bhat BG, Hosea N, Fanjul A, Herrera J, Chapman J, Thalacker F, et al. (2008). Demonstration of proof of mechanism and pharmacokinetics and pharmacodynamic relationship with 4'-cyano-biphenyl-4-sulfonic acid (6-amino-pyridin-2-yl)-amide (PF-915275), an inhibitor of 11-hydroxysteroid dehydrogenase type 1, in cynomolgus monkeys. J. Pharmacol. Exp. Ther. 324(1), 299–305.

76. Courtney R, Stewart PM, Toh M, Ndongo M-N, Calle RA, & Hirshberg B. (2008). Modulation of 11–beta"-hydroxysteroid dehydrogenase (11–beta"HSD) activity biomarkers and pharmacokinetics of PF-00915275, a selective 11–beta"HSD1 inhibitor. J. Clin. Endocrinol. Metab. 93(2), 550–556.

77. Scheen AJ. (2008). CB1 receptor blockade and its impact on cardiometabolic risk factors: Overview of the RIO Programme with Rimonabant. J. Neuroendocrinol. 20(Suppl 1), 139–146.

78. Subauste A, & Burant CF. (2003). DGAT: Novel therapeutic target for obesity and type 2 diabetes mellitus. Curr. Drug Targets Immune Endocr. Metabol. Disord. 3(4), 263–270.

Challenges in Atherosclerosis

John S. Millar

3.1. Introduction

Atherosclerotic cardiovascular disease is the leading cause of death world-wide today.[1] The number of cases of cardiovascular disease is anticipated to increase from 17.5 million to 24.2 million through the year 2030 as rates of obesity and insulin resistance and their associated dyslipidemia (elevated triglycerides and low-density lipoprotein [LDL] cholesterol and reduced high-density lipoprotein [HDL] cholesterol) continue to rise.[1] One proven means of reducing the incidence of cardiovascular disease is through reduction of LDL cholesterol levels.[2–5] Although currently accepted as a way of reducing cardiovascular disease risk, this has not always been the case. Over the past 50 years, the lipid hypothesis, which states that high LDL cholesterol and remnant lipoprotein levels cause atherosclerotic cardiovascular disease, has had its skeptics. Several competing theories have been proposed regarding the factors responsible for the development of atherosclerosis. The following section will provide a brief overview of several theories of atherosclerosis development and show where we stand today. Much of the evidence supporting the lipid hypothesis has recently been reviewed in detail.[6–10]

3.2. Prevailing Hypotheses of Atherosclerosis Development

3.2.1. The Lipid Hypothesis

Early investigations into the structure and composition of atherosclerotic plaque revealed that plaque is enriched in lipid, including cholesterol. How and why it forms was not initially known. Anitschkow and Chalatow made the serendipitous discovery in their studies on dietary protein that feeding egg yolk and brain to rabbits resulted in atherosclerotic plaque formation.[11] They also noted that these animals had an accumulation of lipid in the liver. They hypothesized that it was the cholesterol in the egg yolk and brain that promoted plaque formation when fed to rabbits. Subsequent studies in which rabbits were fed cholesterol[11] were able to reproduce the atherosclerotic plaque formation and lipid accumulation in the liver. These studies were the first to identify cholesterol as a causative agent in the development of atherosclerotic plaque and set the stage for the lipid hypothesis.

Studies by other investigators in the years that followed provided additional evidence that linked plasma cholesterol levels to cardiovascular disease in humans. Some important findings included evidence that

- populations with high plasma cholesterol levels were found to have increased rates of cardiovascular disease,[12]
- dietary fat and cholesterol can influence plasma cholesterol levels and risk of cardiovascular disease independently of genetic background,[13] and
- patients with familial hypercholesterolemia, a genetic predisposition for high plasma cholesterol levels, are at increased risk of developing premature cardiovascular disease.[14]

Although many of these studies suggested that elevated LDL cholesterol levels were responsible for the development of atherosclerosis, there were others that showed no effect (reviewed in reference 15), often due to inadequate sample size.[16] There were also concerns that lowering LDL cholesterol levels could increase the risk of cancer because there was an association between low cholesterol and incidence of cancer.[17] Although this association is likely a confounding effect of low cholesterol resulting from reduced food intake secondary to undiagnosed illness,[18] concerns regarding cholesterol lowering and the development of cancer linger today. In addition to these concerns, some of the early drugs designed to lower LDL cholesterol resulted in adverse effects that made many clinicians question the safety of pharmacologic interventions to lower LDL cholesterol.[16,19] Thus, a great debate ensued as to whether it was worthwhile and safe to pursue a strategy of lowering plasma LDL cholesterol levels as a means of reducing cardiovascular risk. It was during this time that other theories regarding the development of atherosclerosis gained support.

3.2.2. The Response-to-Injury Hypothesis

Originally proposed by Ross, Glomset, and Harker,[20] this hypothesis states that endothelial denudation, injury, or activation is the primary event that promotes the formation of atherosclerotic plaque. This hypothesis was based on studies that showed that experimentally induced endothelial injury could initiate events that lead to plaque formation. Despite using hyperlipidemic animal models in experiments designed to support this hypothesis, the focus was on acute and chronic events, such as shear stress or infection, causing physical damage to the vascular endothelium. The hypothesis states that, in response to injury, a cascade of events that promote platelet and monocyte recruitment to the damaged area ensues. This activity, in turn, promotes smooth muscle cell proliferation, extracellular matrix deposition, and lipoprotein accumulation. Although it was a plausible hypothesis that was supported by ample experimental evidence, it was criticized for the requirement of a rather severe injury to the vascular endothelium, which was not found in most cases of early or advanced atherosclerosis.

3.2.3. The Response-to-Inflammation Hypothesis

This hypothesis is a modification of the response-to-injury hypothesis. The major modification is that the type of injury to the vascular endothelium is less severe than that described in the response-to-injury hypothesis.[21] It was recognized that the endothelial layer in the area of an atherosclerotic plaque is largely intact, indicating that there is no requirement for denudation of the endothelial layer prior to plaque development. Instead, according to this hypothesis, the endothelial injury that leads to atherosclerotic plaque formation is more subtle. This hypothesis states that the vascular endothelium faces a number of insults that elicit an inflammatory response. These insults include elevated lipids, free radicals (from smoking, pollution, antioxidant deficiency, etc.), hyperhomocysteinemia, and infectious microorganisms. If the insult(s) are not effectively eliminated, a chronic inflammatory state develops that initiates events that lead to an early atherosclerotic lesion. Left untreated, this early atherosclerotic lesion can progress to a lipid-enriched plaque and advanced atherosclerosis. Although this hypothesis is supported by both experimental and epidemiological evidence, it does not require hyperlipidemia as a key component involved in the development of atherosclerotic plaque.

3.2.4. The Response-to-Retention Hypothesis

The response-to-retention hypothesis of atherosclerosis development was proposed by Williams and Tabas in 1995.[22] This hypothesis states that retention of apolipoprotein B (apoB)-containing lipoproteins by constituents (primarily proteoglycans and collagen) within the subendothelial matrix is the key event that initiates atherosclerosis. The response-to retention hypothesis is consistent with the lipid hypothesis in that apoB-containing lipoproteins are the key components required for atherosclerotic plaque formation and development. According to this hypothesis, other factors such as hypertension, hyperglycemia, and lipoprotein oxidation can contribute to the development of atherosclerosis but cannot directly result in the formation of atherosclerotic plaque. Only lipoprotein retention within the subendothelial matrix satisfies the criterion of being necessary and sufficient for initiating atherosclerosis. Williams and Tabas suggest that factors that block the retention of lipoproteins within the subendothelial matrix will reduce formation of atherosclerotic plaque. Although this hypothesis places the focus on apoB-containing lipoproteins (very-low-density lipoprotein [VLDL], intermediate-density lipoprotein [IDL], LDL, and lipoprotein(a) [Lp(a)]) in the development of atherosclerotic plaque, and is therefore consistent with the lipid hypothesis, it could be further refined by placing a greater emphasis on the requirement of hyperlipidemia for plaque formation.

3.3. Clinical Trials Supporting the Lipid Hypothesis

Although there were certainly substantial data before 1970 that supported the concept of lowering LDL as a means of reducing the risk of cardiovascular disease, the data were associative and therefore unable to prove definitively that LDL lowering could reduce the risk of atherosclerosis. In an attempt to determine definitively if reducing LDL levels could safely reduce the risk of cardiovascular disease, several large, well-designed studies were conducted. The first study, sponsored by the National Institutes of Health, was the Lipid Research Clinics Coronary Primary Prevention Trial.[2] This trial, initiated in 1973, compared patients treated with the bile acid sequestrant (cholestyramine) to those given placebo. This study, involving 3,806 patients, resulted in a mean LDL reduction of 20% in the cholestyramine treatment group, and this reduction was associated with a significant reduction in nonfatal cardiovascular events. Soon after, the Helsinki Heart study, in which patients were treated with gemfibrozil, showed a significant decrease in cardiovascular events in the treated group.[3] Later, when statin drugs became available, more effective LDL lowering could be achieved, further demonstrating that reducing LDL levels lowers the risk of cardiovascular disease in both primary[4] (Figure 3.1) and secondary prevention studies.[5] Perhaps just as important were the findings from these studies that LDL lowering was safe, being associated with no significant effect on overall mortality or incidence of cancer.

3.4. Where We Stand Today

Epidemiological studies have identified factors such as hypertension, inflammation, increased LDL, and low HDL as being associated with an increase in risk of cardiovascular disease. The question arises as to which factors are important to target to reduce cardiovascular risk. In assessing

Fig. 3.1
Cumulative
cardiovascular events
in patients treated
with either placebo or
pravastatin in the
West of Scotland
Coronary Prevention
Study A. In this study,
baseline LDL
cholesterol levels of
approximately 192
mg/dl were reduced by
26% to approximately
132 mg/dl B. This
change in LDL
cholesterol was
associated with a
significant decrease in
the number of
cardiovascular events
(definite coronary
heart disease death or
nonfatal myocardial
infarction). © 1995
Massachusetts Medical
Society. All rights
reserved.

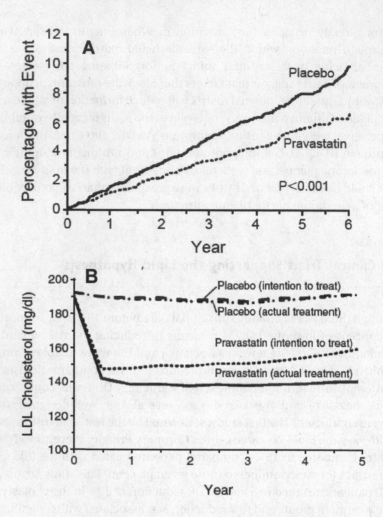

risk of atherosclerosis using data from prospective trials, a number of factors consistently emerge that individually contribute to risk of cardiovascular disease. These factors include smoking status, age, gender, blood pressure, and LDL cholesterol level.[23] Indeed, randomized trials have shown the benefits of smoking cessation,[24] controlling blood pressure,[25] and reducing LDL cholesterol levels.[2-5] The benefit of reducing inflammation and increasing HDL are, thus far, unproven. Statin treatment of patients with normal LDL levels but with elevated levels of the inflammatory biomarker C-reactive protein showed significant reduction in cardiovascular events,[26] although it is not clear if this reduction was due to lowering of LDL levels (50% lower) or improved inflammatory status. The few clinical trials designed specifically to address the questions of whether reducing inflammation and increasing HDL are of benefit in the reduction of cardiovascular risk have been negative,[27,28] likely illustrating the nonspecific nature of inflammation and the complexity of HDL.[29,30]

In contrast to the uncertainty surrounding the relationship between inflammation or HDL levels and the risk of atherosclerosis, evidence for the benefit of reducing LDL cholesterol in reducing the risk of cardiovascular disease continues to grow. This evidence includes findings from studies in subjects with a genetic mutation that predisposes them to low lifelong levels of LDL cholesterol (20–40 mg/dl lower than average) and reduced risk of cardiovascular disease.[31] In addition, recent studies indicate that lowering LDL cholesterol levels below 70 mg/dl is associated with regression of atherosclerosis.[26,32]

3.5. Atherosclerosis and Drug Discovery and Development

This section will discuss the current and future pharmacological approaches to atherosclerosis and the unique challenges in this area where long-term outcomes are the accepted endpoints but development decisions need to be made at a lower cost and on the basis of short-term clinical and biomarker data.

3.5.1. Lipoprotein Metabolism

An understanding of lipoprotein metabolism is important when developing drug candidates to treat dyslipidemia. Although tremendous strides have been made in the past 10 years with regard to our understanding of lipoprotein metabolism, gaps in knowledge still exist, particularly with regard to the significance of HDL cholesterol and reverse cholesterol transport (RCT). This section provides a brief overview of lipoprotein metabolism (depicted in Figures 3.2 and 3.3) and discuss the development of therapies designed to reduce the risk of cardiovascular disease by improving the lipoprotein phenotype.

Triglyceride and cholesterol are necessary for normal growth and metabolism. Being lipophilic substances, these cannot move through the aqueous plasma environment unless they are part of a lipoprotein complex. Despite similarities in their hydrophobicity, the transport of cholesterol and that of triglyceride on lipoproteins is distinctly different. Triglyceride moves through plasma primarily as part of chylomicron and VLDL particles. Its transport is a one-way journey from the intestine (chylomicron) or liver (VLDL) to peripheral tissues, including skeletal muscle and adipose tissue. After being delivered to peripheral tissues, fatty acids from triglyceride are used for energy production or energy storage. Triglyceride stored in adipose tissue can be returned to the liver in the form of nonesterified fatty acids complexed with albumin where they can be repackaged into triglycerides for export on VLDL as needed.

In contrast, cholesterol movement through plasma requires lipoproteins for both the forward transport to peripheral tissues and the reverse

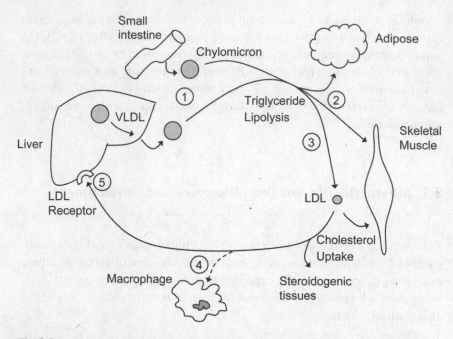

Fig. 3.2 Delivery of triglyceride and cholesterol from the liver and small intestine to peripheral tissues. (1) Triglyceride and cholesterol are packaged into chylomicrons (small intestine) or VLDL (liver) and secreted into plasma as triglyceride-rich particles. (2) When in plasma, these particles are acted on by LPL to release fatty acids from triglyceride. The fatty acids released are taken up by tissues and used for energy production or storage (adipose). (3) Lipolyzed chylomicrons are cleared from plasma by the liver (not shown); lipolyzed VLDL can either be cleared from plasma (not shown) or converted to cholesterol-rich LDL. (4) Modified (oxidized) LDL is a poor ligand for the LDL receptor and is cleared by scavenger receptors on the macrophage. Clearance of modified LDL by scavenger receptors typically represents a minor route of clearance but can be substantial under certain pathological conditions. Normal (unmodified) LDL is taken up by steroidogenic tissues or (5) cleared from plasma by LDL receptors in the liver.

transport back to the liver. In forward cholesterol transport (Figure 3.2), dietary cholesterol on intestinally derived chylomicrons and recycled or endogenously produced cholesterol from liver-derived VLDL (and subsequently LDL) is delivered to peripheral tissues. RCT (Figure 3.3) includes the movement of excess cholesterol from peripheral tissues, including the macrophage, to the liver via transfer to HDL. Some investigators define RCT as the movement of excess cholesterol from peripheral tissues to the liver via HDL,[33] whereas others extend this to include the delivery of cholesterol to the liver with subsequent excretion in feces.[34]

The forward and reverse cholesterol transport pathways function together to maintain normal cellular cholesterol homeostasis. Under pathological conditions, when excess chylomicrons, VLDL, or LDL are produced or when their clearance is impaired, the concentration of these lipoproteins in plasma are elevated. This elevation increases the likelihood of entry and retention of these lipoproteins within the vessel wall, often leading to pathological consequences.

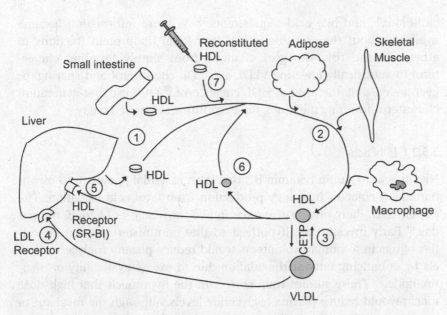

Fig. 3.3 The transport of cholesterol from peripheral tissues to the liver (RCT). (1) Newly synthesized HDL are secreted as free apoA-I or small apoA-I/phospholipid disks from the small intestine and liver. (2) These nascent particles accept free cholesterol from peripheral tissues, a process mediated by the ATP-binding cassette transporter AI (ABCAI) transporter. As HDLs mature and enlarge, the delivery of cholesterol is thought to be mediated by scavenger receptor class B type I (SR-BI) and ATP-binding cassette transporter GI (ABCGI). (3) Cholesterol-enriched HDL unload cholesterol to VLDL and LDL in a process mediated by CETP. (4) The cholesterol in VLDL and LDL obtained by exchange can be delivered to the liver following uptake by the LDL receptor. (5) An alternative route delivery is by uptake of HDL cholesterol by SR-BI. (6) Following delivery of cholesterol from HDL, the cholesterol-depleted HDL can remain in plasma, completing the cycle again. (7) One promising treatment to acutely increase HDL in plasma is to deliver apoA-I/phospholipid complexes that resemble nascent HDL by injection.

Many strategies are being pursued to reduce the risk of atherosclerotic cardiovascular disease through improvement of the lipoprotein phenotype. These strategies include new formulations and combinations of existing drugs as well as development of novel drugs designed to reduce plasma triglyceride and LDL and increase HDL. This next section will focus on current antidyslipidemic therapies that are approved or are in mid- to late-stage clinical development.

3.5.2. Antidyslipidemics

3.5.2.1. First-Generation Antidyslipidemics

Drugs initially used to reduce the risk of cardiovascular disease through alteration of the plasma lipoprotein phenotype were based on their cholesterol-lowering effects. These drugs include niacin,[35] probucol,[36] clofibrate,[37] and bile acid sequestrants.[38] As more information became available about the contribution of individual lipoprotein fractions to atherosclerotic risk, the goal changed from simply lowering cholesterol to specifically lowering VLDL and LDL cholesterol and sparing, or even increasing, the level of HDL cholesterol.[39] Of these first-generation cholesterol-lowering therapies, many continue to be used today.

3.5.2.1.1. Niacin

Niacin is a B vitamin (vitamin B_3) that is an essential precursor to nicotinamide, a cofactor in energy production from fatty acid oxidation. The current U.S. daily dietary reference intake for niacin is 14 to 16 mg per day.[40] Early investigators hypothesized that administering gram quantities of niacin to human volunteers would reduce plasma triglyceride levels by enhancing fatty acid oxidation due to excess availability of nicotinamide.[35] These studies were correct in the hypothesis that high-dose niacin would reduce plasma triglyceride levels, although the mechanism turned out to be different from what was initially thought. We now know that, at high doses (1–2 grams per day), niacin can activate the G-protein-coupled receptor HM74α (known as PUMA G in mice),[41] which is primarily expressed at the cell surface in adipose tissue. Upon ligand binding, HM74α triggers a G-protein-mediated signaling pathway that inhibits hormone-sensitive lipase, which is responsible for fatty acid release from adipose into plasma. The result of inhibiting the activity of hormone-sensitive lipase is a decrease in fatty acid release from adipose into plasma. The natural ligand for HM74α is thought to be β-hydroxybutyrate,[42] and activation of this receptor by high plasma concentrations of niacin appears to be a desirable nonspecific effect. High-dose niacin treatment can also increase HDL levels, although the mechanism for this is not known. Common side effects associated with high-dose niacin include pruritus, facial flushing, and gastrointestinal disturbances, which have been attributed to activation of the prostaglandin D2 (PGD2) receptor.[43] These side effects can be reduced when niacin is administered with aspirin (300 mg).

An extended-release version of niacin is available that minimizes the side effects associated with use of the acute-release formulation.[44] Extended-release niacin has been approved for use in combination with simvastatin. The combination is designed to lower LDL cholesterol levels by reducing endogenous cholesterol synthesis through inhibition of 3-hydroxy-3-methylglutaryl-coenzyme A (HMG CoA) reductase (simvastatin) and to reduce triglyceride and increase HDL levels (extended-release niacin). In clinical studies, the combination was superior to simvastatin alone in reducing triglyceride and LDL levels and increasing HDL levels.[45]

The subcutaneous flushing effects of niacin have been attributed to activation of the PGD2 receptor. Laropiprant (Tredaptive; Merck, Whitehouse Station, NJ) is an antagonist of the PGD2 receptor that was developed for use in combination with extended-release niacin to reduce triglyceride and increase HDL levels while minimizing the flushing associated with extended-release niacin. In clinical studies, the combination was associated with improved tolerance as compared with extended-release niacin alone.[46] This combination is currently approved for use in the European Union and is under development in the United States.

3.5.2.1.2. Fibrates

Fibrates were initially approved for use in reducing high triglyceride levels associated with primary hypertriglyceridemia and mixed dyslipidemia. These drugs were shown to be effective in promoting lipolysis of triglyceride, which was eventually shown to be due to activation of the nuclear receptor peroxisome proliferator-activated receptor-α (PPAR-α).[47] Activation of PPAR-α promotes transcription of lipoprotein lipase (LPL) and apoC-II while repressing expression of apoC-III, a lipase inhibitor. Fibrates have also been shown to increase HDL levels by promoting apoA-I and apoA-II transcription,[47] and they probably act in other ways to increase HDL levels. Fibrates that are currently approved include gemfibrozil, which was shown to reduce the risk of atherosclerosis in a large study of men with low HDL cholesterol levels (Veterans Affairs High-Density Lipoprotein Intervention Trial [VA-HIT] study),[48] fenofibrate, ciprofibrate, and bezafibrate. Trilipix, formerly ABT335 (Abbott Labs, North, Chicago, IL/Solvay, Brussels, Belgium), is a new fenofibrate molecule recently approved and developed as a monotherapy and for use in combination with statins.

3.5.2.1.3. Under Development

Other fibrate/statin combination drugs under development include LCP-AtorFen (LifeCycle Pharma, Hørsholm, Denmark) and fenofibrate/pravastatin (Sciele Pharma, Florham Park, NJ). These drugs are intended to exploit the fibrate effects of reducing plasma triglyceride levels and increasing HDL cholesterol levels and the statin effects of reducing LDL cholesterol levels.

3.5.2.1.4. Fish Oil/Purified Eicosapentaenoic Acid and Docosahexaenoic Acid

Fish oil and standardized preparations of purified eicosapentaenoic acid (EPA) and docosahexaenoic acid (DHA) ethyl esters have been shown to be effective therapies for reducing elevated plasma triglyceride levels.[49] The mechanism responsible for these changes is activation of the PPAR family of nuclear receptors, including PPAR-α, of which long-chain polyunsaturated fatty acids are natural ligands. Fish oil/purified EPA/DHA can also be safely used in combination with statins in patients with mixed dyslipidemia (elevated plasma triglyceride and LDL).[49,50] In clinical studies, purified EPA has been determined to be effective in reducing multiple risk factors for cardiovascular disease.[50]

3.5.2.1.5. Statins

Development of the statins was pursued with the goal of specifically lowering LDL cholesterol through upregulation of the LDL receptor. Studies showed that inhibiting cholesterol synthesis in the liver resulted in an increase in the number of LDL receptors in liver leading to increased LDL clearance from plasma.[51] These findings led to the search for a compound to inhibit cholesterol synthesis.[52] The first agent found to be a safe and effective inhibitor of HMG CoA reductase was a naturally occurring inhibitor, compactin (lovastatin).[52,53] Since that time, approximately 10 other drugs of this class have been developed and approved for use in humans and have become the most prescribed medications worldwide. It is worth noting that at least one statin under development was discontinued in the preclinical stage due to adverse side effects in an animal model[54] and that another was pulled from the market following approval for use in humans because of an increased incidence of rhabdomyolysis.[55] In these cases it was clearly the specific molecule rather than the mechanism of inhibiting cholesterol synthesis that was responsible for the adverse effects.

3.5.2.1.6. Cholesterol Absorption Inhibitors

Cholesterol absorption inhibitors include ezetimibe (Merck, Whitehouse Station, NJ) and phytosterols. Ezetimibe is an inhibitor of the cholesterol transporter, Niemann-Pick type C1-like 1 protein (NPC1L1).[56] NPC1L1 is located on the luminal face of the enterocyte and is responsible for absorption of the majority of cholesterol by the small intestine. Inhibition of NPC1L1 in the small intestine leads to reduced delivery of dietary cholesterol to the liver which, in turn, stimulates upregulation of the LDL receptor. Inhibition of NPC1L1 with ezetimibe has been shown to reduce cholesterol absorption by 54% when compared with placebo.[57] This reduction in cholesterol absorption has been associated with a decrease in LDL cholesterol levels of 18%.

Ezetimibe has also been marketed as a combination therapy with simvastatin. The combination is designed to lower LDL cholesterol levels by reducing endogenous cholesterol synthesis through inhibition of HMG CoA reductase (simvastatin) and to block dietary and biliary cholesterol absorption (ezetimibe). Although the combination has been demonstrated to be more efficacious with regard to LDL lowering than either drug alone,[58] the benefit of ezetimibe with regard to reducing risk of cardiovascular disease is currently controversial. Recently, two smaller trials have reported no benefit of ezetimibe in reducing cardiovascular risk.[58,59] A conclusive answer as to whether ezetimibe reduces risk of cardiovascular disease may be had when the results from The Improved Reduction of Outcomes: Vytorin Efficacy International Trial (IMPROVE-IT) study (ClinicalTrials.gov Identifier: NCT00202878), which is designed to measure cardiovascular events in patients with acute coronary syndrome treated with simvastatin alone or in combination with ezetimibe, are announced. The target enrollment for the study is 18,000 patients with results expected in 2013.

Phytosterols are plant-derived sterols absorbed by the small intestine but rapidly excreted by the liver in bile.[60] In the small intestine, phytosterols can compete with cholesterol for absorption, resulting in reduced cholesterol absorption. The U.S. Food and Drug Administration (FDA) has reviewed clinical studies in which the cholesterol-lowering effect of phytosterols was examined and has concluded that phytosterols in a dose ≥300 mg/day were effective in reducing LDL cholesterol levels.[61] This official recognition of phytosterol efficacy at this dose allows companies whose foods and supplements contain at least 300 mg of phytosterols to make the claim that these products are able to lower plasma cholesterol levels.

3.6. The Future Generation of LDL-Lowering Drugs

3.6.1. Thyroid Receptor-β Agonism

Thyroid hormone has long been known to have beneficial effects on plasma lipoproteins, particularly with regard to reducing LDL cholesterol.[62] Thyroid hormone has been shown to enhance LDL clearance in patients with hypothyroidism via upregulation of the LDL receptor.[63] Due to its metabolic effects, particularly on increasing heart rate, its use as a lipid-lowering agent in the general population is not feasible, however. The discovery that there are two thyroid hormone receptor subtypes, α and β, that differentially affect heart rate and LDL cholesterol levels[64] opened the door for development of specific agonists that could activate thyroid hormone receptor β, which is responsible for LDL cholesterol lowering, while leaving thyroid receptor α, which stimulates heart rate, unaltered. Eprotirome/KB2115 (Karo Bio AB, Huddinge, Sweden) is one such agonist. Initial studies have shown that the compound can safely be used to lower LDL cholesterol levels alone and in combination with statins.[65]

3.6.2. Lipoprotein-Associated-Phospholipase A2 Inhibitors

Lipoprotein-associated-phospholipase A2 (Lp-PLA2) is an enzyme secreted by platelets and macrophages that can associate with lipoproteins, primarily LDL, where it can hydrolyze surface phospholipids.[66] This hydrolysis of LDL surface phospholipids produces a modified LDL particle that is more likely to be retained by proteoglycans in the subendothelial space and be taken up by macrophages.[67] This could result in an increased binding of LDL to artery walls and lead to the formation of atherosclerotic plaque. Inhibition of Lp-PLA2 would be expected to reduce the formation of modified LDL and therefore lower LDL uptake by macrophages. Lp-PLA2 inhibitors under development include darapladib and rilapladib (both from GlaxoSmithKline, Brentford, United Kingdom).

3.6.3. Secretory Phospholipase A2 Inhibitors

Secretory phospholipase A2 (sPLA2), an enzyme that is distinct from Lp-PLA2, is produced by endothelial cells and is capable of hydrolyzing phospholipids on the surface of lipoproteins.[68] sPLA2 is thought to specifically modify LDL and possibly HDL, increasing the likelihood that these modified lipoproteins will be retained by proteoglycans[68] in the subendothelial space and be taken up by macrophages, leading to the formation of atherosclerotic plaque. Inhibition of sPLA2 should prevent these modifications of LDL and HDL, thus decreasing the likelihood of uptake of these lipoprotein particles by macrophages. Varespladib (Anthera Pharmaceuticals, Hayward, CA) is an sPLA2 inhibitor that is currently undergoing clinical development.

3.6.4. Microsomal Triglyceride Transfer Protein Inhibitors

Microsomal triglyceride transfer protein (MTP) is a lipid transfer protein that is essential for the production of chylomicrons and VLDL.[69] Inhibition of MTP results in reduced chylomicron and VLDL synthesis, leading to decreased secretion of these lipoproteins into the blood.[70] This decrease, in turn, leads to lower triglyceride, VLDL, and LDL levels in plasma. MTP inhibitors have been reported to be effective in reducing LDL cholesterol levels as a monotherapy[70] and in combination with statins and ezetimibe.[71] An expected side effect of MTP inhibition is fat accumulation in the enterocytes and hepatocytes[70] caused by the inhibition of triglyceride export from these cell types on chylomicrons and VLDL. These effects, as well as gastrointestinal effects resulting from reduced fat absorption, can be minimized if patients adhere to a low fat diet.[70] Treatment with MTP inhibitors is also associated with weight loss – possibly as a result of stimulation of neuropeptide Y production by fat-engorged enterocytes.[72] Neuropeptide Y is a hormone that signals satiety in the brain, leading to reduced food intake. MTP inhibitors undergoing clinical development include lomitapide (AEGR-733; Aegerion Pharmaceuticals, Bridgewater, NJ) and SLx-4090 (Surface Logix, Inc., Brighton, MA).

3.6.5. Antisense/RNA Interference of apoB mRNA

Antisense oligonucleotides (ASOs) are mRNA binding molecules that can be used to lower the expression of a specific gene.[73] ASOs contain nucleotide sequences that are complementary to a specific target mRNA sequence. After being bound to the target mRNA, the ASO/mRNA complex is degraded, resulting in decreased transcription of the protein product. An ASO being developed with the treatment of hyperlipidemia is mipomersen (formerly ISIS-301012) (ISIS Pharma, Carlsbad, CA/Genzyme, Cambridge, MA). Mipomersen targets apoB mRNA for degradation, resulting in reduced VLDL apoB production.[74] This reduction in VLDL production, in turn, leads to reduced VLDL, LDL, and Lp(a) levels in plasma. As with MTP inhibitors, mipomersen reduces lipid export from the liver, and there is the potential for hepatic fat accumulation. To date, patients treated with mipomersen have been reported to tolerate the drug well[74] with modest increases in hepatic fat reported in some patients.[75] One potential problem with ASO therapies is that, because the drugs are sequence specific, surrogate ASOs must be used in preclinical animal studies in which the mRNA sequence differs from the human mRNA sequence. Because there is the possibility of an off-target mRNA/ASO complex formation, a surrogate ASO that is used in preclinical animal studies may not reveal off-target effects that occur when the candidate ASO is used in humans.

3.7. Therapies to Increase HDL Cholesterol Levels and Improve HDL Function

The initial focus of pharmacologic treatments for dyslipidemia was drugs that reduced LDL cholesterol and triglycerides. This focus changed in 2000 with the appearance of the first cholesterol ester transfer protein (CETP) inhibitor.[76] LDL lowering with statins is effective in reducing the risk of atherosclerosis, although the risk is not entirely eliminated. Further reductions in LDL levels, expected to reduce the risk of atherosclerosis, may not be safely accomplished in the vast majority of patients. An alternate, yet unproven, strategy for reducing the risk of atherosclerosis is to increase the amount of HDL cholesterol, a key component of the RCT pathway. In 2002, the Adult Treatment Panel III, charged with making recommendations regarding treatment of dyslipidemia, recognized that low levels of HDL cholesterol are associated with increased risk of atherosclerosis.[39] The panel made the recommendation to increase HDL levels in patients at high risk of cardiovascular disease. At the time this recommendation was made, however, niacin and fibrates were the only drugs available to increase HDL levels by any appreciable amount (10%–30%).[77,78] Since that time, new therapies have developed that have the potential to increase HDL levels dramatically, making HDL another therapeutic target available for the treatment of dyslipidemia.

3.7.1. CETP Inhibitors

The appearance of the first CETP inhibitor, JTT-705, in mid-2000 provided a way to increase HDL above and beyond what could be achieved with either niacin or fibrates.[76] A second, more potent CETP inhibitor, torcetrapib, appeared late in 2003[79] and quickly moved into human trials. JTT-705 was reported to increase HDL in humans by up to 35% [80] whereas torcetrapib resulted in increases in HDL of up to 100%.[81] The enthusiasm surrounding the potential of CETP inhibition to increase HDL and reduce cardiovascular risk was short-lived, however. Torcetrapib was found to result in an increase in blood pressure.[82] A study testing the effect of torcetrapib on cardiovascular risk was discontinued in late 2006 because of an increase in cardiovascular events in the torcetrapib treatment group,[28] resulting in discontinuation of the drug. The question of whether this result was due to an off-target effect of torcetrapib or an effect of CETP inhibition has still not been resolved.

Dalcetrapib (also known as RO4607381, R1658, or JTT-705; Hoffman-LaRoche, Basel, Switzerland) was the first CETP inhibitor to enter human trials. Since 2000, clinical development of dalcetrapib has been proceeding at a cautious pace. Although less potent than either torcetrapib or anacetrapib (see next paragraph), dalcetrapib has been shown to reduce atherosclerosis in an animal model.[76] Recent studies have focused on demonstrating the absence of adverse blood pressure effects from the drug and on clinical benefit in reducing cardiovascular events.

Development of a third CETP inhibitor, anacetrapib (MK-0859; Merck, Whitehouse Station, NJ), was announced late in 2006. Results from Phase 1 studies have been reported,[83] and the drug is currently in Phase 2. Anacetrapib appears to be more potent than torcetrapib and RO4607381 with regard to HDL raising, with increases in HDL reported up to 139%. Initial reports with anacetrapib indicate that the drug has no effect on blood pressure.

Two other CETP inhibitors under development, DRL-17822 (Dr. Reddy's Laboratories, Hyderabad, India) and LY2484595 (Eli Lilly & Co., Indianapolis, IN) are currently in Phase 2, although no results with these compounds have been released.

3.7.2. PPAR-α Agonists

PPAR-α, the nuclear receptor targeted by fibrate drugs, is an attractive target for treatment of hypertriglyceridemia and low HDL. Activation of PPAR-α results in changes in gene expression that promote transcription of LPL, which enhances lipolysis, represses transcription of the lipase inhibitor apoC-III, and promotes transcription of apoA-I and apoA-II. Specific activation of PPAR-α would be expected to improve the lipid phenotype over what can be achieved with fibrate drugs, which are less specific activators of PPAR-α. Recently, the PPAR-α agonist LY518674 was tested in patients with primary hyperlipidemia and those with mixed dyslipidemia.[84] The results from this trial were somewhat surprising in that the change in plasma lipid levels, and in particular HDL, in these patients was no better than what was achieved with fenofibrate. A separate study showed that the drug resulted in a potent increase in apoA-I and apoA-II production that was counteracted by an increase in clearance of these proteins.[85]

3.7.3. Reconstituted and Recombinant HDL/apoA-I Mimetic Peptides

These drugs were developed as a way to increase RCT from peripheral tissues by increasing the number of cholesterol acceptor particles in plasma. Initial human studies using a phospholipid complex containing recombinant apoA-I$_{Milano}$ were promising because treatment significantly reduced atherosclerotic plaque area (Figure 3.3.)[86] This treatment never progressed very far into development, however, due to difficulties in producing large amounts of recombinant apoA-I$_{Milano}$ protein.[87] These difficulties have apparently been overcome, and continued development of apoA-I$_{Milano}$ is planned by The Medicines Company (Parsippany, NJ). Subsequent studies using a phospholipid complex containing apoA-I recovered from human plasma (CSL111; CSL Limited, Victoria, Australia) were not as promising as the results with apoA-I$_{Milano}$ and showed no change in atherosclerotic plaque volume.[88] A backup phospholipid complex containing apoA-I recovered from human plasma (CSL112; CSL Limited, Victoria, Australia) is currently in Phase 1.[88]

3.8. Biomarkers Linked to Clinical Outcomes

The goal of treatment with antidyslipidemic agents is to reduce atherosclerotic plaque within coronary arteries to decrease cardiovascular events and improve clinical outcomes. Whereas this goal is straightforward, assessing the efficacy of antidyslipidemic treatment is more complicated. The initial stages of antidyslipidemic drug development demonstrate long-term safety and effectiveness with regard to improving the lipoprotein phenotype. An improvement in the lipoprotein phenotype is expected to be associated with a reduction in cardiovascular risk. Because there is not always a clear-cut association between efficacy and cardiovascular risk reduction, however, other plasma markers (biomarkers) of atherosclerotic risk are often measured in an attempt to best evaluate the clinical effectiveness of a drug candidate.

3.8.1. Biomarkers

In a general sense, biomarkers are measures that can be used to predict a clinical outcome. Biomarkers have recently been formally defined as "characteristics that are objectively measured and evaluated as indicators of normal biological processes, pathogenic processes, or pharmacological responses to a therapeutic intervention."[89] A biomarker that is accepted as a substitute for a clinical endpoint is defined as a surrogate endpoint.[89] Common biomarkers in use to evaluate the efficacy of antidyslipidemics include the following: total cholesterol, LDL, HDL, LDL/HDL ratio, apoB, apoA-I, apoA-II, triglycerides, VLDL remnant lipoproteins, oxidized LDL, LDL size, HDL size, apoB, ex vivo cholesterol efflux, in vivo RCT, blood pressure, free fatty acids, inflammatory cytokines, adipokines, glucose, and insulin, among others.[90] The adage, "association does not prove causation" should be kept in mind when using biomarkers to evaluate the clinical benefits and risks of a drug. In the vast majority of cases, biomarkers do not provide a clear-cut indication of clinical benefit or harm of drug treatment, and a decision regarding clinical efficacy must be made based on the weight of evidence from several biomarkers and clinical endpoints.

3.8.2. Measures of Vascular Function and Atherosclerosis

Although biomarkers are useful early in dyslipidemic drug development for assessing the potential benefit of a drug for reducing the risk of cardiovascular disease, the best measure of benefit is a clinical study with decreased morbidity and mortality from cardiovascular events being the outcome. These studies typically involve multiple sites that recruit several thousand patients studied over a 5-year (or longer) period. The cost of such studies may be $10 to $20 million (U.S. dollars), depending on the study design and location. Due to the high cost associated with such studies, developing more cost-effective measures of atherosclerosis may enable more efficient evaluation of new drugs. Studies that directly measure atherosclerosis typically enroll fewer patients followed over a shorter period of time (and at a lower cost) than do studies measuring a clinical event as an outcome. Several measures of atherosclerosis are available today. These vary in the level of invasiveness, ease of use, and amount of radiation exposure. A few of the more commonly used clinical measures of atherosclerosis are described in the next section. A more comprehensive list of what is currently available has recently been reviewed.[91]

3.8.2.1. Angiography

Perhaps the most frequently used method to assess plaque formation in the coronary arteries is angiography, which is an invasive procedure during which the clinician introduces contrast medium into the coronary artery and images of the coronary arteries are taken under x-ray. Because the method allows visualization of vessel lumen, it is useful in assessing advanced plaque but is unable to detect early and moderate plaque that has formed but has not yet begun to encroach on the vessel lumen. Given these limitations, this technique is no longer commonly used as an outcome measure in studies measuring progression of atherosclerosis.

3.8.2.2. Carotid Intima-Media Thickness

Carotid intima-media thickness (CIMT) is a noninvasive measure of the carotid artery that is used as an in vivo surrogate for atherosclerosis. The method involves taking ultrasound images of the right and left carotid arteries. These images allow for the measurement of the CIMT as well as the measure of blood flow, which are influenced by the presence of plaque. Studies using CIMT as an outcome generally are compared after 1 to 2 years of treatment.[92]

3.8.2.3. Flow-Mediated Dilatation

Flow-mediated dilatation is an in vivo measure of endothelial dysfunction that is used as a measure of cardiovascular risk. This technique uses ultrasound to measure blood flow through a brachial artery. Measurements are taken at rest and following occlusion of the artery with a blood pressure cuff. Following deflation of the cuff, the sudden increase in blood flow results in release of nitric oxide by endothelial cells. This release causes an acute vasodilatation of the artery. The change in flow is obtained by ultrasound as a measure of endothelial function. Studies using CIMT as an outcome generally are compared after approximately 1 year of treatment.[93]

3.8.2.4. Intravascular Ultrasound

Intravascular ultrasound (IVUS), like angiography, is a method to assess plaque formation directly within the coronary arteries. It is similar to angiography in that a catheter with an ultrasound probe is placed in the coronary artery. When the catheter is in place, images of plaque can be obtained. The technique is powerful and can be conducted in the same subject before, during, and after an intervention. The lack of standardized procedures and the inherent difficulty in placing a catheter in the identical position within a coronary artery several months apart make the method subject to error. Stringent criteria must be in place at the start of a study to define images that are acceptable. In one infamous study, a negative result, suggesting progression of atherosclerosis in response to a drug, was obtained. Upon reanalysis of the same images by a different group of investigators, the conclusion that the drug was beneficial was reached. One IVUS study involving <50 patients treated with a phospholipid complex containing apoA-I$_{Milano}$ (ETC-216) had positive results indicative of plaque regression in 5 weeks.[86] These results, however, appear to be exceptional. Other trials using IVUS measurements compare measurements following 1 to 2 years of treatment.[94]

3.8.2.5. PET/Computer-Assisted Tomography

PET/Computer-assisted tomography (CAT) is a potentially powerful technique designed to identify unstable plaque that is at risk of rupture. The dual technique involves conducting a PET scan using radioactive fluorodeoxyglucose (FDG). This FDG will be transported to plaque that is populated with activated macrophages that take up glucose owing to their increased energy requirements. This image is superimposed over a CAT scan that allows localization of the PET image. An added benefit of this technique is the ability to compare multiple areas prone to atherosclerosis within a single individual so that the areas that appear to be most susceptible to rupture can be identified. This technique is minimally invasive, although it does involve radiation exposure and specialized equipment and thus cannot be offered at many facilities. A study currently under way that is using PET/CAT as a clinical endpoint is comparing measurements over a 2-year period.[95]

Although these techniques can be useful in assessing the risk of atherosclerosis, they are not always able to replicate the results of an adequately powered study designed to measure an outcome of cardiovascular events. Examples of where measures of atherosclerosis did not correspond to clinical outcome are the two reports that were published shortly after torcetrapib was discontinued (see Section 3.9). One study measured changes in atherosclerotic plaque using IVUS measurements,[96] and the other measured CIMT.[97] Both studies showed that torcetrapib treatment had no effect on the progression of atherosclerotic plaque. Neither study, however, would have provided any indication that torcetrapib treatment would increase the risk of cardiovascular events – a result ultimately found in a study with cardiovascular events as the primary outcome.[28]

3.9. Case Study: CETP Inhibition with Torcetrapib – Mechanism versus Molecule

A drug that is first in its class is in a unique position. If successful in being approved, it stands first among all competitors as the gold standard.

If it has undesirable effects, however, then the question is immediately raised of whether these undesirable effects are due to the drug's mechanism of action or due to an off-target effect. A timely example of a drug that was first in class but had undesirable effects is the CETP inhibitor torcetrapib, a drug designed to raise HDL cholesterol levels. Raising HDL cholesterol is an attractive yet unproven strategy for reducing cardiovascular risk. A successful candidate would not only provide evidence that raising HDL is of benefit with regard to reducing cardiovascular risk but might also prove to be the drug of choice to be used alone or in combination with other antidyslipidemic drugs prescribed to decrease cardiovascular risk.

Torcetrapib was identified through drug screening as an inhibitor of CETP. Preclinical studies showed that the drug was safe in animals, and it was eventually moved into Phase 1 human trials where its short-term safety in humans was demonstrated.[81] Phase 2 trials were done, again showing short-term safety and efficacy with regard to increasing HDL cholesterol levels.[98] Although not the first in its class to enter clinical trials, torcetrapib was taken through the first two phases of clinical development rapidly without any safety concerns and eventually led the CETP inhibitor drug class in clinical development. Animal models treated with torcetrapib were reported to have reduced development of atherosclerosis.[99] Human trials showed that the drug was well tolerated and could effectively raise the antiatherogenic HDL cholesterol to unprecedented levels (up to 100%). Torcetrapib also had the added benefit of lowering the proatherogenic LDL.

A Phase 3 study (the Investigation of Lipid Level Management to Understand its Impact on Atherosclerotic Events (ILLUMINATE) trial) was designed and undertaken to determine the effect of torcetrapib on cardiovascular events in patients with coronary heart disease or those at high risk of coronary heart disease. Because it would be unethical to withhold standard treatment to these high-risk patients during the trial, all patients were to be studied on the background of standard atorvastatin treatment. Whereas data pooled from earlier phase clinical trials indicated that torcetrapib could modestly increase blood pressure in some study subjects,[82] it was thought that this risk could be managed and would be far outweighed by the significant improvement in the lipoprotein profile. Approximately halfway into the 5-year, Phase 3 study, however, the Data Safety Monitoring Board (DSMB) identified a statistically significant increase in the number of cardiovascular events in patients treated with the combination of torcetrapib plus atorvastatin as compared with atorvastatin monotherapy. The DSMB recommended discontinuation of the trial. On the basis of this recommendation, the company suspended all ongoing trials involving torcetrapib and development of two backup CETP inhibitors that did not raise blood pressure.

Subsequent studies showed that the drug acutely stimulated an increase in aldosterone,[100] although the precise mechanism by which it promotes an increase in blood pressure has yet to be identified. It has also not been possible to say with any certainty that the increase in cardiovascular risk by the drug is entirely attributable to an increase in blood pressure.

Thus the jury is still out as to whether CETP inhibition is of any benefit or risk to patients with regard to altering risk of cardiovascular disease. Development of CETP inhibitors (dalcetrapib, anacetrapib, DRL-17822, and LY2484595) is ongoing. None of these drugs has shown evidence of increasing blood pressure. Because it is not clear at this time if there are other harmful direct or off-target effects of CETP inhibition, development is proceeding cautiously. Because studies in animal models often do not identify human safety concerns but do show benefit in reducing experimentally induced atherosclerosis, studies in humans are the only way to determine definitively if these drugs safely reduce the risk of cardiovascular disease. The challenge will be to conduct studies in humans using reliable biomarkers and endpoints that will determine efficacy and clinical benefit while ensuring the safety of participating subjects.

3.10. Conclusion

The lipid hypothesis has been tested over the past several decades and has held up under scrutiny. Treatments designed to lower LDL cholesterol and remnant lipoproteins have become the standard therapy to reduce the risk of cardiovascular disease. Future therapies designed to enhance RCT through an increase in HDL are attractive and have potential to provide a new means of reducing cardiovascular risk. There are a number of promising drugs under development designed to reduce levels of LDL and remnant lipoproteins and specifically to increase HDL. Plasma biomarkers and noninvasive and invasive measures of atherosclerosis will be useful in evaluating the clinical effectiveness of these treatments. Those biomarkers that hold the most promise will ultimately need to be tested in clinical trials with cardiovascular and noncardiovascular morbidity and mortality as the primary endpoints, the current gold standard of clinical efficacy.

3.11. References

1. MacKay J, & Mensah GA. (2004). The Atlas of Heart Disease and Stroke. Geneva, Switzerland: World Health Organization.
2. (1984). The Lipid Research Clinics Coronary Primary Prevention Trial results. I. Reduction in incidence of coronary heart disease. JAMA. 251, 351–364.
3. Frick MH, Elo O, Haapa K, Heinonen OP, Heinsalmi P, Helo P, et al. (1987). Helsinki Heart Study: Primary prevention trial with gemfibrozil in middle aged

men with dyslipidemia: Safety of treatment, changes in risk factors, and incidence of coronary heart disease. N. Engl. J. Med. 317, 2137–2145.

4. Shepherd J, Cobbe SM, Ford I, Isles CG, Lorimer AR, MacFarlane PW, et al. (1995). Prevention of coronary heart disease with pravastatin in men with hypercholesterolemia. West of Scotland Coronary Prevention Study Group. N. Engl. J. Med. 333, 1301–1307.

5. (1994). Randomised trial of cholesterol lowering in 4444 patients with coronary heart disease: The Scandinavian Simvastatin Survival Study (4S). Lancet. 344, 1383–1389.

6. Steinberg D. (2004). Thematic review series: The pathogenesis of atherosclerosis. An interpretive history of the cholesterol controversy: Part I. J. Lipid Res. 45, 1583–1593.

7. Steinberg D. (2005). Thematic review series: The pathogenesis of atherosclerosis. An interpretive history of the cholesterol controversy: Part II: The early evidence linking hypercholesterolemia to coronary disease in humans. J. Lipid Res. 46, 179–190.

8. Steinberg D. (2005). Thematic review series: The pathogenesis of atherosclerosis. An interpretive history of the cholesterol controversy: Part III: Mechanistically defining the role of hyperlipidemia. J. Lipid Res. 46, 2037–2051.

9. Steinberg D. (2006). The pathogenesis of atherosclerosis. An interpretive history of the cholesterol controversy: Part IV: The 1984 coronary primary prevention trial ends it–almost. J. Lipid Res. 47, 1–14.

10. Steinberg D. (2006). Thematic review series: The pathogenesis of atherosclerosis. An interpretive history of the cholesterol controversy: Part V: The discovery of the statins and the end of the controversy. J. Lipid Res. 47, 1339–1351.

11. (1983). Classics in arteriosclerosis research: On experimental cholesterin steatosis and its significance in the origin of some pathological processes by N. Anitschkow and S. Chalatow, translated by Mary Z. Pelias, 1913. Arteriosclerosis. 3, 178–182.

12. Keys A, Aravanis C, Blackburn HW, Van Buchem FS, Buzina R, Djordjević BD, et al. (1966). Epidemiological studies related to coronary heart disease: Characteristics of men aged 40–59 in seven countries. Acta Med. Scand. Suppl. 460, 1–392.

13. Kato H, Tillotson J, Nichaman MZ, Rhoads GG, & Hamilton HB. (1973). Epidemiologic studies of coronary heart disease and stroke in Japanese men living in Japan, Hawaii and California. Am. J. Epidemiol. 97, 372–385.

14. Thompson GR, Miller JP, & Breslow JL. (1985). Improved survival of patients with homozygous familial hypercholesterolaemia treated with plasma exchange. Br. Med. J. (Clin. Res. Ed.) 291, 1671–1673.

15. Levy RI. (1985). Primary prevention of coronary heart disease by lowering lipids: Results and implications. Am. Heart J. 110, 1116–1122.

16. Shepherd J. (1998). A tale of two trials: The West of Scotland Coronary Prevention Study and the Texas Coronary Atherosclerosis Prevention Study. Atherosclerosis. 139, 223–229.

17. Keys A, Aravanis C, Blackburn H, Buzina R, Dontas AS, Fidanza F, et al. (1985). Serum cholesterol and cancer mortality in the Seven Countries Study. Am. J. Epidemiol. 121, 870–883.

18. Law MR, Thompson SG, & Wald NJ. (1994). Assessing possible hazards of reducing serum cholesterol. BMJ. 308, 373–379.

19. Brest AN. (1964). Treatment of coronary occlusive disease: Critical review. Dis. Chest. 45, 40–45.

20. Ross R, Glomset J, & Harker L. (1977). Response to injury and atherogenesis. Am. J. Pathol. 86, 675–684.

21. Ross R. (1999). Atherosclerosis–an inflammatory disease. N. Engl. J. Med. 340, 115–126.

22. Williams KJ, & Tabas I. (1995). The response-to-retention hypothesis of early atherogenesis. Arterioscler. Thromb. Vasc. Biol. 15, 551–561.

23. Wilson PWF, D'Agostino RB, Levy D, Belanger AM, Silbershatz H, & Kannel WB. (1998). Prediction of coronary heart disease using risk factor categories. Circulation. 97, 1837–1847.

24. Reid RD, Quinlan B, Riley DL, & Pipe AL. (2007). Smoking cessation: Lessons learned from clinical trial evidence. Curr. Opin. Cardiol. 22, 280–285.

25. Williams B. (2005). Recent hypertension trials: Implications and controversies. J. Am. Coll. Cardiol. 45, 813–827.

26. Ridker PM, Danielson E, Fonseca FA, Genest J, Gotto AM Jr, Kastelein JJ, et al. (2008). Rosuvastatin to prevent vascular events in men and women with elevated C-reactive protein. N. Engl. J. Med. 359, 2195–2207.

27. Tardif JC, McMurray JJ, Klug E, Small R, Schumi J, Choi J, et al. (2008). Effects of succinobucol (AGI-1067) after an acute coronary syndrome: A randomised, double-blind, placebo-controlled trial. Lancet. 371, 1761–1768.

28. Barter PJ, Caulfield M, Eriksson M, Grundy SM, Kastelein JJ, Komajda M, et al. (2007). Effects of torcetrapib in patients at high risk for coronary events. N. Engl. J. Med. 357, 2109–2122.

29. Wu Z, Wagner MA, Zheng L, Parks JS, Shy JM 3rd, Smith JD, et al. (2007). The refined structure of nascent HDL reveals a key functional domain for particle maturation and dysfunction. Nat. Struct. Mol. Biol. 14, 861–868.

30. Van Der Steeg WA, Holme I, Boekholdt SM, Larsen ML, Lindahl C, Stroes ES, et al. (2008). High-density lipoprotein cholesterol, high-density lipoprotein particle size, and apolipoprotein A-I: Significance for cardiovascular risk: The IDEAL and EPIC-Norfolk Studies. J. Am. Coll. Cardiol. 51, 634–642.

31. Cohen JC, Boerwinkle E, Mosley TH Jr, & Hobbs HH. (2006). Sequence variations in PCSK9, low LDL, and protection against coronary heart disease. N. Engl. J. Med. 354, 1264–1272.

32. Ballantyne CM, Raichlen JS, Nicholls SJ, Erbel R, Tardif JC, Brener SJ, et al. (2008). Effect of rosuvastatin therapy on coronary artery stenoses assessed by quantitative coronary angiography: A study to evaluate the effect of rosuvastatin on intravascular ultrasound-derived coronary atheroma burden. Circulation. 117, 2458–2466.

33. Glomset, JA. (1968). The plasma lecithin: cholesterol acyltransferase reaction. J. Lipid Res. 9, 155–167.

34. Cuchel M, & Rader DJ. (2006). Macrophage reverse cholesterol transport: Key to the regression of atherosclerosis? Circulation. 113, 2548–2555.

35. Altschul R, Hoffer A, & Stephen JD. (1955). Influence of nicotinic acid on serum cholesterol in man. Arch. Biochem. 54, 558–559.

36. Barnhart JW, Sefranka JA, & McIntosh DD. (1970). Hypocholesterolemic effect of 4,4'-(isopropylidenedithio)-bis(2,6-di-t-butylphenol) (probucol). Am. J. Clin. Nutr. 23, 1229–1233.

37. Konttinen A, & Paloheimo J. (1963). The effects of atromid on serum lipids, proteins and some liver function tests in hypercholesterolaemic patients. J. Atheroscler. Res. 3, 525–532.

38. Blacket RB, Woodhill J, & Brown WD. (1964). The effect of cholestyramine ("MK 135") on the serum cholesterol level in man. Med. J. Aust. 2, 15–19.

39. Expert Panel on Detection, Evaluation, and Treatment of High Blood Cholesterol in Adults. (2001). Executive summary of the third report of the National Cholesterol Education Program (NCEP) Expert Panel on Detection, Evaluation, and Treatment of High Blood Cholesterol in Adults (Adult Treatment Panel III). JAMA. 285, 2486–2497.

40. National Academy of Sciences. Institute of Medicine. Food and Nutrition Board. (1998). Dietary Reference Intakes for Thiamin, Riboflavin, Niacin, Vitamin B6, Folate, Vitamin B12, Pantothenic Acid, Biotin, and Choline. Washington, DC: The National Academies Press.

41. Tunaru S, Kero J, Schaub A, Wufka C, Blaukat A, Pfeffer K, et al. (2003). PUMA-G and HM74 are receptors for nicotinic acid and mediate its anti-lipolytic effect. Nat. Med. 9, 352–355.

42. Taggart AK, Kero J, Gan X, Cai TQ, Cheng K, Ippolito M, et al. (2005). (D)-beta-hydroxybutyrate inhibits adipocyte lipolysis via the nicotinic acid receptor PUMA-G. J. Biol. Chem. 280, 26649–26652.

43. Cheng K, Wu TJ, Wu KK, Sturino C, Metters K, Gottesdiener K, et al. (2006). Antagonism of the prostaglandin D2 receptor 1 suppresses nicotinic acid-induced vasodilation in mice and humans. Proc. Natl. Acad. Sci. U. S. A. 103, 6682–6687.

44. Guyton JR, Goldberg AC, Kreisberg RA, Sprecher DL, Superko HR, & O'Connor CM. (1998). Effectiveness of once-nightly dosing of extended-release niacin alone and in combination for hypercholesterolemia. Am. J. Cardiol. 82, 737–743.

45. Ballantyne CM, Davidson MH, McKenney J, Keller LH, Bajorunas DR, & Karas RH. (2008). Comparison of the safety and efficacy of a combination tablet of niacin extended release and simvastatin vs. simvastatin monotherapy in patients with increased non-HDL cholesterol (from the SEACOAST I Study). Am. J. Cardiol. 101, 1428–1436.

46. Paolini JF, Mitchel YB, Reyes R, Kher U, Lai E, Watson DJ, et al. (2008). Effects of laropiprant on nicotinic acid-induced flushing in patients with dyslipidemia. Am. J. Cardiol. 101, 625–630.

47. Schoonjans K, Staels B, & Auwerx J. (1996). Role of the peroxisome proliferator-activated receptor (PPAR) in mediating the effects of fibrates and fatty acids on gene expression. J. Lipid Res. 37, 907–925.

48. Robins SJ, Collins D, Wittes JT, Papademetriou V, Deedwania PC, Schaefer EJ, et al. (2001). Veterans Affairs High-Density Lipoprotein Intervention Trial. Relation of gemfibrozil treatment and lipid levels with major coronary events: VA-HIT: A randomized controlled trial. JAMA. 285, 1585–1591.

49. Harris WS, Miller M, Tighe AP, Davidson MH, & Schaefer EJ. (2008). Omega-3 fatty acids and coronary heart disease risk: Clinical and mechanistic perspectives. Atherosclerosis. 197, 12–24.

50. Maki KC, McKenney JM, Reeves MS, Lubin BC, & Dicklin MR. (2008). Effects of adding prescription omega-3 acid ethyl esters to simvastatin (20 mg/day) on lipids and lipoprotein particles in men and women with mixed dyslipidemia. Am. J. Cardiol. 102, 429–433.

51. Bilheimer DW, Goldstein JL, Grundy SM, & Brown MS. (1975). Reduction in cholesterol and low density lipoprotein synthesis after portacaval shunt surgery in a patient with homozygous familial hypercholesterolemia. J. Clin. Invest. 56, 1420–1430.

52. Endo A, Kuroda M, & Tanzawa K. (1976). Competitive inhibition of 3-hydroxy-3-methylglutaryl coenzyme A reductase by ML-236A and ML-236B fungal metabolites, having hypocholesterolemic activity. FEBS. Lett. 72, 323–326.

53. Mabuchi H, Haba T, Tatami R, Miyamoto S, Sakai Y, Wakasugi T, et al. (1981). Effect of an inhibitor of 3-hydroxy-3-methyglutaryl coenzyme A reductase on serum lipoproteins and ubiquinone-10-levels in patients with familial hypercholesterolemia. N. Engl. J. Med. 305, 478–482.

54. Gerson RJ, Allen HL, Lankas GR, MacDonald JS, Alberts AW, & Bokelman DL. (1991). The toxicity of a fluorinated-biphenyl HMG-CoA reductase inhibitor in beagle dogs. Fundam. Appl. Toxicol. 16, 320–329.

55. SoRelle R. (2001). Baycol withdrawn from market. Circulation. 104, E9015–E9016

56. Altmann SW, Davis HR Jr, Zhu LJ, Yao X, Hoos LM, Tetzloff G, et al. (2004). Niemann-Pick C1 Like 1 protein is critical for intestinal cholesterol absorption. Science. 303, 1201–1204.

57. Sudhop T, Lütjohann D, Kodal A, Igel M, Tribble DL, Shah S, et al. (2002). Inhibition of intestinal cholesterol absorption by ezetimibe in humans. Circulation. 106, 1943–1948.

58. Kastelein JJ, Akdim F, Stroes ES, Zwinderman AH, Bots ML, Stalenhoef AF, et al. (2008). Simvastatin with or without ezetimibe in familial hypercholesterolemia. N. Engl. J. Med. 358, 1431–1443.

59. Taylor AJ, Villines TC, Stanek EJ, Devine PJ, Griffen L, Miller M, et al. (2009). Extended-release niacin or ezetimibe and carotid intima-media thickness. N. Engl. J. Med. 361, 2113–2122.

60. Balmer J, & Zilversmit DB. (1974). Effects of dietary roughage on cholesterol absorption, cholesterol turnover and steroid excretion in the rat. J. Nutr. 104, 1319–1328.

61. U.S. Food and Drug Administration, Department of Health and Human Services. (2000). Food labeling: Health claims; plant sterol/stanol esters and coronary heart disease. Interim final rule. Fed. Regist. 65, 54686–54739.

62. Hansson P, Valdemarsson S, & Nilsson-Ehle P. (1983). Experimental hyperthyroidism in man: Effects on plasma lipoproteins, lipoprotein lipase and hepatic lipase. Horm. Metab. Res. 15, 449–452.

63. Packard CJ, Shepherd J, Lindsay GM, Gaw A, & Taskinen MR. (1993). Thyroid replacement therapy and its influence on postheparin plasma lipases and apolipoprotein-B metabolism in hypothyroidism. J. Clin. Endocrinol. Metab. 76, 1209–1216.

64. Grover GJ, Mellstrom K, & Malm J. (2005). Development of the thyroid hormone receptor beta-subtype agonist KB-141: A strategy for body weight reduction and lipid lowering with minimal cardiac side effects. Cardiovasc. Drug Rev. 23, 133–148.

65. Erion MD, Cable EE, Ito BR, Jiang H, Fujitaki JM, Finn PD, et al. (2007). Targeting thyroid hormone receptor-beta agonists to the liver reduces cholesterol and triglycerides and improves the therapeutic index. Proc. Natl. Acad. Sci. U. S. A. 104, 15490–15495.

66. Tsimikas S, Tsironis LD, & Tselepis AD. (2007). New insights into the role of lipoprotein(a)-associated lipoprotein-associated phospholipase A2 in atherosclerosis and cardiovascular disease. Arterioscler. Thromb. Vasc. Biol. 27, 2094–2099.

67. Schissel SL, Jiang X, Tweedie-Hardman J, Jeong T, Camejo EH, Najib J, et al. (1998). Secretory sphingomyelinase, a product of the acid sphingomyelinase gene, can hydrolyze atherogenic lipoproteins at neutral pH. Implications for atherosclerotic lesion development. J. Biol. Chem. 273, 2738–2746.

68. Hurt-Camejo E, & Camejo G. (1997). Potential involvement of type II phospholipase A2 in atherosclerosis. Atherosclerosis. 132, 1–8.

69. Wetterau JR, Aggerbeck LP, Bouma ME, Eisenberg C, Munck A, Hermier M, et al. (1992). Absence of microsomal triglyceride transfer protein in individuals with abetalipoproteinemia. Science. 258, 999–1001.

70. Cuchel M, Bloedon LT, Szapary PO, Kolansky DM, Wolfe ML, Sarkis A, et al. (2007). Inhibition of microsomal triglyceride transfer protein in familial hypercholesterolemia. N. Engl. J. Med. 356, 148–156.

71. Samaha FF, McKenney J, Bloedon LT, Sasiela WJ, & Rader DJ. (2008). Inhibition of microsomal triglyceride transfer protein alone or with ezetimibe in patients

with moderate hypercholesterolemia. Nat. Clin. Pract. Cardiovasc. Med. 5, 497–505.

72. Wren JA, Gossellin J, & Sunderland SJ. (2007). Dirlotapide: A review of its properties and role in the management of obesity in dogs. J. Vet. Pharmacol. Ther. 30(Suppl 1), 11–16.

73. Stein CA, & Cohen JS. (1988). Oligodeoxynucleotides as inhibitors of gene expression: A review. Cancer Res. 48, 2659–2668.

74. Kastelein JJ, Wedel MK, Baker BF, Su J, Bradley JD, Yu RZ, et al. (2006). Potent reduction of apolipoprotein B and low-density lipoprotein cholesterol by short-term administration of an antisense inhibitor of apolipoprotein B. Circulation. 114, 1729–1735.

75. Visser ME, Akdim F, Tribble DL, Nederveen AJ, Kwoh TJ, Kastelein JJ, et al. (2010). Effect of apolipoprotein-B synthesis inhibition on liver triglyceride content in patients with familial hypercholesterolemia. J. Lipid Res. 51, 1057-62.

76. Okamoto H, Yonemori F, Wakitani K, Minowa T, Maeda K, & Shinkai H. (2000). A cholesteryl ester transfer protein inhibitor attenuates atherosclerosis in rabbits. Nature. 406, 203–207.

77. Brown BG, & Zhao XQ. (2008). Nicotinic acid, alone and in combinations, for reduction of cardiovascular risk. Am. J. Cardiol. 101, 58B–62B.

78. Barter PJ, & Rye KA. (2008). Is there a role for fibrates in the management of dyslipidemia in the metabolic syndrome? Arterioscler. Thromb. Vasc. Biol. 28, 39–46.

79. Reinhard EJ, Wang JL, Durley RC, Fobian YM, Grapperhaus ML, Hickory BS, et al. (2003). Discovery of a simple picomolar inhibitor of cholesteryl ester transfer protein. J. Med. Chem. 46, 2152–2168.

80. Kuivenhoven JA, de Grooth GJ, Kawamura H, Klerkx AH, Wilhelm F, Trip MD, et al. (2005). Effectiveness of inhibition of cholesteryl ester transfer protein by JTT-705 in combination with pravastatin in type II dyslipidemia. Am. J. Cardiol. 95, 1085–1088.

81. Clark RW, Sutfin TA, Ruggeri RB, Willauer AT, Sugarman ED, Magnus-Aryitey G, et al. (2004). Raising high-density lipoprotein in humans through inhibition of cholesteryl ester transfer protein: An initial multidose study of torcetrapib. Arterioscler. Thromb. Vasc. Biol. 24, 490–497.

82. Davidson MH, McKenney JM, Shear CL, & Revkin JH. (2006). Efficacy and safety of torcetrapib, a novel cholesteryl ester transfer protein inhibitor, in individuals with below-average high-density lipoprotein cholesterol levels. J. Am. Coll. Cardiol. 48, 1774–1781.

83. Krishna R, Anderson MS, Bergman AJ, Jin B, Fallon M, Cote J, et al. (2007). Effect of the cholesteryl ester transfer protein inhibitor, anacetrapib, on lipoproteins in patients with dyslipidaemia and on 24-h ambulatory blood pressure in healthy individuals: Two double-blind, randomised placebo-controlled phase I studies. Lancet. 370, 1907–1914.

84. Nissen SE, Nicholls SJ, Wolski K, Howey DC, McErlean E, Wang MD, et al. (2007). Effects of a potent and selective PPAR-alpha agonist in patients with atherogenic dyslipidemia or hypercholesterolemia: Two randomized controlled trials. JAMA. 297, 1362–1373.

85. Millar JS, Duffy D, Gadi R, Bloedon LT, Dunbar RL, Wolfe ML, et al. (2009). Treatment with a potent and selective PPAR-α agonist, LY518674, significantly increases apoA-I and apoA-II production rates in patients with metabolic syndrome despite no change in HDL. Arterioscler. Thromb. Vasc. Biol. 29, 140–146.

86. Nissen SE, Tsunoda T, Tuzcu EM, Schoenhagen P, Cooper CJ, Yasin M, et al. (2003). Effect of recombinant ApoA-I Milano on coronary atherosclerosis in

patients with acute coronary syndromes: A randomized controlled trial. JAMA. 290, 2292–2300.

87. Hunter AK, Suda EJ, Herberg JT, Thomas KE, Shell RE, Gustafson ME, et al. (2008). Separation of recombinant apolipoprotein A-I(Milano) modified forms and aggregates in an industrial ion-exchange chromatography unit operation. J. Chromatogr. A. 1204, 42–47.

88. Tardif JC, Grégoire J, L'Allier PL, Ibrahim R, Lespérance J, Heinonen TM, et al. (2007). Effect of rHDL on Atherosclerosis-Safety and Efficacy (ERASE) Investigators. Effects of reconstituted high-density lipoprotein infusions on coronary atherosclerosis: A randomized controlled trial. JAMA. 297, 1675–1682.

89. Tardif JC, Heinonen T, Orloff D, & Libby P. (2006). Vascular biomarkers and surrogates in cardiovascular disease. Circulation. 113, 2936–2942.

90. Marcovina SM, Crea F, Davignon J, Kaski JC, Koenig W, Landmesser U, et al. (2007). Biochemical and bioimaging markers for risk assessment and diagnosis in major cardiovascular diseases: A road to integration of complementary diagnostic tools. J. Intern. Med. 261, 214–234.

91. Sanz J, & Fayad ZA. (2008). Imaging of atherosclerotic cardiovascular disease. Nature. 451, 953–957.

92. Lorenz MW, Markus HS, Bots ML, Rosvall M, & Sitzer M. (2007). Prediction of clinical cardiovascular events with carotid intima-media thickness: A systematic review and meta-analysis. Circulation. 115, 459–467.

93. Patel S, & Celermajer DS. (2006). Assessment of vascular disease using arterial flow mediated dilatation. Pharmacol. Rep. 58(Suppl), 3–7.

94. De Franco AC, & Nissen SE. (2001). Coronary intravascular ultrasound: Implications for understanding the development and potential regression of atherosclerosis. Am. J. Cardiol. 88, 7M–20M.

95. Aziz K, Berger K, Claycombe K, Huang R, Patel R, & Abela GS. (2008). Noninvasive detection and localization of vulnerable plaque and arterial thrombosis with computed tomography angiography/positron emission tomography. Circulation. 117, 2061–2070.

96. Nissen SE, Tardif JC, Nicholls SJ, Revkin JH, Shear CL, Duggan WT, et al. (2007). Effect of torcetrapib on the progression of coronary atherosclerosis. N. Engl. J. Med. 356, 1304–1316.

97. Kastelein JJ, van Leuven SI, Burgess L, Evans GW, Kuivenhoven JA, Barter PJ, et al. (2007). Effect of torcetrapib on carotid atherosclerosis in familial hypercholesterolemia. N. Engl. J. Med. 356, 1620–1630.

98. Brousseau ME, Schaefer EJ, Wolfe ML, Bloedon LT, Digenio AG, Clark RW, et al. (2004). Effects of an inhibitor of cholesteryl ester transfer protein on HDL cholesterol. N. Engl. J. Med. 350, 1505–1515.

99. Morehouse LA, Sugarman ED, Bourassa PA, Sand TM, Zimetti F, Gao F, et al. (2007). Inhibition of CETP activity by torcetrapib reduces susceptibility to diet-induced atherosclerosis in New Zealand White rabbits. J. Lipid Res. 48, 1263–1272.

100. Forrest MJ, Bloomfield D, Briscoe RJ, Brown PN, Cumiskey AM, Ehrhart J, et al. (2008). Torcetrapib-induced blood pressure elevation is independent of CETP inhibition and is accompanied by increased circulating levels of aldosterone. Br. J. Pharmacol. 154, 1465–1473.

Obesity: New Mechanisms and Translational Paradigms

Gregory Gaich and David E. Moller

4.1. Introduction

4.1.1. Medical Need and History of Failure

From 1985 through 2005, the prevalence of obesity doubled in the United States. In 2005, only four states had obesity prevalence rates less than 20%, whereas 17 states had prevalence rates of at least 25%, with several exceeding 30% (Centers for Disease Control and Prevention's [CDC's] Behavioral Risk Factor Surveillance System [BRFSS]). Obesity is a growing health epidemic outside the United States as well. Conditions of overweight and obesity are the sixth most important risk factor contributing to the overall global disease burden. According to the International Obesity Task Force and the World Health Organization (WHO), globally more than 1.7 billion adults are overweight, including more than 312 million who are obese.[1] The disease burden of excess adiposity contributes to increased risk of additional diseases, including hypertension, type 2 diabetes, atherosclerosis, osteoarthritis, and some cancers.

Lifestyle interventions are the first-line treatments for obesity, yet this precipitous increase in the prevalence of obesity has occurred despite many years of lifestyle intervention as the primary mode of therapy. The underlying reason may be that survival is dependent on avoiding a negative energy balance, and both eating and activity behaviors required to maintain a neutral or positive energy balance are regulated by hundreds of genes in scores of biochemical and neural pathways.[2] The active regulation of energy balance of both energy intake and energy expenditure is extremely precise with the average adult maintaining energy balance to within 0.3% over several decades.[3]

Approved pharmacotherapy for obesity was available in the United States as early as 1944 with the initial U.S. Food and Drug Administration (FDA) approval of desoxyephedrine. Subsequent recognition of the abuse potential of amphetamines and amphetamine-like drugs (e.g., phentermine, diethylpropion) led to the withdrawal of the obesity indications of the amphetamines and restriction of the amphetamine-like drugs to short-term (a few weeks) treatment.[4] Over the last 40 years, serious safety issues have also resulted in the withdrawal of aminorex (pulmonary hypertension), dexfenfluramine (valvulopathy), phenylpropanolamine (stroke), and ephedra-containing supplements (serious palpitations, tremor, and insomnia).[4,5] Currently approved obesity pharmacotherapies provide only modest (3%–5% compared with placebo), but clinically significant, weight loss and are limited by gastrointestinal, cardiovascular, or psychiatric adverse effects.[6] Thus, despite promising animal efficacy data for a number of central and peripheral targets, there are no approved pharmacotherapies that can provide the magnitude of weight loss desired by patients and eliminate the morbidity and mortality associated with obesity.

4.1.2. Pathophysiology and Principles of Energy Balance

Energy storage is one of the most important roles of adipose tissue, and every aspect of energy intake, expenditure, and storage is regulated by an interrelated, complex, highly redundant homeostatic system of energy regulation. Several elegant studies illustrate the interaction between intake and energy expenditure. In the experimental obesity studies of Ethan Sims,[7] normal weight volunteers were overfed to achieve and maintain an at least 20% increase in body weight. Maintenance of this higher body weight required consumption of almost twice the calories of chronically obese subjects matched for body weight. Studies of subjects in the National Weight Control Registry have shown that formerly obese subjects who maintained a healthy body weight had the same caloric intake as matched never-obese subjects but required 500 kcal/day more energy expenditure through moderate- to high-intensity exercise than the never-obese to maintain their weight.[8,9] The interrelationship between intake and expenditure is closely linked temporally, with rats reducing nonambulatory activity almost immediately after removal of food.[10] Studies in humans have also shown that changes in nonexercise activity thermogenesis (NEAT) in response to excess energy intake vary among individuals, are responsible for the differences in propensity to gain weight with overeating, and are genetically determined.[11,12] As these studies illustrate, adipose accumulation, and therefore obesity, are strongly influenced by complex homeostatic mechanisms, many of which are still not well understood.

4.2. Molecular Pathways and Associated Drug Targets

As we have described earlier in the text, a compelling need for new therapeutic approaches designed to favorably influence energy balance exists.

Over the past decade, virtually dozens of new molecular pathways and individual drug targets have been suggested to have potential therapeutic utility – to reduce caloric intake, enhance energy expenditure or both (or to modulate nutrient absorption).[13] The explosion in preclinical science in this field was in large measure fueled by the discovery of leptin – a major adipose-derived, energy-sensing hormone – in 1994.[14] It is noteworthy that this discovery resulted from a concerted positional cloning effort to identify the genetic basis for the *ob/ob* murine obesity trait and that subsequent studies have identified rare human mutations involving precisely the same gene.[15] The identification of many additional potential obesity "players" derived from the application of modern biology techniques, including the study of other mouse genetic traits, the identification of additional rare human monogenic obesity genes, pathway "mining" based on the availability of annotated human and rodent genome sequence databases, a substantial number of mouse gene knockout experiments, other molecular techniques such as DNA microarrays, and even the study of model lower organisms (e.g., *Caenorhabditis elegans*). Despite these substantial advances, our understanding of the physiology of energy regulation is still in its infancy. Moreover, only a handful of newer putative antiobesity mechanisms have yet to be rigorously tested in clinical trials.

A summary of recent developments in the ongoing search for new obesity drug targets is provided later in text. It is useful to characterize these potential new approaches into one of three general classes: (1) mechanisms confined largely to the central nervous system (CNS; e.g., receptors for hypothalamic neuropeptides or CNS neurotransmitters); (2) mechanisms involving the ability to modulate the actions of gut-derived peptides; and (3) mechanisms targeting other peripheral pathways that may affect thermogenesis, lipid metabolism, nutrient absorption, or partitioning (Figure 4.1).

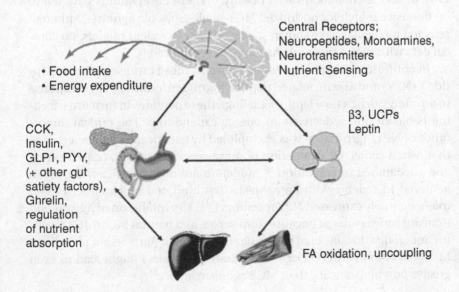

- Food intake
- Energy expenditure

Central Receptors;
Neuropeptides, Monoamines,
Neurotransmitters
Nutrient Sensing

β3, UCPs
Leptin

CCK,
Insulin,
GLP1, PYY,
(+ other gut
satiety factors),
Ghrelin,
regulation
of nutrient
absorption

FA oxidation, uncoupling

Fig. 4.1
Organ systems involved in integrated regulation of energy homeostasis are depicted along with selected pathways and drug targets that have potential value if modulated by specific drugs designed to treat obesity and related disorders. CCK, cholecystokinin; FA, fatty acid; GLP-1, glucagon-like peptide-1; PYY, peptide YY; UCP, uncoupling protein.

4.2.1. Central Regulation of Satiety—Thermogenesis

Regulation of feeding behavior and energy expenditure occurs predominantly via integrated signals (neural, hormonal, visual, taste, and direct sensing of nutrient levels) that are sensed by the CNS and responses that are in turn mediated via neural and hormonal pathways.[16] As listed in Table 4.1, a number of specific G-protein coupled receptors (GPCRs) or enzymes that are expressed in the CNS have been implicated as potential targets for brain-penetrant, small-molecule agonists or antagonists (GPCRs) or inhibitors (enzymes). Modulating these CNS targets is envisioned as a way to affect one or more of the following physiologic processes: direct sensing of nutrients within the hypothalamus, satiety perception, food reward, and neuronal sensing of longer term (adiposity) energy stores.

Leptin levels reflect adipose stores; leptin's actions are mediated via a specific receptor expressed in several hypothalamic nuclei.[16] Unfortunately, recombinant exogenous leptin has not been shown to cause significant weight loss in obese humans. Moreover, the leptin receptor is not amenable (to date) to direct activation via small-molecule ligands. Thus, key hypothalamic pathways downstream from the leptin receptor have preoccupied drug discovery scientists for a decade or more.

Neurons expressing proopiomelanocortin (POMC) are activated by leptin (and insulin, which also serves as a signal of excessive energy stores). Alpha-melanotropin (αMSH) is the major POMC gene product that in turn signals via the melanocortin 4 (MC4) receptor, and, to a lesser extent, the MC3 receptor. Validation of MC4 as an attractive target for specific peptide or small-molecule agonists is derived from several lines of compelling data.[17] First, MC4-null mice are hyperphagic and overtly obese; second, pharmacologic manipulation of this pathway with specific peptides in rodents causes either weight loss (agonists) or gain (antagonists); finally, and most importantly, human loss-of-function MC4 mutations cause a rare form of severe childhood-onset obesity.[18] These observations have led to an intensive search for optimized MC4 small-molecule agonists. Although selected molecules have shown strong efficacy in rodent models, no clinical data with such a molecule have yet been reported.

In contrast to POMC-expressing neurons, those expressing Neuropeptide Y (NPY) and Agouti-related peptide (Agrp) sense and signal in response to an energy deficit (low leptin signaling); these peptides in turn drive feeding behavior and a decrease in energy expenditure. The critical importance of NPY/Agrp action was exemplified by genetically engineered mice that, when subjected to ablation of these specific neurons, ceased eating and succumbed to starvation.[19] Moderate antiobesity efficacy has been achieved in rodents with antagonists that bind and block either of two major centrally expressed NPY receptors (Y1, Y5). Inhibition of Agrp action is an attractive concept because Agrp serves as a natural MC4/MC3 receptor antagonist. Ideally, dual molecular inhibition of Agrp action plus direct MC4 activation (with one or two separate molecules) might lead to even greater potential efficacy than MCR agonism alone.

Table 4.1. Selected Newer Obesity Drug Targets

Molecular Target(s)	Proposed Function(s) and Validation	Reference(s)
Central Regulation of Satiety–Thermogenesis		
CB-1	Central regulation of food reward behavior; Knockout mice have lean phenotype; Inverse agonist compounds produce inhibition of feeding and weight loss in rodents and humans	(24)
MC4	Hypothalamic control of satiety and thermogenesis; Loss-of-function MC4 mutations in rodents and humans produce obesity	(16–18)
Leptin; Leptin receptor	Fat-derived hormone that acts centrally (hypothalamus); Control of satiety and thermogenesis via numerous pathways, including MC4 and NPY; Leptin or leptin receptor mutations cause obesity in rodents and humans	(16,18)
NPY; NPY1 and NPY5 receptors	Major neuropeptide that promotes feeding via NPY1/NPY5 receptors	(16,19)
MCH; MCH1 and MCH2 receptors	Central regulation of food intake (and energy expenditure); MCH1R knockout mice have lean phenotype	(16,20)
Agrp	Antagonist of melanocortin receptors MC3R, MC4R	(16,17)
fat/fat gene product	Carboxypeptidase E Δ (hormone processing defects)	(99)
Tubby *tub/tub* pathway	Probably phosphodiesterase defect (apoptosis proposed as mechanism)	(100)
Bombesin receptor 3 (BRS-3)	Regulation of metabolic rate (+/– feeding); BRS3-null mice have moderate obesity	(101,102)
5 Hydroxytryptophan receptor 2c	CNS 5-HT receptor subtype; 5-HT2c-null mice are obese; 5-HT2c agonists promote weight loss in preclinical species (and humans)	(23)
Gut-Derived Peptides		
CCK, CCK1 receptor	Satiety inducing by action on vagal afferents and in CNS	(30,31)
Enterostatin	Proteolytic product derived from procolipase; mechanism of action unknown; causes satiety	(103)
GLP-1; GLP-1 receptor	Satiety via unknown mechanism	(32)
Oxyntomodulin	Lowers food intake and body weight in humans; Actions may be mediated by GLP-1 receptor	(33,34)
Ghrelin; Ghrelin receptor	Ghrelin is a stomach-derived peptide hormone that promotes feeding (in rodents and humans) via its receptor (predominantly CNS)	(33,36)
GOAT	Enzyme required for conversion of inactive → active ghrelin via covalent addition of 8-carbon fatty acid	(36,38,39)

(continued)

Table 4.1 (*continued*)

Molecular Target(s)	Proposed Function(s) and Validation	Reference(s)
PYY; NPY2 receptor	Reduces food intake in humans (lowers body weight and food intake in rodents); Effects are principally mediated by NPY2 receptor in mice	(33,35)
Pancreatic polypeptide; NPY4 receptor	Reduces food intake in humans and rodents; Effects are principally mediated by NPY4 receptor in mice	(33)
Neuromedin U (NMU); NMU1 and NMU2 receptors	Peptide with both central (NMU2r predominant) and peripheral (NMU1r predominant) satiety and thermogenic effects	(104)
Peripheral Thermogenesis; Adipose Differentiation/Function; Nutrient Partitioning		
β3 adrenergic receptor	Stimulation of lipolysis; Regulation of brown adipocyte function	(47,105)
AMPK (activator – peripheral; inhibitor – central)	AMPK activation inactivates ACC, HSL, mtGPAT (see below); Peripheral AMPK activators induce favorable metabolic effects	(27,29,40)
UCP1 and UCP3	Ablation of brown fat results in obesity; transgenic overexpression of selected UCPs has beneficial metabolic effects	(46)
Targeting proapoptotic peptides to adipose tissue	A specific peptide that binds to prohibin (selectively expressed in adipose tissue vasculature) and induces selective adipose ablation	(49)
ACC	ACC2-null mice are lean; ACC inhibitors ameliorate aspects of metabolic syndrome in rodents	(27)
Perilipin	Regulation of lipolysis and adiposity	(106)
Lipoprotein lipase	Regulation of fat accretion	(27)
DGAT1	Lipogenic enzyme with major actions in intestine and adipose; DGAT1-null mice have lean phenotype	(41)
11β-HSD1	Peripheral (predominant) enzyme that catalyzes the conversion of cortisone to active glucocorticoid (cortisol)	(48)

ACC, Acyt CoA carboxylase; AMPK, adenosine monophosphate-activated protein kinase; DGAT-1, diacylglycerol acyltransferase 1; CCK, cholecystokinin; GLP-1, glucagon-like peptides; GOAT, ghrelin O-acyl transferase.

Another key example of a CNS drug target that may have a role in hypothalamic regulation involves melanin concentrating hormone (MCH), a lateral hypothalamic neuropeptide that stimulates food intake and positive energy balance. In rodents, MCH actions are mediated by a single GPCR (MCHR1), whereas higher species, including humans, have two MCH receptors, MCHR1 and MCHR2.[20] A role for MCH in regulating energy balance was initially implicated in 1996 based on observed upregulation of this pathway in obese rodents.[21] Chronic central infusion of MCH to mice on a high-fat diet results in a large increase in food intake and body weight, producing increases in glucose, insulin, and leptin levels similar to those observed in human metabolic syndrome. Deletion of the MCH gene in mice reduces weight gain and increases metabolic rate when the mice are placed on a high-fat diet, whereas deletion of MCHR1 results in lean mice. Moreover, specific MCHR1 antagonists reduce food consumption and body weight in rodents.[20] Although at least two MCH1R antagonist molecules have been reported to have entered early clinical testing,[20] no results have been described to date.

In contrast to MCH, two alternative CNS pathways that clearly modulate feeding behavior and energy balance in rodents have recently also translated into observed clinical weight-loss efficacy. Serotoninergic pathways have been implicated as major regulators of food intake because serotonin (5-HT) reuptake inhibitors and agonists (e.g., dexfenfluramine) are known to cause decreased food intake and increased metabolism. 5-hydroxytryptamine (5-HT) reuptake inhibitors and agonists have been proposed to involve the suppression of NPY release[22] Importantly, a knockout mouse model lacking the 5-HT2c receptor revealed hyperphagia, suggesting that specific 5-HT2c agonists could be beneficial in the treatment of obesity.[23] Indeed, subsequent research has demonstrated that selective 5-HT2c agonists do indeed mediate weight loss in rodents; with one particular molecule, antiobesity efficacy was also evident in clinical trials as discussed (see later in the text) in Section 4.3. As we have also discussed, modulation of the endocannabinoid system via cannabinoid receptor subtype 1 (CB-1) inverse agonists, which suppress CNS cannabinoid action, have been extensively studied preclinically and in clinical trials in which several molecules (e.g., rimonabant) have been shown to produce moderate weight loss efficacy.[24] Some evidence also suggests that peripheral CB-1 receptors may mediate selected effects of CB-1 inverse agonist molecules;[25] this evidence implies that peripherally restricted molecules may also exert antiobesity efficacy while avoiding CNS-based adverse effects (see later in the text).

Whereas longer term sensing of energy stores and leptin action is fairly well understood, pathways involved in more acute direct CNS sensing of nutrients are less well defined at present. It is now clear, however, that direct sensing of fatty acids, glucose, and even amino acids does occur. Fatty acid sensing by the CNS appears to involve locally mediated mitochondrial oxidation; carnitine palmitoyl transferase (CPT1) is a key mediator of mitochondrial fatty acid import in all tissues, including those of the CNS.[26] New insights into the therapeutic potential of modulating CNS fatty acid sensing came from the use of a known fatty acid synthase (FAS) inhibitor C75, which strongly suppressed appetite and produced weight loss in rodents (reviewed in [27]). Additional data suggested that C75 regulated appetite through the central regulation of malonyl-conenzyme A (CoA) concentrations. Because malonyl-CoA is the major FAS substrate, FAS inhibition would be expected to increase malonyl-CoA levels, which in turn would lead to inhibition of CPT1.[27] Other lines of evidence also strongly suggest that selectively inhibiting fatty acid oxidation in the brain, hypothalamus, or both, might result in suppression of appetite or increased thermogenesis via cross-talk with leptin signaling.[26] Hypothalamic activation of adenosine monophosphate (AMP)–activated protein kinase (AMPK) presents an alternative to direct inhibition of FAS (or of central CPT1). AMPK is a general intracellular fuel-sensing enzyme that is activated by a reduction in the cellular adenosine triphosphate/adenosine diphosphate (ATP/ADP) ratio. Hypothalamic AMPK activity is enhanced by fasting and is suppressed in response to leptin.[28] Thus, AMPK activity is implicated as a key integrator of divergent signals – leptin and nutrients – in the hypothalamus. In theory, an approach to AMPK inhibition in the hypothalamus might be desirable. It is well known, however, that AMPK has critical roles in peripheral tissues such as the heart, liver, and skeletal muscle.[29] Inhibition of AMPK in these tissues is likely to have profound adverse consequences.

4.2.2. Modulating the Actions of Gut-Derived Peptide Hormones

Over the past decade, an increasing number of peptide hormones expressed in, and secreted by, the gastrointestinal tract have been implicated as potential therapeutic approaches to treating obesity (Table 4.1). Cholecystokinin (CCK) has a prominent role in mediating acute satiety after eating.[30] The satiety-inducing effects of CCK are believed to be mediated via activation of CCK-A receptors within the vagus nerve or brainstem, leading to CNS signals that impede further eating. A number of small-molecule, CCK-A receptor selective agonists have been synthesized and have been shown to exert potent satiety effects in preclinical models.[31] Although at least one such CCK-A agonist has apparently advanced into human clinical testing, detailed results have yet to be described.

Glucagon-like peptide-1 (GLP-1) was initially discovered to be a key "incretin" hormone that is secreted from intestinal cells and acts to augment insulin secretion in response to orally ingested nutrients. It is now quite clear that GLP-1 actions also include substantial inhibition of gastric emptying, increased satiety, and net reductions in body weight. These effects have clearly translated from preclinical species to humans following the development of multiple peptide agonists targeting the GLP-1 receptor, including exenatide, liraglutide, and others as agents to treat type 2 diabetes.[32] The full therapeutic potential of GLP-1 agonists for the treatment of obesity, however, has yet to be realized because there are no reported clinical trials that have examined weight loss effects in nondiabetic obese patients to date. In addition, precise mechanisms that underlie GLP-1's effects to modulate feeding behavior and energy balance have yet to be defined.

The experience with the GLP-1 pathway has contributed to an emerging understanding of alternative gut-derived factors that may serve as satiety signals via receptors that may be present on vagal afferents or within the brainstem and hypothalamus. Oxyntomodulin (OXM) is an intriguing candidate satiety factor that is also a product of the same gene (preproglucagon) as GLP-1.[33] Although this peptide appears to act via GLP-1 receptors to mediate suppression of feeding behavior, OXM's effects may differ from GLP-1 with respect to its precise sites of action or the relative effects on body weight versus nausea. Recent early clinical testing with native human OXM has demonstrated that it exerts GLP-1-like antiobesity efficacy.[34] A second important member of this family is peptide YY (PYY). Like GLP-1 and OXM, PYY is secreted by intestinal L cells in a postprandial fashion.[35] PYY appears to act principally via activation of another NPY receptor subtype, Y2, although it can also activate Y1 and Y5. Because systemic exogenous PYY suppresses food intake (in both rodents and humans), it appears likely that access to central Y1 and Y5 receptors is limited compared with Y2, which may be the major in vivo pathway that produces an anorectic effect.[35] As discussed in Section 4.3, further clinical testing of PYY has been recently attempted in obese patients. Pancreatic polypeptide represents a satiety factor that is primarily expressed in and secreted by pancreatic islets in response to food intake.[33] Like PYY, pancreatic polypeptide has a role in appetite regulation. Anorectic effects have been reported in rodents and after acute administration in humans as well. In contrast to PYY, pancreatic polypeptide activates yet another NPY receptor subtype (Y4) within regions of the CNS, including the area postrema.[33] Clearly, the early clinical experience with PYY, OXM, and pancreatic polypeptide warrants further attention. Therapies based on these findings would include modified (more potent, longer acting) peptides or a range of peptides with altered receptor pharmacology (e.g., PYY analogs with Y2 >> Y1, Y5 selectivity), or both.

Short- and intermediate-term suppression of feeding behavior and appetite appears to involve a range of gut-derived satiety factors, including those noted earlier in the text. In contrast, a single acylated peptide hormone, ghrelin, has been characterized as a potent orexigenic factor. Ghrelin is produced by the stomach and is released in increased amounts during fasting. Its effects are mediated by the growth hormone secretagogue receptor (GHSR). GHSR signaling in the hypothalamus is linked to the induction of NPY and Agrp expression and increased firing of NPY/Agrp neurons, which in turn mediate increased appetite and food intake.[36] Given that ghrelin potently stimulates feeding and weight gain in rodents and that it increases food intake in humans in response to acute infusion, therapies designed to block ghrelin action are desired. This notion is supported by data showing that ghrelin-null mice have a (albeit subtle) phenotype of protection from early-onset obesity.[36] Moreover, neutralizing peripheral ghrelin with a specific oligonucleotide Spiegelmer caused modest weight loss in rodents.[37] Attempts to generate specific small-molecule GHSR antagonists have not yet succeeded in producing molecules with robust efficacy in preclinical models. An additional and potentially attractive approach might be to inhibit enzymatically mediated ghrelin acylation, which is required to generate a bioactive peptide. Recent research from two independent groups[38,39] has identified a single novel acyltransferase – now known as ghrelin O-acyl transferase (GOAT). GOAT may thus represent a new and potentially "drugable" target that can be modulated as a means of attenuating ghrelin action. Table 4.1 summarizes the broad range of gut-expressed peptides that may be considered as targets (or pathways containing targets) that have antiobesity therapeutic potential.

4.2.3. Targeting Other Peripheral Pathways

Several interesting candidate obesity drug targets with predominant expression in peripheral tissues mediate important steps in lipogenesis, lipid oxidation, or both.[27] Among these targets, inhibitors of acyl-CoA carboxylase (ACC) have received considerable attention as a possible approach to treating obesity and related conditions. ACC catalyzes the carboxylation of acetyl-CoA to form malonyl-CoA, which is a key molecule controlling intracellular fatty acid metabolism. ACC exists as two isozymes: ACC1 is a cytosolic enzyme that provides malonyl-CoA to FAS for subsequent de novo lipogenesis. ACC2 mediates local malonyl-CoA on the mitochondrial surface. As noted earlier in the text, this action of ACC would thus impede fatty acid oxidation. Inhibition of ACC1 is therefore predicted to reduce de novo lipogenesis, whereas inhibition of ACC2 (in peripheral tissues) is predicted to enhance fat oxidation. An ACC2-null mouse model has been reported to exhibit beneficial metabolic phenotypes, including resistance to diet-induced obesity. Subsequently, several compounds that act to inhibit both ACC1 and ACC2 have been described to exert antiobesity effects in rodent models in addition to triglyceride lowering and a reduction in hepatic steatosis.[27] Because ACC is coupled to FAS in a linear lipogenic pathway, it is plausible that FAS inhibition may represent an additional peripheral antiobesity target; however, as described earlier in the text, FAS inhibitors appear to have predominant effects within the CNS to modulate nutrient-sensing pathways as a means of inducing weight loss. It is also noteworthy that AMPK acts to directly phosphorylate and thus inactivate ACC. Therefore, allosteric activators of AMPK have been described to result in inhibition of peripheral ACC.[40] This inhibition of peripheral ACC suggests that peripherally restricted AMPK activators might represent an additional approach to obesity; in contrast, inhibition of AMPK would be desired within the CNS as noted earlier in the text.[27]

Several additional candidate drug targets exist within the biochemical pathways mediating lipogenesis. Acyl-CoA:diacylglycerol acyltransferase 1 (DGAT1) catalyzes the final step in triglyceride synthesis. Following the creation of a DGAT1 knockout mouse, this model was noted to have reduced adiposity and to be resistant to diet-induced weight gain and insulin resistance.[41] Importantly, transplantation of white adipose tissue from DGAT1-deficient into wild-type mice also decreases adiposity and increases insulin sensitivity.[41] Potential mechanisms might include an increase in the secretion of adiponectin from DGAT1-deficient adipose because adiponectin can promote fatty acid oxidation and enhance insulin sensitivity.[42] Clearly, DGAT1 deficiency imparts favorable changes in the characteristics of white adipose; other aspects include smaller sized adipocytes and altered gene expression profiles, which suggest increased local energy expenditure.[41] In addition to adipose effects, DGAT1 inhibition should impede chylomicron formation within the gut, leading to markedly reduced postprandial lipemia. Downsides of DGAT1 inhibition might include some degree of alopecia or impairment of lactation, for these effects are also observed in DGAT1 knockout mice. Another compelling drug target that modulates long-chain fatty acid synthesis is stearoyl-CoA desaturase 1 (SCD1). SCD1 mediates de novo synthesis of monounsaturated fatty acids (MUFAs) from saturated fatty acids by introducing cis-double bonds at the Δ9 position. SCD1 was initially implicated as a drug target for obesity following the observation that leptin deficiency produced a marked increase in liver SCD1 expression; moreover, cross-breeding of SCD1-null mice with leptin-deficient ob/ob mice ameliorated obesity in the double mutant mice.[43] An additional line of investigation showed that pharmacologic inhibition of SCD1 expression with antisense oligonucleotides could also impart resistance to diet-induced weight gain in mice.[44] Other results suggest that inhibition of SCD1 can induce energy expenditure and increase fatty acid oxidation[27]; however, precise mechanisms for these effects are not defined. Adverse effects of total SCD1 deficiency in mice are noteworthy and may temper the enthusiasm for pursuit of this target; these effects include skin abnormalities, alopecia, and atrophic changes in sebaceous and meibomian glands.

By targeting uncoupling protein (UCP) activation in peripheral tissues, one might also be able to augment thermogenesis and thereby favor increased energy expenditure. This concept has been validated via several genetic mouse models in which UCPs have been overexpressed or deleted or in which brown adipose tissue (BAT) – a site of UCP-mediated thermogenesis – has been ablated.[45,46] Although attractive in principle, no specific allosteric UCP activators have been identified that can induce energy expenditure in vivo. An alternative to direct UCP activation involves targeting β3 adrenergic receptors, which are specifically expressed in adipose tissue and mediate thermogenesis (in part via strong induction of UCP1 expression). Thus, agonists for this receptor have been shown to promote BAT accumulation, stimulate UCP1 expression, and induce weight loss in rodent models of obesity.[47] Subsequent translation of the β3 agonist concept into humans has been attempted and will be discussed in Section 4.3

Table 4.1 presents several additional peripheral therapeutic approaches to treating obesity and its complications. One attractive concept involves selective inhibition of 11β-hydroxysteroid dehydrogenase type 1 (11β-HSD1), the enzyme that catalyzes the conversion of cortisone to the active glucocorticoid cortisol. 11β-HSD1-null mice have metabolic improvements in the context of diet-induced obesity, and small-molecule 11β-HSD1 inhibitors have also been implicated as causing weight loss in pre-clinical models.[48] A more ambitious and potentially risky approach that has been piloted in rodents involves selective ablation of white adipose tissue by using a proapoptotic peptide that selectively targets adipose tissue vascular beds.[49] These recent developments underscore the potential for an even broader range of innovative drug targets and therapeutic approaches that may emerge in the coming years.

4.3. Clinical Paradigm and Recent Clinical Experience

Although scores of pharmacotherapies for obesity have been tested in humans after sibutramine was removed recently from the US market due to increased cardiovascular risk, only two treatments remain approved for chronic use in either Europe or the United States – orlistat and rimonabant. Even those two have not achieved full potential and illustrate some of the challenges in translating promising treatments for obesity from the laboratory into the clinic.

For CNS targets, the clinical experience has been marked by dose-limiting adverse effects that have prevented approval or limited the doses to well below the maximally effective level. Fenfluramine and dexfenfluramine as monotherapies were modestly effective, and dosing was limited by somnolence. There was, however, a clear exposure–response relationship with weight loss, for patients who could tolerate high exposures were able to achieve substantial weight loss.[50] The combination with phentermine (an amphetamine-like CNS stimulant approved for short-term treatment) was proposed as a way to reduce the CNS-depressant side effects of fenfluramine and improve tolerability while maintaining efficacy.[51] Fenfluramine and dexfenfluramine were both ultimately withdrawn from the market following the observation of valvulopathy in some patients, an adverse effect not observed in animal studies.[4] Likewise, maximal clinical efficacy of both sibutramine (a serotonin, norepinephrine, and dopamine reuptake inhibitor) and the CB-1 inverse agonists rimonabant and taranabant has not been achieved due to dose-limiting adverse effects. With sibutramine, weight loss in Phase 2 studies was significantly greater with a 30-mg dose than with the maximum approved dose of 15 mg, but doses higher than 15 mg were associated with an unacceptable increase in heart rate and blood pressure.[52] Both rimonabant and taranabant are limited by increased anxiety and depression at high doses.[53–55] The depressive effects were not predicted by animal models, for rimonabant exhibited antidepressant effects in common models such as the forced-swim test.[56] Although increased anxiety and depression may be an on-target effect of CB-1 antagonists, they are probably not mediated by the same pathways as energy balance; a peripherally restricted CB-1 antagonist has been hypothesized to avoid the adverse CNS effects observed with the centrally acting CB-1 inverse agonists.[25]

The fenfluramine–phentermine combination spurred interest in combination therapy, and several combinations of approved drugs are now in clinical development. Bupropion, in combination with naltrexone or zonisamide, is in development based on observations of synergistic activation of the POMC neurons in preclinical models. Although all three components are approved drugs, none is approved for obesity, and each has its own significant potential toxicity. Early efficacy studies with naltrexone–bupropion have shown modest efficacy.[57] The zonisamide–bupropion combination was initially dose limited by adverse effects, which seem to have lessened with the development of sustained-release formulations.[57–59] Both combinations have demonstrated weight loss that is at least additive compared with each component alone. A combination of phentermine and topiramate is also under current development. Phentermine is currently approved for short-term use and is a controlled substance. Topiramate was investigated as monotherapy for obesity and was abandoned because of substantial adverse effects at high doses. The combination under investigation uses lower doses to avoid the adverse effects, and the early efficacy studies have indicated acceptable tolerability and modest, but clinically relevant, weight loss.[60]

As noted earlier in the text, early experiments with i.c.v. injection of NPY showed increased food consumption leading to the development of NPY-Y1 and Y5 receptor antagonists. Although Y5 antagonists have reduced body weight in animal models, they have failed to provide meaningful weight loss in clinical trials.[61] Of the gut hormones, there is the most clinical experience with PYY and pancreatic polypeptide and with the incretins, such as exenatide and GLP-1 analogs. In short-term studies using i.v. infusion, PYY has been shown to reduce ad lib caloric intake substantially for as long as 12 to 24 hours after the infusion.[35,62,63] A 12-week weight loss study using intranasal delivery of PYY3-36, however, failed to produce significant weight loss even though pharmacologically relevant plasma concentrations were documented. Prior to the study, the investigators hypothesized that the potential for direct CNS transport via the nasal route might be advantageous. In light of the negative results, and given that PYY3-36 has affinity for the orexigenic Y1 and Y5 receptors, enhanced central penetration may have resulted in diminished efficacy[64] and rendered the study invalid for testing the effects of peripherally administered PYY3-36.

Exenatide, an incretin that acts through the GLP-1 receptor, has been approved for the treatment of type 2 diabetes. In clinical studies in patients with diabetes, progressive weight loss was observed in exenatide-treated patients, which resulted in small weight reduction at the end of 2 years.[65] Similar results have been observed with other GLP-1 agonists in patients with diabetes. Recently, a 52-week study of liraglutide in obese patients without diabetes showed a 5.5- to 6.0-kg weight loss compared with placebo.[66] All of the GLP-1 agonists appear to slow gastric emptying and cause mild to moderate nausea (the most common adverse effect).

β3 agonists have been extensively studied[46] in clinical trials. Early attempts were hampered by optimization for the rat β3 receptor and resulted in only partial agonists to the human β3 receptor – an unfortunate fact that was discovered only retrospectively following the successful cloning of both rat and human receptors. Several other potent and selective β3 agonists have been tested in humans[46,67,68] in short-term studies of body weight and energy expenditure and have failed to demonstrate the desired effects, although there were small, but encouraging, trends. Compared with rodents, adult humans have much less BAT, the target tissue for a β3 agonist, which may explain the failure of the β3 agonists to translate to humans. BAT can be induced in humans, however, by exposure to cold temperatures and in animals by β3 agonists. Seasonal differences in human BAT mass and activity have been observed in autopsy studies of cold-exposed workers and more recently by the use of fluorodeoxyglucose–positron emission tomography (FDG-PET) imaging.[67,69] Although the exact time course of cold-induced BAT activation is not known, it is unlikely that a 4-week study was adequate to allow maximal activation of BAT with a β3 agonist.

In summary, the clinical experience has illustrated several major challenges to successful translation of promising obesity treatments from animal experiments to clinical use. CNS targets have commonly been associated with CNS adverse effects probably mediated by the same receptors in different pathways than those regulating energy balance. Unsuspected differences among species in receptor affinities or target tissue distribution, as in the case of the β3 agonists, or limitation in study design, as with the β3 agonists or PYY3-363, have all hampered successful translation. In addition, limited tools to assess target engagement and downstream pharmacology have impaired our ability to fully understand the differences in the physiology of energy balance among species. Finally, as noted earlier in the text, obesity is a heterogeneous disease – and there are hundreds of genes associated with obesity – yet the clinical approach has been to test new drugs in broad populations rather than to seek out more homogenous populations that might be best suited to treatment directed at a specific target. The large number of redundant mechanisms to maintain energy balance may also limit the efficacy of any approach that does not target multiple pathways. Approaches to overcome these challenges are discussed in Section 4.4.5.

4.4. Translational Approaches

As new mechanisms of energy balance are discovered in animal models, translation of that knowledge into clinical therapeutics depends on those mechanisms also being operative and important in humans. Therefore, one of the key objectives of a translational approach to new mechanisms for the treatment of obesity is a robust assessment of target validation in the clinic. The initial steps of target validation are to ensure that the drug is engaged with its target, be it a receptor, an enzyme, or an ion channel. The second step is to confirm that target engagement results in the expected pharmacology, and the third is to determine if that pharmacology results in a change in the disease process such as an increase in energy expenditure, a decrease in caloric intake, a decrease in lipogenesis, or an increase in lipolysis. The final step, of course, is the clinical outcomes of reduced fat mass, improved metabolic and cardiovascular outcomes, and improved quality of life. Without thorough assessment of target engagement and validation early in development, however, the ultimate outcomes studies are unlikely to succeed. By definition, the clinical validation of novel targets is unprecedented. Therefore, this section can only describe the general approach to target validation and provide a few illustrative examples from previous clinical experience or highlight new technologies that might be useful in future studies of novel targets. Furthermore, although target validation progresses in a logical order from engagement through pharmacology and disease process evaluations, in reality the availability of methods and the study requirements usually dictate a different order or an incomplete evaluation. For example, it may be feasible to measure pharmacology in a single-ascending-dose safety study prior to direct assessment of target engagement in a PET study.

4.4.1. Target Engagement

Ensuring target engagement is the only way to ascertain that the mechanisms tested in humans have been adequately studied. Particularly for CNS targets, where passage across the blood–brain barrier may be limited or the drug may be actively transported from the CNS compartment by P-glycoprotein and related transporters, assessing target engagement is vital to the interpretation of subsequent pharmacology and efficacy studies.

Strictly speaking, a target engagement biomarker directly measures only the interaction of the compound with its target (receptor, enzyme, ion channel, etc.) and does not rely on detection of downstream signal transduction to establish target engagement. Because downstream signals may be different in animals and humans, any downstream pharmacology must be validated in humans before it can be used to evaluate target engagement. For novel targets, well-characterized active controls are commonly available for use in nonclinical models, but, in clinical studies, they are rare. Two target engagement biomarkers for novel targets are useful in the absence of a positive control: PET and agonist reversal for antagonist drugs.

PET ligands for some targets of interest (such as D2 or opioid receptors) already exist. For novel targets, the use of PET requires the discovery, development, and human validation of a suitable ligand, which is a costly and lengthy process with no guarantee of success. Nevertheless, PET is currently the only way to assess the degree of target engagement for CNS-active agents directly.

Agonist reversal can occasionally be useful to evaluate target engagement even without positive controls. Cannabinoid- and opioid-receptor antagonists have been evaluated by using agonist reversal[70,71] because agonists for both targets are readily available and well characterized (cannabis sativa or dronabinol for cannabinoid antagonists and many opiate analgesics for opioid antagonists).

Despite its importance in evaluating the translation of mechanisms from animals to humans, direct assessment of engagement of novel targets remains a major limitation of many clinical development programs.

4.4.2. Drug Pharmacology or Mechanism Biomarkers

Assessment of drug pharmacology in humans can be vital in successful translation as confirmation both that the compounds are engaging the target and that the proximal downstream effects are comparable to those in the preclinical models. The development and validation of pharmacology or mechanism biomarkers will be specific for each target, but similar methods may be leveraged across targets, and the methods can be refined in animal models. (See Chapter 1 for biomarker classification.) For CNS-active targets, agonist reversal, such as that described earlier in the text for cannabinoid receptor inverse agonists and opioid receptor antagonists, has been demonstrated. Effects on sleep electroencephalography (EEG) has been described for cannabinoids as well as 5-HT-2c agonists and can be used to confirm central penetration and drug action.[72] Functional magnetic resonance imaging (fMRI) provides the ability to measure changes in blood flow secondary to altered neuronal activity in specific areas of the brain in real time following drug administration. Although it is not yet widely used, it has the potential to evaluate drug action in the target nuclei of the hypothalamus, which may be the most direct assessment of CNS-active drug action currently possible in humans.

Pharmacological evaluation of gut peptide action, particularly for peptides that work via hypothalamic receptors such as PYY3-36 and pancreatic polypeptide, is as challenging as for the intrinsic CNS-active targets. Pharmacology of other peptide targets with peripheral action may be more straightforward but may not be related to the mechanisms by which they work in obesity. For example, inhibition of ghrelin action can be assessed by evaluation of the growth hormone axis, but the stimulation of food intake by ghrelin is independent of its effects on growth hormone secretion.[73] Likewise, the pharmacology of GLP-1 analogs can be assessed via effects on insulin secretion in a glucose tolerance test,[74] but the mechanism by which they produce weight loss is not well understood let alone directly measurable.

The pharmacology of peripheral targets, such as lipogenic or lipolytic enzymes, lends itself to a different set of methods. Sensitive measures of both de novo lipogenesis, lipid recycling, and lipolysis using stable-labeled palmitate or endogenous labeling with deuterated water have been developed[75] and could be used as pharmacology or mechanism biomarkers for peripheral targets. Fecal fat excretion has been used as a nonclinical pharmacology biomarker for lipase inhibitors or other drugs that reduce energy absorption[76] and is readily translated to humans. As described earlier in the text, the evaluation of β3 agonists' pharmacology using energy expenditure as a mechanism biomarker has not been particularly successful, although humoral markers of drug effect, such as increased insulin action and fat oxidation, have been observed in some studies.[77] The biomarker approach to β3 agonists also needs to take into account the time course of BAT induction in humans as well as the most sensitive methods. The same is true for other targets, particularly as they apply to disease process biomarkers, which are discussed next.

4.4.3. Disease Process or Outcome Biomarkers and Mechanism Biomarkers Linked to Efficacy Outcomes

The third leg of the human validation package after the confirmation that the target is engaged and that the pharmacology has translated from animals to the clinic is to confirm that the pharmacology has the expected impact on the disease process and on clinical outcomes. For central anorexigenic targets, reduction in ad lib caloric intake is a well-established and reproducible methodology that can quantitatively evaluate the target mechanism over a wide range of doses.[78] The specific methods used have varied from single- to repeated-dose assessments, single-meal to 24-hour measurements, and fixed- or variable-meal composition (through use of a buffet or vending machine). Excluding highly restrained eaters and rigorously controlled eating environments and allowing subjects to self-select portions from an excess of available food are important elements common to all methods.[62,79–81] Reduced food intake as a mechanism biomarker has at least medium linkage to clinical outcomes (weight loss).

Short weight loss studies have also been widely used as an early assessment of efficacy. Four-week studies have been widely used, and a weight loss of approximately 0.9 to 1.5 kg compared with placebo has been reported with several different classes of drug. This paradigm works well for central anorexigenic targets, where weight loss is most rapid at the initiation of therapy, and studies as short as 3 months may be able to predict final weight loss reasonably.[52] For other targets, such as GLP-1 analogs or β3 agonists, the time course of weight loss is different, and 4-week studies may not be suitable as a measure of early efficacy. In fact, given the seasonal induction/regression of BAT in humans, a study of 6 to 12 months may be the minimum needed to establish proof of concept for a β3 agonist.

Short caloric intake or weight loss studies can identify targets having pharmacology that does not affect the obesity disease process. Even if positive, however, the target may not translate into long-term weight loss. Naltrexone, for example, showed significant reduction in a single-dose ad lib caloric intake study but had no effect on weight in 4- or 8-week weight loss studies.[78,82–84] At the other end of the spectrum, in a 12-month study, fluoxetine (60 mg) resulted in weight loss at least as great as any currently approved obesity drug through 6 months, but the effect completely reversed during the second 6 months of treatment.[85]

Because most of the targets evaluated in the past have been central anorexigenic targets, most of the effort at developing disease process or outcome biomarkers has been focused on caloric intake and short-term weight loss. For peripheral targets, pharmacology or mechanism biomarkers may have at least medium linkage to outcome and also serve as disease process biomarkers. Mechanism biomarkers of lipogenesis or lipolysis also have some linkage to outcome for drugs such as ACC or DGAT-1 inhibitors that affect that pathway, and energy expenditure is a mechanism biomarker with medium linkage to outcome for β3 agonists. Even for peripheral targets, caloric intake may be a valuable adjunct in understanding the full mechanism of peripheral targets or in identifying counterregulatory mechanisms that may limit the efficacy of the target. For example, microsomal transfer protein inhibitors have been reported to reduce food intake in animal models[86] and may contribute to the efficacy of those targets. In contrast, targets that increase energy expenditure may also increase caloric intake, and reducing food intake typically results in reduced energy expenditure.

4.4.4. Subject Selection

Another major objective of the translational approach to new obesity targets is the identification of a suitable population of subjects for each mechanism or drug target. As described earlier in the text, there are hundreds of different genes and scores of known pathways that have been associated with obesity. It is unlikely that targeting one pathway will be uniformly effective in all patients. Careful evaluation of pharmacology and disease process biomarkers in different subgroups may contribute immensely to our understanding of the pathophysiology and pharmacotherapy of human obesity. Clear a priori hypotheses can be defined for targets with polymorphisms in the pathway that may affect function, such as those described in the β3 receptor[87] or the μ-opioid receptor,[88] or that may affect endogenous tone such as the fatty acid amide hydrolase (FAAH) polymorphisms in the endogenous cannabinoid synthesis pathway.[89] Less apparent are differences in pathophysiology or drug response resulting from developmental influences, behavioral phenotypes, or comorbid conditions. Many attempts have been made to identify phenotypic predictors of weight loss,[90] but most have been hampered by small sample size and are limited to lifestyle interventions. Nevertheless, several studies have identified behavioral or biochemical prognostic markers of weight loss.[91-93] Two studies of determinants of response to pharmacotherapy also identified several significant factors in drug response, including binge eating behaviors[94] and high-state anxiety scores.[95] Preclinical evaluation of ancillary effects of the target mechanisms may suggest hypotheses that could be evaluated in the translational paradigm. For example, a population with comorbid anxiety may be more responsive to an MCH-R1 antagonist, which has ancillary anxiolytic effects in animal models.[96]

4.4.5. Combination Therapy

Often, a third major objective of the translation approach is to begin to evaluate the feasibility of combination therapy. Given the exponentially increasing number of combinations that become available as novel targets are evaluated clinically, a sound translational biomarker strategy can expeditiously evaluate combination hypotheses. As described in Section 4.2, several combination therapies are now being evaluated clinically. All are combinations of currently approved drugs, although only one component of a combination is used clinically to treat obesity (phentermine), and all are CNS-active targets. As additional CNS, gut hormone, and peripheral targets enter clinical development, the potential for combination therapies with complementary mechanisms may lead to substantial improvements in efficacy.

4.5. Concluding Comments

The collective understanding of molecular pathways and discrete proteins that contribute to obesity pathophysiology in humans is expanding at a rapid pace. Gains in our knowledge base to date have largely been fueled by the availability of complete genome sequences and the application of modern molecular techniques, including mouse genetics, the use of transgenic and knockout mice, gene expression profiling, and so forth. Key insights have also been provided via the identification of single-gene obesity syndromes in humans – such as MC4 loss-of-function mutations.[97] We are now on the verge of a second wave of discoveries emanating from the advent of genome-wide association studies that include the determination of body weight and adiposity as primary clinical endpoints. The recent completion of one such series of studies has revealed a totally novel obesity gene (FTO) that may represent a new pathway harboring novel obesity drug targets that heretofore have not been considered.[98]

Translating basic discoveries into clinical trial results that are informative and meaningful has proven to be difficult as evidenced by the paucity of obesity mechanisms that have been rigorously tested over the past decade or so. In addition, it is apparent that the majority of specific mechanisms that appear to result in attractive efficacy in preclinical models (principally rodents) have not translated into significant (i.e., clinically meaningful) human efficacy. What accounts for these discrepancies and the apparent lack of success? Clearly, body weight regulation is complex, and the relative contribution of individual molecules and pathways is likely to differ greatly among species. In addition, many compounds advancing into clinical trials have been hampered by off-target adverse effects or toxicity in preclinical safety studies that may have precluded adequate testing (with doses sufficient to engage the target fully). It is also apparent in selected instances that mechanism-based adverse effects can preclude the achievement of maximal efficacy in humans. Importantly, few obesity translational medicine experiments have included an adequate measure (a biomarker or receptor occupancy test) to verify that sufficient target engagement and downstream pharmacology was, in fact, achieved.

How can advances in biomarker technologies and translational medicine models and development strategies assist in testing additional putative antiobesity mechanisms with greater frequency, shorter duration clinical testing, and greater fidelity so that clear go–no go decisions for given mechanisms can be efficiently achieved? As we have described in this chapter, biomarker approaches and imaging technologies that allow for direct clinical measurement of target (or pathway) engagement have advanced to the point that nearly every mechanism being tested initially in humans can and should include these measures. These maneuvers will ensure that proof of concept clinical trials involve the use of molecules at relevant doses, exposure, and duration. In addition, earlier and more sensitive measures of altered energy homeostasis can now be easily used; these human translational models include sensitive measures of food consumption, metabolic rate, and body composition. Finally, we acknowledge that obesity is not a homogeneous disease state; rather, it is a syndrome (or series of syndromes) resulting from a broad range of etiologies. Thus, the selection of subjects and clinical parameters to be measured is critical. It is therefore likely that further efforts to characterize disease subphenotypes and specific genetic markers will translate into selective therapies that can be tailored to the treatment of distinct subgroups of patients.

4.6. References

1. Haslam DW, & James WP. (2005). Obesity. Lancet. 366, 1197–1209.
2. Rankinen T, Zuberi A, Chagnon C, Weisnagel SJ, Argyropoulos G, Walts B, et al. (2006). The human obesity gene map: The 2005 update. Obesity. 14, 529–644.

3. Rosenbaum M, Leibel RL, & Hirsch J. (1998). Obesity. N. Engl. J. Med. 338, 555.

4. Colman E. (2005). Anorectics on trial: A half century of federal regulation of prescription appetite suppressants. Ann. Intern. Med. 143, 380–385.

5. Department of Health and Human Services, Food and Drug Administration, Final rule declaring dietary supplements containing ephedrine alkaloids adulterated because they present an unreasonable risk, Federal Register, 21 CFR, Part 119, (2004).69,6787–6854.

6. Li Z, Maglione M, Tu W, Mojica W, Arterburn D, Shugarman L, et al. (2005). Meta-analysis: Pharmacologic treatment of obesity. Ann. Intern. Med. 142, 532–546.

7. Sims EAH. (1976). Experimental obesity, dietary-induced thermogenesis, and their clinical implications. Clin. Endocrinol. Metab. 5, 377–395.

8. Phelan S, Roberts M, Lang W, Raynor H, & Wing R. (2006). Initial results of the LITE (Living Lean in a Toxic Environment) Study: Successful weight losers work harder than never overweight individuals to maintain a normal body weight. Obesity. 14(Suppl), A32.

9. Wing RR, & Phelan S. (2005). Long-term weight loss maintenance. Am. J. Clin. Nutr. 82(Suppl), 222S–225S.

10. Heinrichs SC. (2003). Nonexercise muscle tension and behavioral fidgeting are positively correlated with food availability/palatability and body weight in rats. Physiol. Behav. 79, 199–207.

11. Bouchard C, Tremblay A, Despres JP, Nadeau A, Lupien PJ, Theriault G, et al. (1990). The response to long-term overfeeding in identical twins. N. Engl. J. Med. 322, 1477–1482.

12. Levine JA, Eberhardt NL, & Jensen MD. (1999). Role of nonexercise activity thermogenesis in resistance to fat gain in humans. Science. 283, 212–214.

13. Moller DE. (2001). New drug targets for type 2 diabetes and the metabolic syndrome. Nature. 414, 821–827.

14. Zhang Y, Proenca R, Maffei M, Barone M, Leopold L, & Friedman JM. (1994). Positional cloning of the mouse obese gene and its human homologue. Nature. 372, 425–432.

15. Montague CT, Farooqi IS, Whitehead JP, Soos MA, Rau H, Wareham NJ, et al. (1997). Congenital leptin deficiency is associated with severe early-onset obesity in humans. Nature. 387, 903–908.

16. Morton G, Cummings D, Baskin D, Barsh G, & Schwartz MW. (2006). Central nervous system control of food intake and body weight. Nature. 443, 289–295.

17. Jobst E, Enriori P, Sinnayah P, & Cowley M. (2006). Hypothalamic regulatory pathways and potential obesity treatment targets. Endocrine. 29, 33–48.

18. O'Rahilly S, & Farooqi I. (2006). Genetics of obesity. Phil. Trans. R. Soc. B. 361, 1095–1105.

19. Luquet S, Perez F, Hnasko T, & Palmiter R. (2005). NPY/AgRP neurons are essential for feeding in adult mice but can be ablated in neonates. Science. 310, 683–685.

20. Rivera G, Bocanegra-García V, Galiano S, Cirauqui N, Ceras J, Pérez S, et al. (2008). Melanin-concentrating hormone receptor 1 antagonists: A new perspective for the pharmacologic treatment of obesity. Curr. Med. Chem. 15, 1025–1043.

21. Qu D, Ludwig DS, Gammeltoft S, Piper M, Pelleymounter MA, Cullen MJ, et al. (1996). A role for melanin-concentrating hormone in the central regulation of feeding behaviour. Nature. 380, 243–247.

22. Dryden S, Wang Q, Frankish HM, Pickavance L, & Williams G. (1995). The serotonin (5-HT) antagonist methysergide increases neuropeptide Y (NPY) synthesis and secretion in the hypothalamus of the rat. Brain Res. 699, 12–18.

23. Tecott LH, Sun LM, Akana SF, Strack AM, Lowenstein DH, Dallman MF, et al. (1995). Eating disorder and epilepsy in mice lacking 5-HT2c serotonin receptors. Nature. 374, 542–546.

24. Kyrou I, Valsamakis G, & Tsigos C. (2006). The endocannabinoid system as a target for the treatment of visceral obesity and metabolic syndrome. Ann. New York Acad. Sci. 1083, 270–305.

25. Horvath T. (2006). The unfolding cannabinoid story on energy homeostasis: Central or peripheral site of action. Int. J. Obesity. 30, S30–S32.

26. Lam TKT, Schwartz GJ, & Rossetti L. (2005). Hypothalamic sensing of fatty acids. Nat. Neurosci. 8, 579–584.

27. Kusunoki J, Kanatani A, & Moller DE. (2006). Modulation of fatty acid metabolism as a potential approach to the treatment of obesity and the metabolic syndrome. Endocrine. 29, 91–100.

28. Minokoshi Y, Alqular T, Furukawa N, Kim Y-B, Lee A, Xue B, et al. (2004). AMP-kinase regulates food intake by responding to hormonal and nutrient signals in the hypothalamus. Nature. 428, 569–574.

29. Winder W, & Hardie D. (1999). AMP-activated protein kinase, a metabolic master switch: Possible roles in type 2 diabetes. Am. J. Physiol. 40, E1–E10.

30. Liddle RA. (1997). Cholecystokinin cells. Ann. Rev. Physiol. 59, 221–242.

31. Sherrill R, Berman J, Birkemo L, Croom D, Dezube M, Ervin G, et al. (2001). 1,4-Benzodiazepine peripheral cholecystokinin (CCK-A) receptor agonists. Bioorg. Med. Chem. Lett. 11, 1145–1148.

32. Drucker D. (2006). The biology of incretin hormones. Cell Metab. 3, 153–165.

33. Stanley S, Wynne K, & Bloom S. (2003). Gastrointestinal satiety signals III. Glucagon-like peptide I, oxyntomodulin, peptide YY and pancreatic polypeptide. Am. J. Physiol. 286, G693–G697.

34. Wynne K, Park A, Small C, Patterson M, Ellis S, Murphy K, et al. (2005). Subcutaneous oxyntomodulin reduces body weight in overweight and obese subjects. Diabetes. 54, 2390–2395.

35. Renshaw D, & Batterham R. (2005). Peptide YY: A potential therapy for obesity. Curr. Drug Targets. 6, 171–179.

36. Wortley K, del Rincon J-P, Murray J, Garcia K, Iida K, Thorner M, et al. (2006). Absence of ghrelin protects against early-onset obesity. J. Clin. Invest. 115, 3573–3578.

37. Shearman L, Wang S, Helmling S, Stribling D, Mazur P, Ge L, et al. (2006). Ghrelin neutralization by a ribonucleic acid-SPM ameliorates obesity in diet-induced obese mice. Endocrinol. 147, 1517–1526.

38. Yang J, Brown M, Liang G, Grishin N, & Goldstein J. (2008). Identification of the acyltransferase that octanoylates ghrelin, an appetite-stimulating peptide hormone. Cell. 132, 387–396.

39. Gutierrez J, Solenberg P, Perkins D, Willency J, Knierman M, Jin Z, et al. (2008). Ghrelin octanoylation mediated by an orphan lipid transferase. Proc. Natl. Acad. Sci. U. S. A. 105, 6320–6325.

40. Zhou G, Myers R, Li Y, Chen Y, Shen X, Fenyk-Melody J, et al. (2001). Role of AMP-activated protein kinase in mechanism of metformin action. J. Clin. Invest. 108, 1167–1174.

41. Chen H, & Farese R. (2000). DGAT and triglyceride synthesis: A new target for obesity treatment? Trends Cardiovasc. Med. 10, 188–192.

42. Nawrocki A, & Scherer P. (2005). Keynote review: The adipocyte as a drug discovery target. Drug Discovery Today. 10, 1219–1230.

43. Cohen P, Miyazaki M, Socci N, Hagge-Greenberg A, Liedtke W, Soukas A, et al. (2002). Role for stearoyl-CoA desaturase-1 in leptin-mediated weight loss. Science. 297, 240–243.

44. Jiang G, Li Z, Liu F, Ellsworth K, Dallas-Yang Q, Wu M, et al. (2005). Prevention of obesity in mice by anti-sense oligonucleotide inhibitors of stearoyl-CoA desaturase-1. J. Clin. Invest. 115, 1030–1038.

45. Lowell BB, S-Susulic V, Hamann A, Lawitts J, Himms-Hagen J, Boyer BB, et al. (1993). Development of obesity in transgenic mice after genetic ablation of brown adipose tissue. Nature. 366, 740–742.

46. Lowell B, & Spiegelman B. (2000). Towards a molecular understanding of adaptive thermogenesis. Nature. 404, 652–660.

47. Grujic D, Susulic VS, Harper ME, Himms-Hagen J, Cunningham BA, Corkey BE, et al. (1997). Beta3-adrenergic receptors on white and brown adipocytes mediate beta3-selective agonist-induced effects on energy expenditure, insulin secretion, and food intake. J. Biol. Chem. 272, 17686–17693.

48. Walker BR, & Seckl JR. (2003). 11 β-hydroxysteroid dehydrogenase type 1 as a novel therapeutic target in metabolic and neurodegenerative disease. Expert Opin. Ther. Targets. 7, 771–783.

49. Kolonin M, Saha P, Chan L, Pasqualini R, & Arap W. (2004). Reversal of obesity by targeted ablation of adipose tissue. Nat. Med. 10, 625–632.

50. Innes JA, Watson ML, Ford MJ, Munro JF, Stoddart ME, & Campbell DB. (1977). Plasma fenfluramine levels, weight loss, and side effects. Br. Med. J. 2, 1322–1325.

51. Weintraub M, Hasday JD, Mushlin AI, & Lockwood DH. (1984). A double-blind clinical trial in weight control. Use of fenfluramine and phentermine alone and in combination. Arch. Intern. Med. 144, 1143–1148.

52. Bray GA, Blackburn GL, Ferguson JM, Greenway FL, Jain AK, Mendel CM, et al. (1999). Sibutramine produces dose-related weight loss. Obes. Res. 7, 189–198.

53. Addy C, Wright H, Van Laere K, Gantz I, & Erondu N. (2008). The acyclic CB1R inverse agonist taranabant mediates weight loss by increasing energy expenditure and decreasing caloric intake. Cell Metab. 7, 68–78.

54. Scheen AJ. (2008). CB1 receptor blockade and its impact on cardiometabolic risk factors: Overview of the RIO programme with rimonabant. J. Neuroendocrinol. 20(Suppl 1), 139–146.

55. Christensen R, Kristensen PK, Bartels EM, Bliddal H, & Astrup A. (2007). Efficacy and safety of the weight-loss drug rimonabant: A meta-analysis of randomised trials. Lancet. 370, 1706–1713.

56. Steiner MA, Marsicano G, Nestler EJ, Holsboer F, Lutz B, & Wotjak CT. (2008). Antidepressant-like behavioral effects of impaired cannabinoid receptor type 1 signaling coincide with exaggerated corticosterone secretion in mice. Psychoneuroendocrinol. 33, 54–67.

57. Greenway F, Fujioka K, Anderson J, Raj YP, Gupta A, O'Neil P, et al. (2007). A double-blind, placebo-, bupropion-, naltrexone-controlled study of the efficacy and safety of 3 doses. Obesity. 15, A85.

58. Fujioka K, Greenway F, Cowley M, Guttadauria M, Robinson J, Landbloom R, et al. (2007). The 24-week experience with a combination sustained release product of zonisamide and bupropion: Evidence of an encouraging benefit:risk profile. Obesity. 15, A85.

59. Greenway F, Fujioka K, Gupta A, Smith S, Guttadauria M, Tollefson G, et al. (2007). A double-blind, placebo-, bupropion- and naltrexone-controlled study of the efficacy and safety of 3 doses of naltrexone-bupropion SR combination therapy in obesity: Effects on total and visceral adipose tissue and CV risk markers. Obesity. 15, A85.

60. Gadde KM, Yonish GM, Foust MS, Tam PY, & Najarian T. (2006). A 24-week randomized controlled trial of VI-0521, a combination weight loss therapy, in obese adults. Obesity. 14, A17.

61. Erondu N, Gantz I, Musser B, Suryawanshi S, Mallick M, Addy C, et al. (2006). Neuropeptide Y5 receptor antagonism does not induce clinically meaningful weight loss in overweight and obese adults. Cell Metab. 4, 275–282.

62. Batterham RL, Cohen MA, Ellis SM, Le Roux CW, Withers DJ, Frost GS, et al. (2003). Inhibition of food intake in obese subjects by peptide YY3–36. N. Engl. J. Med. 349, 941–948.

63. Batterham RL, Le Roux CW, Cohen MA, Park AJ, Ellis SM, Patterson M, et al. (2003). Pancreatic polypeptide reduces appetite and food intake in humans. J. Clin. Endocrinol. Metab. 88, 3989–3992.

64. Gantz I, Erondu N, Mallick M, Musser B, Krishna R, Tanaka W, et al. (2007). Efficacy and safety of intranasal peptide YY3–36 for weight reduction in obese adults. J. Clin. Endocrinol. Metab. 92, 1754–1757.

65. Riddle MC, Henry RR, Poon TH, Zhang B, Mac SM, Holcombe JH, et al. (2006). Exenatide elicits sustained glycaemic control and progressive reduction of body weight in patients with type 2 diabetes inadequately controlled by sulphonylureas with or without metformin. Diabetes Metab. Res. Rev. 22, 483–491.

66. Significant weight loss sustained in obese people treated with liraglutide for one year. (2008). Novo Nordisk. Available at: http://www.novonordisk.com

67. de Souza CJ, & Burkey BF. (2001). Beta 3-adrenoceptor agonists as anti-diabetic and anti-obesity drugs in humans. Curr. Pharm. Des. 7, 1433–1449.

68. Redman LM, de Jonge L, Fang X, Gamlin B, Recker D, Greenway FL, et al. (2007). Lack of an effect of a novel beta3-adrenoceptor agonist, TAK-677, on energy metabolism in obese individuals: A double-blind, placebo-controlled randomized study. J. Clin. Endocrinol. Metab. 92, 527–531.

69. Cohade C, Mourtzikos KA, & Wahl RL. (2003). "USA-Fat": Prevalence is related to ambient outdoor temperature-evaluation with 18F-FDG PET/CT. J. Nucl. Med. 44, 1267–1270.

70. Wilson DM, Varvel SA, Harloe JP, Martin BR, & Lichtman AH. (2006). SR 141716 (rimonabant) precipitates withdrawal in marijuana-dependent mice. Pharmacol. Biochem. Behav. 85, 105–113.

71. Verebey K, Volavka J, Mule SJ, & Resnick RB. (1976). Naltrexone: disposition, metabolism, and effects after acute and chronic dosing. Clin. Pharmacol. Ther. 20, 315–328.

72. Fairchild MD, Jenden DJ, Mickey MR, & Yale C. (1980). EEG effects of hallucinogens and cannabinoids using sleep-waking behavior as baseline. Pharmacol. Biochem. Behav. 12, 99–105.

73. Tschop M, Smiley DL, & Heiman ML. (2000). Ghrelin induces adiposity in rodents. Nature. 407, 908–913.

74. Cervera A, Wajcberg E, Sriwijitkamol A, Fernandez M, Zuo P, Triplitt C, et al. (2008). Mechanism of action of exenatide to reduce postprandial hyperglycemia in type 2 diabetes. Am. J. Physiol. Endocrinol. Metab. 294, E846–E852.

75. Vedala A, Wang W, Neese RA, Christiansen MP, & Hellerstein MK. (2006). Delayed secretory pathway contributions to VLDL-triglycerides from plasma NEFA, diet, and de novo lipogenesis in humans. J. Lipid Res. 47, 2562–2574.

76. Ahnen DJ, Guerciolini R, Hauptman J, Blotner S, Woods CJ, & Wargovich MJ. (2007). Effect of orlistat on fecal fat, fecal biliary acids, and colonic cell proliferation in obese subjects. Gastroenterol. Hepatol. 5, 1291–1299.

77. Weyer C, Tataranni PA, Snitker S, Danforth EJ, & Ravussin E. (1998). Increase in insulin action and fat oxidation after treatment with CL 316,243, a highly selective beta3-adrenoceptor agonist in humans. Diabetes Metab. Res. Rev. 47, 1555–1561.

78. Yeomans MR, & Gray RW. (1997). Effects of naltrexone on food intake and changes in subjective appetite during eating: Evidence for opioid involvement in the appetizer effect. Physiol. Behav. 62, 15–21.

79. Chapelot D, Marmonier C, Thomas F, & Hanotin C. (2000). Modalities of the food intake-reducing effect of sibutramine in humans. Physiol. Behav. 68, 299–308.

80. Rolls BJ, Shide DJ, Thorwart ML, & Ulbrecht JS. (1998). Sibutramine reduces food intake in non-dieting women with obesity. Obes. Res. 6, 1–11.

81. Gregersen NT, Flint A, Bitz C, Blundell JE, Raben A, & Astrup A. (2008). Reproducibility and power of ad libitum energy intake assessed by repeated single meals. Am. J. Clin. Nutr. 87, 1277–1281.

82. Atkinson RL, Berke LK, Drake CR, Bibbs ML, Williams FL, & Kaiser DL. (1985). Effects of long-term therapy with naltrexone on body weight in obesity. Clin. Pharmacol. Ther. 38, 419–422.

83. Malcolm R, O'Neil PM, Sexauer JD, Riddle FE, Currey HS, & Counts C. (1985). A controlled trial of naltrexone in obese humans. Int. J. Obes. 9, 347–353.

84. Mitchell JE, Morley JE, Levine AS, Hatsukami D, Gannon M, & Pfohl D. (1987). High-dose naltrexone therapy and dietary counseling for obesity. Biol. Psychiatr. 22, 35–42.

85. Goldstein DJ, Rampey AH, Enas GG, Potvin JH, Fludzinski LA, & Levine LR. (1994). Fluoxetine: A randomized clinical trial in the treatment of obesity. Int. J. Obes. 18, 129–135.

86. Wren JA, Gossellin J, & Sunderland SJ. (2007). Dirlotapide: A review of its properties and role in the management of obesity in dogs. J. Vet. Pharmacol. Ther. 30(Suppl 1), 11–16.

87. Lipworth BJ. (1996). Clinical pharmacology of beta 3-adrenoceptors. Br. J. Clin. Pharmacol. 42, 291–300.

88. Grosch S, Niederberger E, Lotsch J, Skarke C, & Geisslinger G. (2001). A rapid screening method for a single nucleotide polymorphism (SNP) in the human MOR gene. Br. J. Clin. Pharmacol. 52, 711–714.

89. Monteleone P, Tortorella A, Martiadis V, Di Filippo C, Canestrelli B, & Maj M. (2008). The cDNA 385C to A missense polymorphism of the endocannabinoid degrading enzyme fatty acid amide hydrolase (FAAH) is associated with overweight/obesity but not with binge eating disorder in overweight/obese women. Psychoneuroendocrinol. 33, 546–550.

90. Teixeira PJ, Going SB, Sardinha LB, & Lohman TG. (2005). A review of psychosocial pre-treatment predictors of weight control. Obes. Rev. 6, 43–65.

91. Astrup A, Buemann B, Gluud C, Bennett P, Tjur T, & Christensen N. (1995). Prognostic markers for diet-induced weight loss in obese women. Int. J. Obes. 19, 275–278.

92. Wadden TA, Foster GD, Wang J, Pierson RN, Yang MU, Moreland K, et al. (1992). Clinical correlates of short- and long-term weight loss. Am. J. Clin. Nutr. 56(1 Suppl), 271S–274S.

93. Foster GD, Wadden TA, Swain RM, Stunkard AJ, Platte P, & Vogt RA. (1998). The Eating Inventory in obese women: Clinical correlates and relationship to weight loss. Int. J. Obes. 22, 778–785.

94. Weintraub M, Taves DR, Hasday JD, Mushlin AI, & Lockwood DH. (1981). Determinants of response to anorexiants. Clin. Pharmacol. Ther. 30, 528–533.

95. Womble LG, Williamson DA, Greenway FL, & Redmann SM. (2001). Psychological and behavioral predictors of weight loss during drug treatment for obesity. Int. J. Obes. 25, 340–345.

96. Shimazaki T, Yoshimizu T, & Chaki S. (2006). Melanin-concentrating hormone MCH1 receptor antagonists: A potential new approach to the treatment of depression and anxiety disorders. CNS Drugs. 20, 801–811.

97. Farooqi I, Keogh J, Yeo G, Lank E, Cheetham T, & O'Rahilly S. (2003). Clinical spectrum of obesity and mutations in the melanocortin 4 receptor. N. Engl. J. Med. 348, 1085–1095.

98. Loos R, & Bouchard C. (2008). FTO: The first gene contributing to common forms of human obesity. Obes. Rev. 9, 246–250.

99. Naggert JK, Fricker LD, Varlamov O, Nishina PM, Rouille Y, Steiner DF, et al. (1995). Hyperproinsulinaemia in obese fat/fat mice associated with a carboxypeptidase E mutation which reduces enzyme activity. Nat. Genet. 10, 135–142.

100. Noben-Trauth K, Naggert JK, North MA, & Nishina PM. (1996). A candidate gene for the mouse mutation tubby. Nature. 380, 534–538.

101. Ohki-Hamazaki H, Watase K, Yamamoto K, Ogura H, Yamano M, Yamada K, et al. (1997). Mice lacking bombesin receptor subtype-3 develop metabolic defects and obesity. Nature. 390, 165–169.

102. Ladenheim E, Hamilton N, Behles R, Bi S, Hampton L, Battey J, et al. (2008). Factors contributing to obesity in bombesin receptor subtype-3-deficient mice. Endocrinol. 149, 971–978.

103. Erlanson-Albertsson C, & York D. (1997). Enterostatin–a peptide regulating fat intake. Obes. Res. 5, 360–372.

104. Doggrell S. (2005). Neuromedin U–a new target in obesity. Expert Opin. Ther. Targets. 9, 875–877.

105. Charon C, Dupuy F, Marie V, & Bazin R. (1995). Effect of the b-adrenoceptor agonist BRL-35135 on development of obesity in suckling Zucker (fa/fa) rats. Am. J. Physiol. 268, E1039–E1045.

106. Greenberg AS, Egan JJ, Wek SA, Garty NB, Blanchette-Mackie EJ, & Londos C. (1991). Perilipin, a major hormonally regulated adipocyte-specific phosphoprotein associated with the periphery of lipid storage droplets. J. Biol. Chem. 266, 11341–11346.

Bone Disorders: Translational Medicine Case Studies

S. Aubrey Stoch

5.1. Introduction

In the United States, about 10 million Americans have osteoporosis (8 million women and 2 million men), whereas another 34 million individuals have osteopenia and are considered at risk for osteoporosis. Osteoporosis contributes to substantial disease burden with an excess of 2 million osteoporosis-related fractures in the United States in 2005.[1] Osteoporosis is characterized by low bone mass with skeletal fragility and increased occurrence of fractures. Bone loss results from an imbalance between bone resorption and formation. The field has witnessed the emergence of an array of new treatments providing physicians and patients a much enriched range of therapeutic options. Existing agents are not without their challenges, including significant safety issues for estrogens, bisphosphonates, and the combination of bisphosphonates with parathyroid hormone (PTH). Despite a wide range of existing therapies from which to choose, most patients remain untreated.

The major current antiosteoporotic therapies include bisphosphonates (alendronate [ALN], risedronate, ibandronate, and zoledronate), estrogens, selective estrogen receptor modulators (raloxifene, bazedoxifene), and PTH. Other niche treatments include calcitonin, vitamin D derivatives, and strontium (in some countries). Except for PTH and strontium, these drugs inhibit bone resorption. In addition, the anti-RANK-ligand monoclonal antibody (denosumab) was recently recommended for approval by a U.S. Food and Drug Administration (FDA) advisory committee (August 13, 2009) and was approved on June 1, 2010, for the treatment of postmenopausal osteoporosis and for the treatment of bone loss in patients undergoing hormone ablation for prostate cancer.

5.2. Challenges in Translational Research

Translational science supporting drug discovery and development for osteoporosis has many advantages over some other therapeutic areas. Not only are there a number of predictive preclinical models, but there are also qualified predictive biomarkers of bone turnover and bone mineral density (BMD) that can be used for benchmarking from bedside-to-bench and back again. This chapter will focus on the role of translational medicine in approaching several novel therapeutic mechanisms for osteoporosis and review the current status of these emerging mechanisms.

Novel agents target either the osteoclast (the principal bone resorbing cell) or the osteoblast (the key bone forming cell). Consequently, osteoporosis therapies can generally be grouped into two main categories: (1) antiresorptives (those agents targeting the osteoclast) and, (2) anabolics (agents that specifically target the osteoblast). Furthermore, bone resorption and formation are coupled, and agents that influence one principal cell usually have a modulating influence on the others involved in the homeostatic pathway.

5.3. Osteoporosis: Biomarker Considerations

Biomarkers provide a key translatable link between an intended drug target and the activity of molecules designed to engage with these targets. Some biomarkers also predict clinical outcomes and can be used to assess the efficacy of novel agents. In the next few sections, biomarkers will be formally presented, and their use during osteoporosis drug development will be illustrated as each case study is presented.

5.3.1. Biochemical Biomarkers of Bone Turnover

Many drugs developed to treat osteoporosis and other metabolic bone disorders reduce bone metabolic activity referred to as "bone turnover." Bone turnover is characterized both by bone resorption and bone formation – processes that reflect osteoclast and osteoblast activity, respectively. Osteoclasts and osteoblasts are tightly coupled, and the measurement of markers of bone turnover allows for a more precise quantitative estimate. Biochemical markers of bone turnover can be grouped into two categories: (1) enzymes and proteins secreted by osteoclasts and osteoblasts, and (2) products of bone type I collagen degradation and formation. Markers of bone resorption reflect osteoclast activity, whereas markers of bone formation capture the activity of osteoblasts (Table 5.1).

Table 5.1. Major Biomarkers of Bone Turnover

Biomarker	Type	Source	Measurement	Precision
CTx	Resorption	Type I collagen degradation	ELISA (urine, serum), RIA (urine)	3%–5.8% (serum) 19%–23% (urine)
NTx	Resorption	Type I collagen degradation	ELISA (urine, serum)	13% (serum) 16%–23% (urine)
DPD	Resorption	Type I collagen degradation	ELISA (urine) HPLC (serum)	23% (urine)
TRACP5b	Resorption	Enzyme secreted by osteoclasts	ELISA (serum)	2.2%
BSAP	Formation	Enzyme secreted by osteoblasts	ELISA (serum)	4.4%
PINP	Formation	Type I collagen synthesis	ELISA (urine) HPLC (serum)	7.2%–4.4%
OC	Formation	Bone matrix components synthesized by osteoblasts	ELISA (serum)	8%–63%

Notes: ELISA: enzyme-linked immunosorbent assay; RIA: radioimmunoassay; HPLC: high-performance liquid chromatography.
Source: Reproduced with permission from Tesch G, Amur S, Schousboe JT, Siegel JN, Lesko LJ, Bai JPF. Successes achieved and challenges ahead in translating biomarkers into clinical applications. The AAPS Journal 2010 (published online).

5.3.1.1. Biomarkers of Bone Resorption

When bone is resorbed, peptide products of type I collagen are released and can be measured in either the serum or urine.[2–4] The N- and C-telopeptides of the cross-links of type I collagen are termed NTx and CTx, respectively.[4] NTx and CTx are generated by the direct action of cathepsin (Cat) K on collagen. Cat K cleaves the N-telopeptide of collagen to generate NTx and also degrades the serum C-terminal telopeptide of type I collagen (1-CTP), a larger C-terminal fragment of type I collagen produced by the action of matrix metalloproteinases,[5,6] to generate CTx (Figure 5.1).[7,8] Deoxypyridinoline (DPD), another biomarker released during bone resorption, forms cross-links between collagen peptides, stabilizes collagen molecules, and provides a direct measure of the mass of resorbed collagen.[9] The enzyme tartrate-resistant acid phosphatase 5b (TRACP5b) is a good indicator of osteoclast number.[10] Serum and urinary levels of resorption markers show a circadian rhythm and are highest in the early morning and at their nadir in the afternoon hours.[5,11]

5.3.1.2. Biomarkers of Bone Formation

Markers of bone formation reflect direct and indirect products of active osteoblasts. Bone-specific alkaline phosphatase (BSAP) is one of the

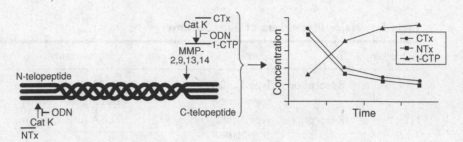

Fig. 5.1
Schematic representation of collagen with Cat K cleavage sites. CatK cleaves the N-telopeptide of collagen to generate NTx. A number of matrix metalloproteinases (MMPs) cleave collagen at the C-telopeptide, releasing the C-terminal telopeptide of type I collagen (1-CTP) epitope, which is further digested by Cat K to generate CTx. Inhibition of Cat K with odanacatib (ODN) results in a decrease in CTx and NTx levels and an accumulation of 1-CTP. From Stoch SA, Zajic S, Stone J, et al. (2009). Effect of the cathepsin K inhibitor odanacatib on bone resorption biomarkers in healthy postmenopausal women: Two double-blind, randomized, placebo-controlled phase I studies. Clin. Pharmacol. Ther. 86, 175–182.

isoforms of alkaline phosphatase; its exact role is not known. Osteocalcin (OC; bone gla-protein) is a hydroxyl-apatite-binding protein that is synthesized by osteoblasts and is expressed mainly during the osteoid mineralization phase of bone formation.[4] Type 1 procollagen propeptide (procollagen type I N-terminal peptide (P1NP) and procollagen type I C-terminal peptide (P1CP) are the amino- and carboxy-terminal extension propeptides of type I collagen, respectively.[4] The cleavage products are released into the circulation and reflect bone formation. Markers of bone formation are less subject to diurnal or food influences.

Biochemical markers have been used to predict response to drug therapy. They allow for an earlier assessment of effectiveness of pharmacological intervention compared with changes in BMD. Moreover, short-term changes in bone turnover markers appear to predict response to agents used to prevent fractures.[5] Both reductions in serum NTx (sNTx) and serum CTx (sCTx) during the first 6 months of ALN therapy have been associated with a greater increase in BMD.[12] Similarly, reductions in serum OC (sOC) are predictive of BMD changes on ALN.[13] The magnitude of P1NP increase appears to correlate strongly with increases in BMD.[14] Although markers of bone resorption and formation are coupled, markers of bone resorption decrease more quickly following the administration of antiresorptive therapy, whereas bone formation markers lag by several months. By contrast, markers of bone formation (e.g., serum P1NP) increase earlier with the initiation of osteoanabolic therapy with teriparatide (TER), whereas bone resorption markers decrease months later. Markers of bone turnover remain central to assessing early pharmacodynamic (PD) activity in healthy volunteers and postmenopausal women when novel bone-active agents are introduced in the clinic. Furthermore, the direction and magnitude of response are consistent with what is seen in preclinical animal models.

5.3.2. Imaging Biomarkers (BMD)

Although biochemical markers of bone turnover are widely predictive of early PD response and allow more rapid decision making in early drug development, BMD is considered a surrogate endpoint with prognostic value.[15] Decreased BMD is among the most powerful predictors of fracture occurrence. After the relationship between BMD and fracture risk reduction has been established for a particular agent, regulators are willing to extrapolate to other agents within a class of drugs as well as across populations.[15] More recently, there is an opinion that changes in both BMD and biochemical markers of bone turnover (resorption and formation) are integral in predicting changes in fracture risk.[15] With the bisphosphonates, BMD became an accepted surrogate in predicting fracture rates in conjunction with preclinical evidence of bone quality and safety.[16] This acceptance was subsequently revisited in 1994 with the revision of the U.S. draft guidelines for osteoporosis,[17] and BMD lost its surrogate endpoint status largely due to the nonpredictive nature of increases in BMD seen with etidronate and fluoride. Preclinical data, however, showed a reduction in bone quality with both agents, which, despite being available in the literature at the time, were not presented at the FDA advisory committee meetings. Notwithstanding this, BMD remains a predictive and a necessary component for evaluating novel mechanisms, particularly in the Phase 2 setting, and for establishing both proof of concept (POC) and dose ranging.

The combination of preclinical bone strength data, along with appropriate alterations in biochemical markers and BMD (see Table 5.2), allows for a much higher probability of success that a novel mechanism will likely demonstrate fracture risk reduction in the clinic.

5.3.3. Preclinical Models

Animal models (e.g., rats, rabbits, and nonhuman primates) of osteoporosis have been used to evaluate potential novel therapies prior to testing in humans for target engagement and distal effects. The ovariectomized (OVX) rhesus monkey, an estrogen deficiency model of bone loss characterized by accelerated bone resorption and formation, has been used to characterize bone-active compounds and has been a predictive model for human osteoporosis,[18] although all of the aforementioned species may be used for evaluating compounds in vivo.

In addition to using preclinical animal models to define efficacy and pharmacokinetic (PK) and PD correlations to define initial dosing targets for the clinic, animal models are also required from a regulatory standpoint. U.S. and European Union (EU) guidance for the development of antiosteoporosis agents specifically requires demonstration of normal bone quality (architecture, mass, and strength) in two species (rodent and nonrodent; OVX). It is generally agreed that the OVX rat is a useful model of human bone loss because its response to mechanical forces as well as to hormone and drug interventions is similar to that of humans. There is less agreement, however, regarding the relevance of mouse models to postmenopausal bone loss. Although mouse models are readily available and knockout and transgenic mouse models allow for elegant experimentation

Table 5.2. Bone Translational Biomarkers

Name	Mechanism	Linkage to Outcome
Bone Resorption: Mechanism biomarkers related to osteoclast function		
NTx	Cat K cleaves the N-terminal cross-link of type I collagen to release NTx into serum and then urine	Increased BMD with ALN
CTx of type I collagen cross-links	Cat K cleaves the C-terminal fragment of type I collagen that results from metalloprotease digestion of type I collagen, producing CTx in serum and then urine	Increased BMD with ALN
DPD	From collagen cross-links and provides a measure of type I collagen degradation	
Enzyme-resistant phosphatase 5b (TRACP5b)	Derived from osteoclasts; level related to number of functional osteoclasts	
Bone Formation: Mechanism biomarkers related to osteoblast function		
BSAP	Role in bone formation uncertain	
OC (bone gla-protein)	Hydroxy-apatite binding protein produced by osteoblasts during osteoid mineralization	Reduction with ALN predicts increased BMD
PINP	Amino-terminal peptides released after the synthesis of type I collagen	Increase correlated with BMD increase
PICP	Carboxy-terminal peptides released after the synthesis of type I collagen	
Imaging Biomarkers		
BMD	Measured by a variety of radiographic methods, including CT and various photon densitometry methods	Decrease predicts increased fracture risk; increases from drug treatment usually predict lower fracture risk with few exceptions

and genetic analysis, mouse strains differ in peak bone mass and susceptibility to bone loss.[19] Importantly, differences also exist in how the human and mouse skeletons respond to estrogen.[19] Notwithstanding these issues, the mouse model has proven beneficial in the evaluation of new chemical entities and their ability to mitigate bone loss.

Clinical considerations typically include genetic data as well as pharmacological POC in human volunteers. These are described for each molecular target in subsequent sections below. In the subsequent sections, specific translational (nonclinical and clinical) paradigms will be reviewed for each class of drugs in the context of new and emerging targets.

5.4. Antiresorptives

Osteoclast-mediated bone resorption requires two processes: demineralization of the inorganic bone components and degradation of the organic bone matrix (Figure 5.2). These two processes occur in the osteoclast in a coordinated manner by two separate mechanisms.[20] The first phase involves acid secretion by the osteoclast into the resorption lacunae, and the second phase is the organic matrix degradation by cysteine proteases. An acidic microenvironment is required for bone resorption, both to dissolve the mineral component of bone and to aid protein matrix digestion. This unique metabolic milieu is achieved by lowering the pH in the resorption lacunae via acid secretion by the osteoclast.

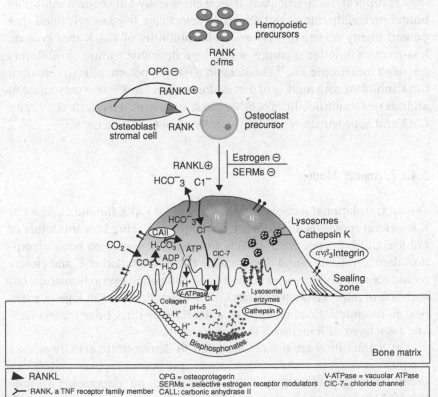

Fig. 5.2
Potential therapeutic targets, including Cat K, for pharmacological manipulation. From Stoch SA & Wagner JA. (2008). Cathepsin K inhibitors: A novel target for osteoporosis therapy. Clin. Pharmacol. Ther. 83, 172–176.

5.4.1. Cat K Inhibitors

5.4.1.1. What Is Known about the Target?

Cat K is the most abundant cysteine protease expressed in the osteoclast and is believed to be instrumental in bone matrix degradation necessary for bone resorption. Cat K is a member of the papain family of cysteine proteases and is both selectively and highly expressed in osteoclasts that mediate bone resorption.[21] Activated Cat K is capable of degrading several components of bone matrix, including type I collagen (which accounts for ~90% of bone matrix), osteopontin, and osteonectin.

Cathepsins have known collagenolytic activity under acidic conditions, and Cat K is capable of degrading type I collagen, the major component of bone matrix.[22] The finding of Cat K deficiency in pycnodysostosis,[23] an osteopetrotic disorder characterized by decreased bone resorption, further highlights the tractability of this enzyme as a potential target for developing agents to treat osteoporosis and other disorders characterized by increased bone resorption.

The designing of specific Cat K inhibitors has recently progressed. Initial Cat K inhibitors bound irreversibly to the cysteine protease, thereby conferring the theoretical possibility of generating antigenic and immunologic complications, particularly if used chronically. Subsequent inhibitors bound reversibly but lacked adequate selectivity. It was envisioned that potent, highly selective, and reversible inhibitors of Cat K that contain less-reactive functional groups would be a desirable feature of inhibitors intended for chronic use.[24] Odanacatib (ODN), a potent, selective, neutral Cat K inhibitor with an IC_{50} of 0.2 nM for human Cat K[25] was developed to address metabolic liabilities of other Cat K inhibitors. It has little activity on Cat L and approximately 400-fold selectivity for Cat F and Cat V.[25]

5.4.1.2. Animal Models

Several translational paradigms are available for Cat K inhibitors. The Cat K knockout mouse is an excellent model for analyzing how inhibitors of Cat K could influence both aspects of osteoclast-mediated bone resorption, demineralization and organic bone matrix degradation,[19] and closely reproduces the phenotype of human Cat K deficiency, pycnodysostosis. Cat K–deficient mice, generated by targeted disruption of the Cat K gene, manifest an osteopetrotic phenotype characterized by thick bone trabeculae[26] and associated with increases in bone strength.[27]

Cat K inhibitors are usually designed to demonstrate activity against the human enzyme and are significantly less potent (approximately two orders of magnitude) against the mouse and rat enzymes.[28] Despite this, Cat K inhibitors have been shown to prevent bone loss in OVX mice[29] without perturbing the anabolic action of PTH, suggesting that the

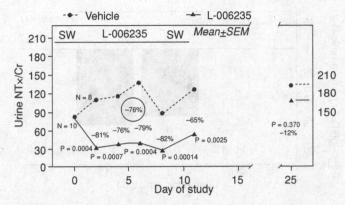

Fig. 5.3
Ratio of NTx to Cr
during dosage (15
mpk, p.o., q.d.) of
L-0006235 in adult
OVX rhesus monkeys.
Reprinted with
permission from
Palmer JT, Bryant C,
Wang DX, Davis DE,
Setti EL, Rydzewski
RM, et al. (2005).
Design and synthesis
of tri-ring P3
benzamide-containing
aminonitriles as
potent, selective,
orally effective
inhibitors of cathepsin
K. J. Med. Chem. 48,
7520–7534. Copyright
2005, American
Chemical Society.

combination of a Cat K inhibitor with an anabolic agent may further increase bone mass when compared with that seen with a bisphosphonate given with an anabolic. The combination of a Cat K inhibitor with PTH enhances the anabolic action of PTH on BMD and bone volume (BV) at both the primary and secondary spongiosa, whereas the bisphosphonate ALN has a similar effect at the primary spongiosa but blunts the remodeling of trabecular bone.[30] Whether this added efficacy will translate to the clinic remains to be demonstrated.

The rat Cat K enzyme is only 88% homologous to the human enzyme, whereas the sequence in the rabbit is 96% identical to human Cat K. The monkey enzyme is identical to the human one.[31] Although the OVX rat model is considered the classic animal model for revaluating bone active compounds, the rat is not the preferred species for testing Cat K inhibitors because of its low homology with the human Cat K. Nevertheless, Cat K inhibitors have demonstrated potent antiresorptive activity when evaluated in established models of acute bone resorption, including the thyroparathyroidectomized (TPTX) rat model[32] and the OVX rat model.[33] Cat K inhibitors have demonstrated increased BMD in the OVX rabbit.[34]

Because monkey Cat K is identical to mature human Cat K both in sequence and kinetics,[35] the monkey is a suitable species for evaluating Cat K inhibitors preclinically. Administration of selective Cat K inhibitors to OVX rhesus monkeys results in robust suppression of biochemical biomarkers of bone resorption. Oral dosing of the potent, selective, benzamide-containing aminonitrile (L-006235) in OVX rhesus monkeys once daily for 7 days resulted in a dose-dependent decrease in urinary N-telopeptide/creatinine (uNTx/Cr; Figures 5.3 and 5.4).[36] Similar decreases in indices of bone resorption have also been observed with the administration of another Cat K inhibitor, relacatib (SB-462795), which decreased bone resorption and increased blood PTH levels.[37] Levels of sCTx and sNTx and levels of uNTx were reduced within 1.5 h after dosing and remained suppressed (~37%) for up to 48 h, depending on the dose administered in OVX and intact monkeys.[37]

Fig. 5.4
Dose-reponse effect of L-0006235 on uNTx/Cr in the OVX monkey model. Reprinted with permission from Palmer JT, Bryant C, Wang DX, et al. (2005). Design and synthesis of tri-ring P3 benzamide-containing aminonitriles as potent, selective, orally effective inhibitors of cathepsin K. J. Med. Chem. 48, 7520–7534. Copyright 2005, American Chemical Society.

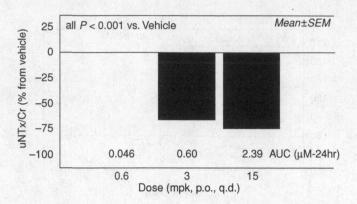

In OVX adult rhesus monkeys treated with vehicle or ODN for 21 months, ODN suppressed biomarkers of bone resorption without negatively affecting bone formation – BMD was increased both at the hip and spine.[38] More recent data from this study suggest that treatment with ODN for 21 months increased cortical thickness without affecting cortical porosity at the central femur.[39] These data support the finding that ODN, unlike bisphosphonates, acts as a bone formation–sparing antiresorptive in the central femur and effectively protects cortical bone. The relative bone formation–sparing properties of Cat K inhibition have been observed with a number of different compounds, suggesting that this Cat K mechanism likely differentiates from traditional antiresorptives (bisphosphonates and estrogens). Human translation of this effect, however, requires confirmation in the clinic.

5.4.1.3. Human Data

Autosomal recessive Cat K deficiency in humans is associated with findings in patients with pycnodysostosis. These individuals (both children and adults) also tend to have a reduction in bone resorption markers (uNTx, sCTx). In a report on 6 affected adults, uNTx measured 16 ± 8 versus 37 ± 16 nmol/l bone collagen equivalents mmol/l creatinine in controls, $P < .01$, and was significantly reduced in 17 affected children ($P < .0003$).[40] No abnormality was seen in markers of bone formation, OC, or P1CP, suggesting preservation of normal osteoblastic activity.[40] Bone biopsies obtained from patients with pycnodysostosis also revealed disturbances in bone remodeling,[41] which may contribute to the increase in fragility in patients with pycnodysostosis. The relevance of these findings in pycnodysostosis patients to patients with osteoporosis treated with Cat K inhibitors is not known, however. Patients with pycnodysostosis have a total absence of Cat K from fetal development to adulthood – a scenario different from partial pharmacological inhibition in patients treated with Cat K inhibitors in osteoporosis.

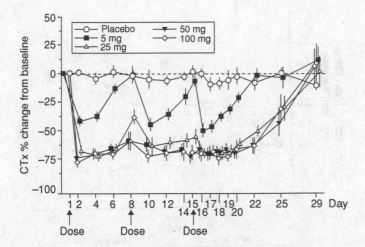

Fig. 5.5
CTx – mean (standard error, SE) percentage change from baseline following 3 weeks of weekly dosing with odanacatib. From Stoch SA, Zajic S, Stone J, et al. (2009). Effect of the cathepsin K inhibitor odanacatib on bone resorption biomarkers in healthy postmenopausal women: Two double-blind, randomized, placebo-controlled phase I studies. Clin. Pharmacol. Ther. 86, 175–182.

The pharmacological POC for the Cat K mechanism in humans has been established. At least two Cat K inhibitors, ODN (MK-0822) and balicatib (AAE581), demonstrated PD activity based on reductions in bone resorption biomarkers and increased BMD in humans. Three doses of ODN (0.5, 2.5, and 10 mg) were administered once daily to 30 postmenopausal female subjects ($N = 10$ per group [8 active, 2 placebo]) for 21 days. Robust reductions in uNTx (~80%) were seen following daily administration of 2.5 and 10 mg of ODN for 21 days, whereas more modest reductions in uNTx (~15%) were seen following administration of 0.5 mg for 21 days.[42] The effects of ODN on sCTx were similar to those seen with uNTx, eliciting a response of ~15%, ~70%, and ~80% reduction following 21 days of dosing ODN at 0.5, 2.5, and 10 mg, respectively. No significant effect was seen on bone-formation markers such as BSAP and OC.[42] It should be noted that, because Cat K specifically cleaves the N-telopeptide of collagen to generate NTx and also degrades serum 1-CTP to generate CTx, for this mechanism, one should also evaluate DPD, a resorption biomarker not influenced by Cat K processing itself.

ODN has a long PK half-life and has shown PD activity with robust sCTx suppression in a once-weekly dosing paradigm in 48 postmenopausal women (Figure 5.5).[42] Data from a multicenter, randomized, placebo-controlled trial in postmenopausal women with low BMD have demonstrated increases in BMD with ODN.[43] Doses administered once weekly included placebo and 3, 10, 25, and 50 mg. In this 1-year dose-finding trial with a 1-year extension performed in 399 postmenopausal women (64.2 ± 7.8 years) with low BMD (mean T-scores ≤ –2.0 and ≥ –3.5) at lumbar spine (LS), femoral neck, trochanter, or total hip, ODN treatment resulted in dose-dependent increases in BMD from baseline (Figure 5.6).

Two categories of adverse events (AEs) involving the skin and upper respiratory tract infections have been observed with the Cat K inhibitor balicatib.[44] A higher incidence of skin AEs (mainly pruritus) was observed in clinical trials with balicatib. Although the precise reason why balicatib

Fig. 5.6
Graphic presentation of the mean percentage change from baseline over 24 months in lumbar spine (LS) BMD in the full-analysis-set population. From Bone HG, McClung MR, Roux C, et al. (2010). Odanacatib, a cathepsin-K inhibitor for osteoporosis: A two-year study in postmenopausal women with low bone density. J. Bone Miner. Res. 25, 937–949. Reprinted with permission of John Wiley, & Sons, Inc.

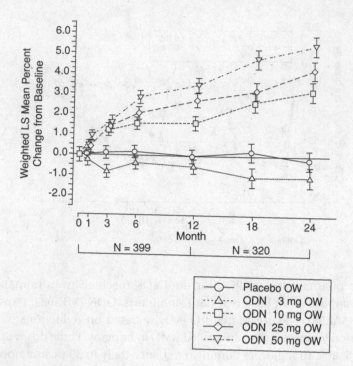

elicited skin lesions is not known, it is known that balicatib exhibits lyso-somotropic behavior as well as increased off-target cysteine Cat activity in vivo.[45] In particular, balicatib may not be sufficiently selective with inhibition of Cats B, L, and S, all of which are expressed in skin fibroblasts.[45,46]

ODN was generally well tolerated with an incidence of clinical and laboratory AEs similar to that of the placebo across treatment groups. There were no dose-related increases in the incidence of skin AEs or upper respiratory infections compared with placebo through 24 months. In contrast to what is seen with bisphosphonates, treatment discontinuation resulted in bone loss from all sites, with higher rates in the initial 6 months and less loss between Months 30 and 36. Biochemical biomarkers of bone remodeling also increased rapidly above baseline following the discontinuation of ODN. Levels of sCTx reached >2-fold above baseline by Month 30 but were only ~10% above baseline by Month 36. ODN has entered Phase 3 development in postmenopausal women in a trial designed to demonstrate fracture risk reduction and is the most advanced Cat K inhibitor in development.

It is increasingly recognized that Cat K is a novel target for osteoporosis and, inherently, there may be gaps in our knowledge to understand the viability of this mechanism. Although Cat K is most abundantly expressed in the osteoclast, lower levels have been demonstrated in other cell types, including synovial and skin fibroblasts, macrophages, dendritic cells, and epithelial cells of different origins.[47] Cat K–deficient mice exhibit characteristics of lung fibrosis in a bleomycin disease model.[48] Patients with pycnodysostosis, a life-long absence of Cat K, have demonstrated accumulation of collagen fibrils in osteoclasts as well as fibroblasts.[47] Although the preceding findings may be consistent with Cat K's affecting type I collagen turnover, the degradation of collagen by fibroblasts appears to be a predominantly lysosomal event.[49] Cat K is also expressed in the thyroid epithelium and is probably involved in thyroglobulin processing for thyroxine liberation.[50,51] No thyroid abnormalities have been described in clinical trials to date.

Thus, the translation of Cat K inhibition from a theoretical novel target to a drug in development was facilitated by animal and human data from genetic deficiency of Cat K, qualified biomarkers, animal PD and disease models, and an early mechanistic POC in human studies.

5.4.2. $\alpha_v\beta_3$ Integrin Antagonists

5.4.2.1. What Is Known about the Target?

Osteoclast adhesion involves several integrins, including $\alpha_v\beta_3$, $\alpha_2\beta_1$, and $\alpha_v\beta_1$.[52] The highest level of physiological expression of $\alpha_v\beta_3$ is on the osteoclast with approximately 15×10^6 receptors/osteoclast.[52] Integrins comprise a family of cell surface receptors constructed from transmembrane heterodimeric glycoproteins that have a pivotal role in numerous developmental, physiological, and pathological processes. They are the principal mediators of cell-to-extracellular matrix anchorage, which is of fundamental importance to cell function and tissue integrity. In a myriad of roles, integrins promote platelet aggregation, bone resorption, immune function, cell fusion, tumor invasion and metastases, programmed cell death, leukocyte homing and activation, and the response of cells to biomechanical forces.[53-58] Importantly, integrins play a critical role in mediating osteoclast attachment at sites of bone resorption. Integrin antagonists interrupt this necessary step for mediating bone resorption and therefore represent a novel approach to treat osteoporosis. Hence, development of $\alpha_v\beta_3$ antagonists represents a sound mechanism-based target for a novel antiresorptive approach to therapy.

The disintegrins are a group of peptides that includes echistatin, a 49-amino-acid peptide that was isolated from snake venom.[59] Echistatin has been found to be a highly potent inhibitor of bone resorption both in vitro[59-61] and in vivo.[32] A 4-week study of in vivo echistatin administration (0.26 µg/kg/h) to OVX rats was shown to prevent bone loss in femur with no evidence of side effects, such as bleeding due to inhibition of platelet aggregation through the $\alpha_{IIb}\beta_3$ integrin.[62] As further POC of the fundamental role that the vitronectin receptor plays in osteoclast-mediated bone resorption, echistatin has been shown to dose dependently reverse PTH-induced hypercalcemia in TPTX rats ($IC_{50} = 100$ nM).[32] Three-day treatment with echistatin (30 µg/kg/min) also prevented bone resorption in mice with low-calcium-diet–induced secondary hyperparathyroidism.[63]

Immunochemistry has shown colocalization of echistatin with the α_v-like subunit at the osteoclast clear zone, suggesting that echistatin blocks bone resorption by interacting with $\alpha_v\beta_3$.[63] Echistatin has several drawbacks, however, including lack of selectivity and its requirement for parenteral administration. In addition, it is only 300-fold more potent as an antiresorptive agent than as an antiplatelet aggregation agent.[59] The lack of selectivity is attributed to the common β-subunit shared by both $\alpha_v\beta_3$ and $\alpha_{IIb}\beta_3$. Nevertheless, studies with disintegrins indicate that integrin selectivity is effected by the amino acids flanking the active site and can be modified by their substitution.[64]

5.4.2.2. Animal Models

In vivo assays that have been used in qualifying preclinical candidates include, among others, the TPTX rat model, the OVX rat model, the rapidly growing rat minipump model, and the OVX rhesus monkey.

In certain instances, mutations of the $\alpha_v\beta_3$ receptor may either exist in nature, albeit rarely, or be established for biological proof of principle (knockout mouse model). Targeted disruption of the β_3 integrin in mice induces progressive osteosclerosis without a detectable reduction in the number of osteoclasts.[65] The β_3-null mice also exhibit a bleeding disorder consistent with the lack of $\alpha_{IIb}\beta_3$ integrin on platelets. $\beta_3^{-/-}$ mice are phenotypically similar to wild-type (WT) mice both at birth and throughout life. As the β_3-null mice age, however, they become osteosclerotic with radiographic evidence of increased bone mass by 4 months.[65] Histological sections of $\beta_3^{-/-}$ bones reveal a marked increase in cortical and trabecular bone but do not show the persistence of cartilaginous bars, reflecting the failure to resorb primary spongiosa characteristically seen in mice with osteopetrosis. Despite increases in bone mass, the number of osteoclasts in homozygous mutant mice is increased when compared with WT animals,[65] and levels of circulating calcium are much lower than levels seen in heterozygous animals. Despite an increase in the number of osteoclasts in $\beta_3^{-/-}$ mice, they do not appear to resorb bone efficiently. Whereas heterozygous animals display a normal, thin villous appearance in their ruffled membranes, the null mice have an abnormal organelle that is thick with blunted projections. Osteoclasts generated from β_3-null mice have a crenated appearance indicative of a cytoskeletal abnormality.[66] Normal bone resorption requires the formation of actin rings to establish the "sealing zone" necessary to isolate the resorption environment. β_3-deficient osteoclasts fail to form actin rings.[67] Mutant osteoclasts also fail to effectively resorb bone when placed on dentine slices. Importantly, the β_3-knockout mouse is also resistant to postmenopausal osteoporosis.[68]

OVX rats experience accelerated bone loss that mimics estrogen-deficiency bone loss seen in postmenopausal women. It is well established that the OVX rat model may be used to profile the in vivo efficacy of bone resorption inhibitors preclinically. This model is widely accepted as predictive of efficacy in the clinic and may be used to establish PK and biomarker targets. Compounds may be dosed orally for 28 days and may be compared with vehicle control and sham-operated rats.[69] Efficacy readouts include BMD measured by dual-energy x-ray absorptiometry (DXA) at both the distal femoral metaphysis (DFM) and the central femur. The results are usually expressed as the ratio of the BMD of the DFM compared with the BMD of the central femur (DFM:central ratio) to compensate for differences in bone size among animals.[69] A potent, selective, nonpeptide propionic acid was dosed orally (10 and 30 mg/kg body weight b.i.d. for 28 days) in the OVX rat model and compared with vehicle and sham-operated rats.[69] Vehicle-treated OVX rats demonstrated a significant decrease in BMD, whereas drug-treated rats exhibited a dose-dependent BMD increase.[69]

A short-term model of thyroid-induced osteopenia has been established in the rat to evaluate vitronectin receptor antagonists. When the $\alpha_v\beta_3$ antagonist, SB-273005, was evaluated in this high turnover model, it demonstrated a dose-dependent inhibition of resorption after only 7 days of treatment.[70] In response to bolus injections of L-thyroxine (T4), robust increases in bone turnover are observed. In the T4-treated group, significant increases in urinary DPD, a bone resorption maker, and sOC, a bone formation marker relative to vehicle-treated animals, are seen. The $\alpha_v\beta_3$ antagonist, SB-273005, when coadministered with T4, decreases urinary DPD levels in a dose-dependent manner. SB-273005 had no significant effect on sOC levels.[70]

The rat Schenk model uses young, rapidly growing male rats in which the growth of long bones is associated with the formation of new bone trabeculae in the metaphysis under the epiphyseal plate. When bone resorption and remodeling are inhibited, increased density of the cancellous bone occurs as measured by BMD. The Schenk assay has been used to evaluate in vivo effects of $\alpha_v\beta_3$ antagonists directly on bone and makes it possible to relate PK and PD. When the ALN or the propionic acid derivative $\alpha_v\beta_3$ antagonist was administered s.c. by minipump infusion for 10 days, both ALN and the $\alpha_v\beta_3$ antagonist demonstrated significant increases in BMD when compared with the vehicle-treated group.[69]

The OVX rhesus monkey model has been used to monitor the effect of antiresorptive agents on urinary markers of bone degradation. Adult female rhesus monkeys are ovariectomized for ~28 months and are used to evaluate antiresorptives for efficacy on uNTx and Cr with results expressed as uNTx/Cr. Once-daily administration of the integrin propionic acid derivative $\alpha_v\beta_3$ antagonist for 2 weeks in this model achieved a 39% reduction in the level of uNTx when compared with vehicle controls. After discontinuing the drug, the uNTx levels returned to baseline after 2 days.[69] Therefore, suppression of uNTx levels by $\alpha_v\beta_3$ antagonists is fully reversible within 1 to 2 days of cessation of treatment. This finding is in striking contrast to those of other antiresorptives, most notably the bisphosphonates, which have sustained PD effects.

5.4.2.3. Human Data

POC for this mechanism has been established in the clinic[71] with L-000845704, which increased LS BMD (2.1%, 3.1%, and 3.5% for the 100-mg-q.d., 400-mg-q.d., and 200-mg-b.i.d. treatment groups, respectively, vs. −0.1% for placebo, $P < .01$ all treatment vs. placebo).[71] Only the b.i.d. regimen, 200 mg of L-000845704, significantly increased BMD at the hip and femur. No increases in total-body BMD were observed. All doses of L-000845704 resulted in a similar, approximately 42% decrease from baseline in uNTx cross-links ($P < .001$ vs. placebo). Similar mean decreases from baseline relative to placebo were also observed for sCTx (~48%). The 200-mg regimen resulted in a significant reduction in the bone formation marker, BSAP (31%), whereas the reductions seen with the 100- and 400-mg q.d. regimens were more modest (~22%). A similar response pattern was observed with sOC. Although both the q.d. and b.i.d. regimens had similar effects on markers of bone resorption, the 200-mg-b.i.d. regimen appeared to have a more pronounced effect on bone formation markers compared with the q.d. regimens (Figure 5.7). L-000845704 was generally well tolerated. Adverse experiences resulting in discontinuation from the study were relatively infrequent. These data are consistent with preclinical data and suggest that $\alpha_v\beta_3$ integrin antagonists may provide promise for the treatment of postmenopausal osteoporosis.

From the translational perspective, however, given the wide expression of integrins, it is plausible that pharmacological inhibition may have undesirable effects. Even though there has been remarkable progress in designing and testing highly potent, orally active $\alpha_v\beta_3$-selective antagonists, the long-term safety of such agents will need to be evaluated. Possible side effects of this mechanism could include bleeding and compromised wound healing. Because the $\alpha_v\beta_3$ integrin is upregulated during myocardial ischemia, it is possible that the vitronectin receptor participates in the cardiac repair process.[72] Notwithstanding these concerns, an antagonist has been administered for at least a year in the clinic[71] and has been generally well tolerated.

5.5. Osteoanabolics

Osteoanabolic agents stimulate bone formation through activation of the osteoblast. Early proof of pharmacology can be confirmed with specific increases in bone formation markers (P1NP, OC, and BSAP). Because bone resorption and formation are coupled, agents that increase bone formation (e.g., PTH) often increase bone resorption along with bone formation. Other agents that stimulate the osteoblast more modestly, however, may increase resorption to a lesser extent. Ultimately, combining anabolic

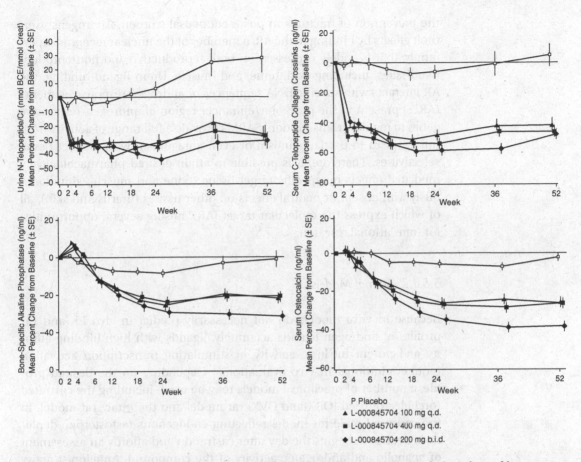

Fig. 5.7 Mean percent change (± standard error [*SE*]) from baseline in four biochemical markers of bone turnover (uNTx/Cr, sCTx, sBSAP, sOC) in postmenopausal women during a 12-month treatment with L-000845704 or placebo. Reprinted with permission from Murphy GM, Cerchio K, Stoch SA, Gottesdiener K, Wu M, & Recker R, for the L-000845704 Study Group. (2005). Effect of L-000845704, an αvβ3 integrin antagonist, on markers of bone turnover and bone mineral density in postmenopausal osteoporotic women. J. Clin. Endocrinol. Metab. 90, 2022–2028. Copyright 2005, The Endocrine Society.

agents with antiresorptive agents that do not suppress the "anabolic window" will facilitate greater increases in BMD.

5.5.1. Selective Androgen Receptor Modulators

5.5.1.1. What Is Known about the Target?

Androgens are considered to be osteoanabolic in men and women, including women with postmenopausal osteoporosis. Androgens, as male sex hormones, can produce androgenizing side effects, however, such as hirsutism, acne, and deepening of the voice and might also adversely affect lipid profiles. Selective androgen receptor modulators (SARMs) are androgen receptor (AR) ligands that provide the beneficial effects of androgens with substantially reduced risks of virilization and thus could be used for the prevention of fractures in postmenopausal women. Androgens exert their effects by binding to the AR, a member of the nuclear receptor super-family, that is widely expressed on both reproductive and nonreproduc-tive tissues, including skin, bone, and muscle. Upon ligand binding, the AR interacts with specific DNA sequences or androgen response elements (AREs) present in the promoter/enhancer region of androgen-responsive genes to regulate transcription. SARMs provide a full range of activity from full agonism to partial agonism or even antagonism with distinct tissue selectivities. Therefore, it is possible to attain desired pharmacologically mediated effects on specific target tissue (bone and muscle) simultane-ously with absent or neutral effects on other tissues (uterus and skin), all of which express the molecular target (AR), raising several opportunities for translational research.

5.5.1.2. Animal Models

Because in vitro models do not necessarily predict in vivo PK and PD profiles of androgen ligands accurately, ligands with high binding affin-ity and potent intrinsic activity in stimulating transcription activation require additional in vivo evaluation.[73] Depending on the desired pro-file, a number of preclinical models may be used, including the castrated (orchidectomized [ORX]and OVX) rat model and the intact rat model. In the castrated male rat model reflecting endogenous testosterone deple-tion, treatment begins the day after castration and affords an assessment of anabolic and androgenic activity of the compound. Antagonist activ-ity is usually assessed in the intact male rat model, which contains nor-mal endogenous testosterone, allowing an evaluation of the test molecule to inhibit the actions of the endogenous ligand.[73] Treatment generally lasts 2 weeks, and the target tissues are weighed to assess androgenic (e.g., prostate and seminal vesicle) and anabolic (e.g., levator ani mus-cle and BMD) activity. Serum gonadotropins (luteinizing hormone/follicle-stimulating hormone) and testosterone are measured to reflect effects of the test ligand on the hypothalamic–pituitary–gonadal axis.

To confirm proof of principle for the efficacy of the SARM mechanism, one may use preclinical models, including OVX rat studies with decreases in BMD. In addition to the OVX rodent, other models, such as nonhuman primates, may be used. The AR knockout (ARKO) mouse serves as an excel-lent model to probe the physiological importance of AR physiology in the skeleton. It may also be used to evaluate the potential for mechanism-based consequences of SARM activity in other tissues. Given the par-ticular challenge of isolating AR function in the skeletal system due to aromatization of androgens to estrogens,[74] the ARKO mouse model was generated using the Cre-loxP system, which can circumvent the problem of male infertility.[75] It has been suggested that AR function is essential for male-type bone mass and bone remodeling. A study conducted in 8-week-old male ARKO ($AR^{L-/Y}$) mice demonstrates osteopenia with retarded growth curves, but otherwise mice are phenotypically indistinguishable from WT female littermates. Whereas male $AR^{L-/Y}$ mice experience high bone turnover (bone resorption exceeding bone formation), female ARKO ($AR^{L-/L-}$) mice appear normal with respect to both bone mass and bone remodeling.[74] Histomorphometric analyses of 8-week-old male ARKO mice showed high bone turnover with increased bone resorption that results in reduced trabecular and cortical bone mass without altering bone shape.[74] Bone loss in ORX ARKO mice is only partially prevented with aromatizable testosterone, highlighting the pivotal role of AR in male-type bone remodeling. Given the lack of bone loss in female ARKO mice, the AR is one of the determining factors in the formation of male-type bone. As opposed to male ARKO mice, no differences in bone phenotype are discernable between female AR-deficient and WT littermates.

SARMs have been evaluated for AR agonist activity (efficacy and safety) in vivo using the ORX and OVX rat models. The sex steroid "deplete model" is necessary because in vitro models cannot accurately predict PK/PD profiles for AR ligands in vivo given the nuances of these high-affinity binders with potent intrinsic activity in stimulating transcription activation.[74] Both of these in vivo models have typically been used to evaluate efficacy of bone-specific compounds in the preclinical context and allow the focusing of PK/PD targets for later clinical development. Moreover, one can more confidently assess the inherent anabolic and androgenic activity of the test agent in the absence of the endogenous ligand. By contrast, antagonistic activity is more often evaluated in the intact male rat model with normal circulating testosterone levels. The ORX model has frequently been used to profile the tissue-selective pharmacologic properties of SARM compounds. This model typically allows a sensitive preclinical assessment of anabolic effects of SARMs on muscle, bone, and body composition as well as the agonist activity of SARMs in the pituitary in the setting of androgen deprivation. Moreover, the ability of SARMs to stimulate prostate growth under these conditions is critical.

It a recent study conducted in 9-month-old ORX rats, 5 months post ORX, a decrease in serum amino-terminal propeptide of collagen type 1 (sP1NP) was observed.[76] This decrease was still evident 11 months postsurgery. There was a corresponding decrease in femoral BMD when compared with sham counterparts. The observation of a decrease in sP1NP in the setting of androgen deficiency is of interest, as P1NP is a known bone formation marker and is expected to increase with the treatment of androgens or SARMs.

A novel SARM, ORM-11984, was recently evaluated for the treatment of established osteopenia in ORX rats.[77] The effects of ORM-11984 were studied both as monotherapy and in combination with ALN. Male Sprague–Dawley rats underwent ORX at 3 months of age and were observed for 3 months thereafter prior to initiation of therapy. Monotherapy with ORM-11984 increased bone mineral content of metaphyseal trabecular bone and mineral density of diaphyseal cortical bone. In the combination arm, ORM-11984 enhanced the therapeutic effects of ALN, especially in the diaphyseal region.[77] These data demonstrate that the SARM, ORM-11984, was sufficient to treat established osteopenia in ORX-treated rats in the monotherapy setting and, furthermore, that it exhibited enhanced efficacy in combination with ALN.

ORM-11984 was also administered to female Sprague–Dawley rats immediately after undergoing ovariectomy at 3 months of age and continued for a 2-month period.[78] The rats were allocated to 5 groups: sham-operated animals and OVX animals receiving vehicle, dihydrotestosterone (DHT) (3.0 mg/kg/day s.c.), and ORM-11984 (0.5 and 3.0 mg/kg/day p.o.). The ORM-11984–treated animals showed anabolic bone effects at cortical bone, including increased cortical thickness, cortical bone area, cortical bone mineral content, periosteal perimeter, polar moment of inertia, and biomechanical properties.[78] Bone formation rate (BFR) was increased at the periosteal surface and decreased at the endocortical surface. The results seen with ORM-11984 were reported as similar but more beneficial than those seen with DHT. Mention was not made as to how ORM-11984 was qualified as a SARM in preclinical species.

ORM-11984 was also evaluated in a rat immobilization model of secondary osteoporosis. Three-month-old Sprague–Dawley rats were divided into 5 groups ($n = 12$/group) with immobilization of the left hind limb by plaster cast in plantar flexion.[79] Immobilization resulted in osteoporotic changes both in the metaphyseal and diaphyseal region of the immobilized bones. Clodronate, as expected, prevented osteoporotic changes in the immobilized limbs, especially in the metaphyseal region. The SARM, ORM-11984, increased the formation of trabecular bone and apposition of mineral within the periosteum without affecting the amount of diaphyseal bone.

5.5.1.3. Human Data

There is little human validation demonstrating the activity of SARMs on bone parameters in humans. There are, however, data demonstrating the activity of androgens, most notably testosterone, in patients with osteoporosis. These data may, in part, be used to project the likely activity of SARMs in the target population – men and women with osteoporosis. To best appreciate the advantages of SARMs in patients (postmenopausal women or hypogonadal men), it is essential to understand biomarkers of androgenization. In postmenopausal women, it is important to recognize what could be considered a clinically meaningful change in skin virilization or endometrial proliferation. To better appreciate the skin effects of androgens, a pilot study was performed to identify skin biomarkers following testosterone administration in postmenopausal women. A double-blind, placebo-controlled, parallel-group study was conducted in 36 healthy postmenopausal female subjects to identify early biomarkers of androgen administration.[80] Subjects were randomized to receive 2.5 mg of transdermal testosterone gel (TTG), 300 μg of TTG, or placebo daily for 6 weeks in a 1:1:1 ratio. Six weeks of treatment with 2.5 mg of TTG increased seba-ceous gland volume on average by 42% ($P = .0410$) and sebum excre-tion rate (SER) by 52% ($P = .0021$) relative to placebo.[80] Microarray and Taqman analyses of skin samples also demonstrated changes in the 2.5-mg-TTG group. These biomarkers appear sufficiently robust to support using them to test androgen-mediated skin effects in postmenopausal women.

The effects of androgens on postmenopausal osteoporosis have not been thoroughly evaluated. Preliminary data are available documenting the effects of androgens on biochemical biomarkers of bone turnover. It is known that ARs are found on bone cells both in men and women.[81,82] Moreover, there is a positive correlation between bone mass and andro-gen levels in women.[83] Recent reports highlight the positive correlation between free testosterone (T) and the bone formation marker, serum P1NP ($P = .031$, $r = 0.451$), in premenopausal exercising women with oligomen-orrhea.[84] Despite an interest in the effects of androgens on bone turnover in postmenopausal women, only limited data are available in the literature. The anabolic-androgenic steroid, nandrolone, has been demonstrated to increase bone formation markers in postmenopausal women.[85] A more recent study evaluated the effects of estrogen (E) with and without small doses of an oral androgen (A; methyltestosterone) on biomarkers of bone turnover in postmenopausal women.[85] Following 9 weeks of therapy, both groups (E and E+A) demonstrated a reduction in urinary excretion of bone resorption biomarkers: DPD, pyridinoline, and hydroxyproline compared with control (C).[85] Increases in markers of bone formation (BSAP, OC, and C-terminal procollagen peptide) were seen in patients treated with E+A, whereas the E-only group demonstrated a decrease in bone forma-tion markers.[85] In this study, differences in bone resorption and formation biomarkers were already evident as early as 3 weeks following the initiation of therapy.[85] The largest change was documented during the first 3 weeks of therapy with only a small decrease thereafter through 9 weeks. The maxi-mum decrease in the bone resorption biomarker, total DPD ($\sim$30%), was evident by Week 9. Whereas bone formation biomarkers decreased with conjugated equine estrogens (CEE), bone formation biomarkers increased with E+A. With CEE, BSAP fell to a low of -26% by Week 3 and remained at this nadir through Week 9, and OC and P1CP reached a nadir of -40% and -15%, respectively, by Week 9. With E+A therapy, BSAP showed a sustained increase of 10%–15%, OC peaked at 24% at Week 9, and P1CP increased by 28% by Week 3 and showed a small increase thereafter. Post-treatment, BSAP remained elevated, whereas OC and P1CP returned to below pretreatment levels.

It remains unclear, however, how a SARM will affect biochemical biomarkers of bone turnover. In particular, there is no reason to expect that E+A will replicate the effects of a nonaromatizable androgen. Despite the lack of specific bone data in patients with SARMs, there is experience with SARMs in the clinic. In a 12-week randomized, double-blind, placebo-controlled, parallel group study performed in 66 healthy postmenopausal women, a SARM (MK-0773) was administered at two doses (25 mg b.i.d. and 100 mg b.i.d.) and compared with placebo.[86] After 12 weeks of treatment, both doses of MK-0773 significantly increased lean body mass from baseline: a mean of 750.6 g (25 mg) and 1410.9 g (100 mg). When compared with placebo, however, the difference in lean body mass was significant only for the 100-mg dose. Twelve weeks of treatment with MK-0773 as compared with placebo did not significantly increase SER or mean sebaceous gland volume. Furthermore, there was no significant increase in gene expression of 6 candidate genes of virilization. No difference in endometrial thickness (as assessed by transvaginal ultrasonography) or vaginal bleeding following progesterone challenge (as assessed by bleeding diary) was observed.[86] Biochemical markers of bone turnover and BMD data were not provided.

Because SARMs most likely target the periosteal bone envelope that comprises a small (~5%) but critical component of the skeleton, demonstrating POC may be more challenging. From a biomechanical perspective, the periosteum is the preferred anatomical location at which new bone should be added in osteoporotic persons. In fact, the amount of new bone needed at periosteal surfaces to affect bone strength positively is relatively small. The most widely used modalities, including bone densitometry and biochemical biomarker approaches, are likely not sufficiently sensitive to discern meaningful changes at this metabolically quiescent anatomical region. The most appropriate modality to demonstrate POC may require the use of histomorphometric analysis of bone tissue obtained by transilial bone biopsy to demonstrate the effect of a SARM on periosteal bone formation. Transilial bone biopsy specimens present three envelopes: trabecular, endocortical, and periosteal. The trabecular envelope is the one most frequently studied because it is most responsive to existing antiosteoporosis drugs, which include antiresorptives such as bisphosphonates and selective estrogen receptor modulators (SERMs) and injectable anabolic agents such as PTH. Data from the estrogen-deficient rat model suggest that SARMs increase BFR at the periosteal surface, the most desired anatomical location (the periosteal envelope).

Given the pleiotropic effects of androgens in both men and women, SARMs may offer promise beyond the treatment of osteoporosis and conditions associated with increased bone loss. Other benefits may include the treatment of male hypogonadism, female sexual dysfunction, muscle wasting, cancer cachexia, anemia, and hormonal male contraception.

5.5.2. Calcium Receptor Antagonists (Calcilytics)

5.5.2.1. What Is Known about the Target?

Anabolic therapies have recently emerged as the primary focus of new approaches to treat osteoporosis. The shift in focus is somewhat driven by the maturity of antiresorptive fields with a reasonable array of mechanisms from which to choose and by a perceived lack of osteoanabolic options. It is widely alleged that antiresorptives mitigate the trajectory of bone loss, and, in many instances, restore bone to a significant extent in patients with extensive bone loss. They do not, however, primarily build new bone by creating "struts and contacts" in the bone microarchitecture, which has highlighted the perceived need for osteoanabolic therapies that can potentially yield a biomechanical advantage. The era of anabolic therapy was shepherded in with PTH analogs, which are approved for limited duration of administration to treat postmenopausal osteoporosis. These agents take advantage of well-described and elegant bone physiology. PTH (1-84) is the endogenous master regulator of calcium and mineral homeostasis. It has long been appreciated, however, that sustained PTH excess is paradoxically responsible for bone loss, whereas PTH administration using an appropriate kinetic profile ("bursts") can actually increase bone formation and reduce fracture occurrence.

Calcium receptor (CaR) antagonists or calcilytics are compounds that specifically block CaR activity and consequently stimulate PTH secretion. Calcilytic compounds came into maturity with the cloning and structural characterization of the Ca^{2+} receptor.[87] Although no calcilytics have found their way to clinical therapeutic use, the activation of CaR with calcimimetics is used to treat hyperparathyroid states, including secondary hyperparathyroidism associated with chronic renal failure. Cinacalcet, the first approved Ca^{2+} receptor activator, sensitizes the CaR to calcium with a left shift in the signaling response in the set-point for PTH secretion, thereby lowering endogenous PTH levels. Cinacalcet has been used in the treatment of primary hyperparathyroidism, secondary hyperparathyroidism, as well as parthyroid cancer.[88–90] Calcilytic compounds, by contrast, seek to stimulate endogenous PTH secretion to yield new bone formation. Given the well-characterized bone loss observed in patients with primary hyperparathyroidism, a state of sustained PTH elevation with loss of optimal feedback control, it would be essential to achieve an ideal PTH kinetic profile to ensure bone formation and minimize bone loss. A rapid and transient pulsatile increase in circulating PTH is preferred.[91] Although one may debate the optimal PTH kinetic profile, it is suggested that a 3- to 4-fold increase in plasma PTH levels lasting ~1 to 2 hours is necessary to stimulate new bone formation without activating bone resorption.[92] Hence, the ideal calcilytic is a short-acting CaR antagonist – orally active, rapidly absorbed, and briskly cleared from the systemic circulation.[92]

The CaR is a member of the superfamily of seven transmembrane, G-protein coupled receptors (GPCRs) that also includes the metabotropic glutamate receptors (mGluRs), the γ-aminobutyric acid (GABA) receptors, as well as GPCRs for sensing pheromones, taste, and odors.[93] CaRs are richly expressed in parathyroid glands, calcitonin-secreting C cells of the thyroid, the kidney, as well as the gut and bone.[94] The receptor possesses five protein kinase C (PKC) phosphorylation sites[95] that are part of a negative feedback system whereby phosphorylation of one or more of the PKC sites inhibits CaR-mediated activation of phospholipase C (PLC), which is responsible for downstream biological response. Studies in human embryonic kidney (HEK) cells stably transfected with the CaR (HEK-CaR) as well as in parathyroid cells have shown that the CaR activates phospholipases (PL) A2, C, and D. PLC hydrolyzes phosphatidylinositol bisphosphate to generate inositol trisphosphate (IP3), which will activate the IP3 receptor in endoplasmic reticulum (ER) to release calcium from internal stores within the ER with a resultant spike in cytosolic free calcium concentration.[93] It has also been demonstrated that the CaR in parathyroid cells and HEK-CaR cells stimulate the activity of mitogen-activated protein kinases (MAPKs) with probable changes in gene expression (i.e., cell cycle regulation and cell membrane changes with peptide secretion).[93]

The physiological relevance of the CaR in humans was proven with the identification of inherited disorders characterized by either loss- or gain-of-function mutations in the CaR. Heterozygous loss-of-function mutations manifest with a disorder termed "familial hypocalciuric hypercalcemia" (FHH), which typically presents with asymptomatic hypercalcemia with hypocalciuria.[96] By contrast, the homozygous state of the inactivating mutation produces neonatal severe primary hyperparathyroidism (NSHPT), which may be lethal if not appropriately treated. This biochemical phenotype is reliably recapitulated in murine models with targeted disruption of one or both CaR genes.[93]

After the existence of the CaR was determined,[96] it was demonstrated that it could be activated by a number of di- and trivalent cations as well as several organic compounds that share the common property of possessing a net positive charge at physiological pH.[92] This category of molecular ligands has been shown to act directly on the CaR and includes polyamines from mammals, spider venoms, aminoglycoside antibiotics, and poly-basic amino acids.[92] Furthermore, the response to extracellular Ca^{2+} and the organic and inorganic polycations is potentiated by phenylalkylamines (e.g., verapamil) or TMB-8, the trimethoxybenzoate derivative.[92] Those ligands that mimic or potentiate the action of extracellular Ca^{2+} at the CaR are termed "calcimimetics"[97] Calcimimetics inhibit the secretion of PTH and lower circulating levels of PTH. They are categorized either as inorganic ions or organic molecules that act as agonists (type I) or allosteric activators (type II) of the receptor.[92] Cinacalcet is an approved type II compound licensed for the treatment of secondary hyperparathyroidism of chronic renal failure. It is remarkable that the identification of CaR antagonists has posed a much larger challenge than the generation of agonists or allosteric activators.[92] This design challenge has been attributed to the manner in which the receptor couples to effector systems, making its activity more difficult to suppress.[92] A number of typical strategies were adopted with little success, including structural modifications to the cognate physiological agonist with the hope of generating a high-affinity ligand devoid of intrinsic activity as well as structural modifications of molecule calcimimetics that generated additional calcimimetics.[92]

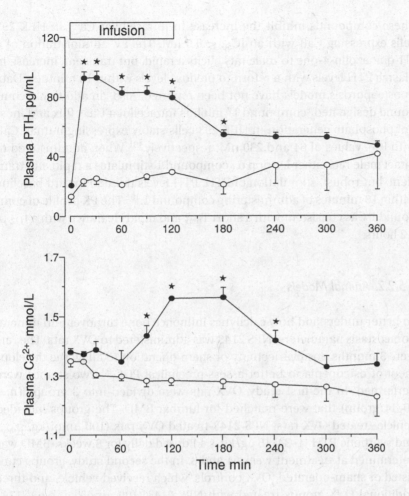

Fig. 5.8
Plasma levels of PTH
and Ca²⁺ in normal
rats infused i.v. with
vehicle (○) or NPS
2143 (●) (0.1 μmol/kg/
min) for 2 hours.
Values are mean ±
standard error (SE), *n*
= 3/group, *P* < .05
vs. vehicle-infused
controls. Reprinted
with permission from
Nemeth EF, DelMar EG,
Heaton WL, Miller MA,
Lambert LD, Conklin
RL, et al. (2001).
Calcilytic compounds:
Potent and selective
Ca2+ receptor
antagonists that
stimulate secretion of
parathyroid hormone.
J. Pharmacol. Exp.
Ther. 299, 323–331.

Moreover, molecular modeling of the receptor and its presumed binding pocket was likewise unhelpful. Initial efforts to identify calcilytics focused on screening compound libraries using bovine parathyroid cells because they retain the parathyroid phenotype.[92] With the cloning of the CaR, efforts shifted to stably transfected cell lines using high-throughput screening. Eventually, compounds that blocked the CaR were identified and have been termed "calcilytics."[92,98] One of the early calcilytic compounds evaluated, NPS 2143, was not a perfect molecule, but it served as an important chemical probe to elucidate understanding of how calcilytics perturb bone physiology (Figure 5.8).

NPS 2143 is not rapidly eliminated from the body following oral administration and results in sustained, rather than transient, increases in circulating PTH levels.[99] Following NPS 2143 there have been new families of calcilytics displaying more favorable PK profiles.[100–103] Calhex 231 exhibited a more optimal profile.[100] Both NPS 2143 and Calhex 231 share an overlapping binding site. A three-dimensional binding model of the CaR was generated based on the template of the x-ray structure of bovine rhodopsin by modeling the seven transmembrane domains of the CaR.[104,105] A new series of the calcilytic template includes the 3H-quinazolin-4-ones.[103]

These compounds inhibit the increase in intracellular Ca^{2+} in HEK 293 cells expressing CaR with an $IC_{50} < 0.5$ μM. The i.v. administration of a 3H-quinazolin-4-one to male rats elicits a rapid, but transient, increase in plasma PTH levels with a return to predose levels within 10 minutes. Data in osteoporosis models have not been reported. Also, an additional compound designated "compound 1" inhibits intracellular Ca^{2+} flux and inositol phosphate generation in HEK 293 cells stably expressing human CaR with IC_{50} values of 64 and 230 nM, respectively.[101] When administered to intact male rats either i.v. or p.o., compound 1 stimulates a rapid and transient, but robust, stimulation of PTH. PTH levels trended toward baseline within 10 minutes of administering compound 1.[101] The PK profile of compound 1 was consistent with a short T_{max} and rapid clearance with a $t_{1/2}$ of ~2 hours.

5.5.2.2. Animal Models

To better understand how calcilytics influence bone turnover and mineral homeostasis parameters, NPS 2143 was administered to OVX rats. The rats were 3 months postovariectomy or sham operation to allow the development of osteopenia to better assess preclinical POC.[99] Two studies were performed. In the first study, OVX rats were divided into 3 groups ($n = 10$–14/group) that were matched for lumbar BMD. The groups included vehicle-treated OVX rats, NPS 2143-treated OVX rats (100 μmol/kg, p.o.), and synthetic PTH (1–34) (5 μg/kg, s.c.) dosed daily for 8 weeks. BMD was determined at treatment weeks 4 and 8. In the second study, groups consisted of sham-operated, OVX controls, which received vehicle, and three additional OVX groups treated with NPS 2143 (100 μmol/kg, p.o.), 17β-estradiol (0.01 mg/90 days, continuous infusion, s.c. implanted pellet), or NPS 2143 together with 17β-estradiol.[99] In Study 1, animals that had undergone ovariectomy 3 months previously demonstrated significantly lower BMD at all three skeletal sites: reductions of 15% at the LS and proximal tibia, and 24% at the distal tibia.[99] BMD at the proximal tibia was unaffected by daily treatment with NPS 2143, and PTH therapy restored BMD to pre-OVX levels after 8 weeks of treatment. Similar changes were noted at the distal femur and LS. Plasma PTH levels were elevated (>100 pg/mL) within 30 minutes of dosing NPS 2143 and remained high for at least 4 hours. By comparison, PTH levels in the animals treated with PTH s.c. were similar to levels in the animals treated with NPS 2143 but returned to baseline within 2 hours of dosing.[99] In a separate experiment, PTH levels were elevated for up to 8 hours after dosing NPS 2143 and were undetectable (<10 ng/mL) at 24 hours.[99]

It should be noted that the different PTH profiles obtained under the two dosing conditions resulted in markedly different effects on bone turnover. Dynamic histomorphometric analysis of cancellous bone at the proximal tibial metaphysis demonstrated increased bone formation above the OVX control level with both PTH and NPS 2143 treatment. Bone resorption was significantly higher, however, in the NPS 2143 compared with both the PTH and OVX control groups.[99] The modest, but sustained elevation in PTH seen with NPS 2143 most likely explains the dramatic increase in both bone formation and resorption, with no net bone gain or loss. PTH injections also increased bone formation and resorption (formation > resorption), resulting in a net increase in bone mass. This observation further underscores the importance of attaining an optimal PTH profile with oral calcilytic administration. Chronic PTH elevations, as seen in hyperparathyroidism, lead to bone loss and abnormal bone histology. Moreover, restoring normal PTH-secretory dynamics in hyperparathyroidism improves BMD.[106] A similar finding has been reproduced in rats with s.c. infusions of high doses of PTH (40 μg/kg and 80 μg/kg) over ≥ 2 h/d for 7 days, which resulted in weight loss, hypercalcemia, and skeletal abnormalities consistent with hyperparathyroidism.[107] Circulating PTH levels in this study reached 10,000 pg/mL.[107] OVX rats administered PTH (1–34) at doses as low as 1 μg/kg which yields PTH increases of ~3-fold, is sufficient to elicit an anabolic response.[108] Although the data with NPS 2143 do not reveal a hyperparathyroid phenotype, they do underscore the importance of eliciting a sharp PTH increase, but of limited duration. These data established "near" proof of pharmacology for the mechanism, highlighting the need for a shorter-acting compound that can induce more transient increases in PTH levels to elicit a net anabolic effect on bone. One potential concern with calcilytics that would not be evident with exogenous PTH administration is the potential for parathyroid cell hyperplasia. It has been well described that rats fed a low-calcium diet manifest larger parathyroid glands.[109] Whether the glandular enlargement is exclusively related to parathyroid cell hypertrophy rather than to hyperplasia is debated in the literature.[110] There are data showing markedly increased parathyroid cell proliferation in weanling rats fed a low-calcium diet for 3 weeks.[111] A hyperplastic response was not reported with NPS 2143 in the rodent studies as assessed by bromodeoxyuridine staining,[99] and there was no evidence of parathyroid gland hypertrophy.

Given the theoretically superior profile of combining an antiresorptive with anabolic therapy, the second study specifically evaluated the combination of NPS 2143 with 17β-estradiol in OVX rats.[99] The magnitude of the increase in BMD in rats given the combination of estradiol and the calcilytic was significantly greater ($P < .02$) than in rats administered estradiol alone.[99] The rationale behind combination therapy is to augment bone mass and mechanical strength beyond that achieved with either mechanism alone. Taking advantage of the complementary and possibly synergistic approach offered by combining these two fundamental strategies is appealing.

Because it is important to ensure an ideal PTH kinetic profile to realize optimal bone formation, a preclinical study was performed to understand whether fractionating the total daily dose would achieve comparable BMD results. Ten-month-old female Wistar rats received s.c. injections with PTH (1–34) 2.5, 5, or 10 μg/kg per dose daily or b.i.d. for 6 months.[112] BMD, cortical, and trabecular architecture were measured monthly by peripheral quantitative computed tomography (pQCT)/micro-computerized tomography (μCT) in the proximal tibial metaphysis for 6 months. Daily and b.i.d. injections resulted in a rapid dose-dependent increase in total BMD, trabecular BMD, cortical thickness, trabecular BV, and trabecular thickness.[112] The PTH (1–34) dose of 2.5 μg/kg given b.i.d. resulted in a faster onset of the bone anabolic response compared with the 5 μg/kg dose administered once daily. These data suggest that splitting the total daily dose of PTH (1–34) into two injections does not compromise (and could even lead to a more rapid) bone anabolic response. These provocative data highlight the possibility of administering a calcilytic as a b.i.d. regimen to enhanced bone formation, perhaps with better tolerability. Although this concept is provocative, it remains to be seen whether it translates into a preferred clinical profile given that AEs are based on a peak-plasma PTH profile.

5.5.2.3. Human Data

Currently no calcilytics are approved for clinical use. POC, however, has apparently been established for the mechanism. At least two calcilytics, JTT-305 (MK-5442) and ronacaleret (RON; SB-751689), have demonstrated PD activity based on increases in bone formation markers and, in the case of JTT-305, increases in BMD in humans. A randomized, single-blinded, placebo-controlled study was conducted in 154 patients (52–83 years old) with postmenopausal osteoporosis (mean baseline LS T-score = −3.17).[113] Patients were randomized to two doses of JTT-305 (10 mg and 20 mg) and placebo administered once daily for 12 weeks. All patients were supplemented with calcium (610 mg/day) and vitamin D (400 IU/day). After 12 weeks, P1NP increased in a dose-dependent manner in patients treated with JTT-305 (−13.3% in placebo, +19.8% in 10 mg, and +61.2% in 20 mg).[113] Consistent with the administration of exogenous PTH, bone resorption markers tended to increase after the increase in formation markers. Changes in LS BMD from baseline were 0.9%, 2.3%, and 1.8% with placebo, JTT-305 10 mg, and JTT-305 20 mg, respectively. The increase in the 10 mg was significantly greater than that of the placebo group. Mention is made of a dose-dependent increase in serum calcium,[113] although the actual numeric increases are not highlighted.

An interim analysis performed at 6 months in a 1-year double-blind, placebo-controlled, dose-ranging Phase 2 study in 569 postmenopausal women receiving placebo, 1 of 4 doses of RON (100 mg, 200 mg, 300 mg, or 400 mg), ALN (70 mg weekly) or open-label TER (20 μg daily) resulted in early termination of the trial due to lack of efficacy.[114] At Months 10 to 12, RON (200, 300, and 400 mg) effects were not significantly different from those of placebo (~1.4%–1.9%), whereas ALN and TER increased LS BMD 4.7% and 9.2%, respectively. At the total hip, however, RON administration caused a small but significant decrease in BMD (−0.6% to −1.2%), whereas

ALN and TER yielded modest increases of 2.8% and 2.6%, respectively.[114,115] Using QCT, at the LS, vertebral integral volumetric BMD (vBMD) showed a dose-dependent mean increase over baseline with the 400-mg RON dose comparable to ALN.[115] At the total hip, the vBMD followed a similar pattern to the areal BMD (aBMD) with decreases with RON and increases with ALN and TER. The bone formation marker, P1NP, attained maximal increases up to 148% over baseline in RON (200, 300, and 400 mg) dose groups at Month 10 compared with the median maximal 151% increase for TER at Month 6. BSAP showed similar trends for all groups. Importantly, the bone resorption marker, sCTx, showed median increases of >20% starting at 6 months, reaching a maximum of 58% at Month 10 for RON (200, 300, and 400 mg), whereas TER showed a median increase of 57% at Month 3 and reached a maximum of 103% at Month 10. Serum calcium was dose dependently increased in all RON dose groups starting at Week 1. Apparently, the PK data revealed that the PTH 1–84 area under the curve was larger in RON dose groups compared with PTH 1–34 for TER groups, although the actual profiles were not revealed in the report.[114] It was concluded that, based on the elevated serum calcium, the observed PTH profile, and the BMD findings, RON administration may have been associated with a state of mild hyperparathyroidism.

In a study performed to characterize the mechanism of fractional urinary calcium excretion following CaR blockade, RON and TER were administered to a group of postmenopausal women.[116] Fifty-two subjects were randomized to receive RON 100 mg ($n = 15$), RON 400 mg ($n = 19$), or s.c. recombinant human PTH (rhPTH; 1–34) TER 20 µg ($n = 18$). RON increased mean plasma PTH (1–84) levels to a maximum of 5.6 and 9.8 pM for the 100 and 400 mg groups, respectively, after 20 to 40 minutes. TER resulted in a rapid increase in PTH (1–34) with a mean maximal level of 18.4 pM. The 24-hour postdose serum calcium remained slightly elevated in the RON-treated subjects versus the TER-treated subjects. Notably, RON was associated with a marked and prolonged decrease in calcium excretion, with levels returning to near baseline within 12 to 24 hours.[116] A similar pattern was noted for TER, although a more moderate decrease in calcium excretion was observed. Whereas modest increases in urinary cyclic adenosine monophosphate (cAMP) were seen with RON, TER caused a marked increase in urinary cAMP. It was concluded that these data confirm that RON exerts a direct effect on calcium excretion independent of its ability to increase endogenous PTH.

An additional POC study was conducted to determine whether a CaR antagonist would promote fracture healing. In a randomized, double-blind, placebo-controlled study, subjects with a radial fracture were randomized (1:1:1) to one of two doses of RON (200 mg twice daily or 400 mg daily) or matching placebo for 12 weeks.[117] The primary objective was to assess the impact of RON on time to radiographic healing. Due to the lack of efficacy in the osteoporosis trial at the 6-month interim analysis, the trial was terminated for futility. At the time the POC study was terminated, 85 subjects had been randomized: placebo ($N = 27$), RON 200 mg ($N = 28$), and RON 400 mg ($N = 30$). At the time of discontinuation, 73% of the subjects had completed the trial. RON had no significant effect on duration of healing by radiograph or CT scan, time to cast removal, clinical symptoms, grip strength, or range of motion.[117] RON was generally well tolerated with hypercalcemia reported as the most frequently occurring AE.

In summary, attaining the optimal PTH kinetic profile is necessary to achieve osteoanabolism versus increased resorption. Finding the ideal calcilytic would be a boon for treating osteoporosis, for this could realize the "upside" of exogenous PTH administration with oral dosing. Currently, s.c. PTH (1–34) and (1–84) remain the standard of care as osteoanabolics. Although injectables are not preferred, there are recent data demonstrating that transdermal TER delivery may be an alternative to s.c. injection. In a recent publication, Cosman et al. demonstrated that a novel transdermal microneedle patch delivering TER significantly increased LS BMD versus placebo in a dose-dependent manner at 6 months ($P < .001$).[118] As anticipated, bone turnover markers (P1NP and CTx) increased from baseline in a dose-dependent manner in all the treatment groups.[118] Notably, all treatments were well tolerated with no prolonged hypercalcemia.[118]

The success of oral calcilytic administration is contingent on eliciting the optimal kinetic profile of endogenous PTH secretion. Not only is the peak PTH response potentially important, but the duration of the PTH effect is likely more critical. Sustained PTH levels could convert a net osteoanabolic phenotype into a resorption phenotype characteristic of that seen in states of hyperparathyroidism. The theoretical possibility of sustained PTH stimulation and potential parathyroid hyperplasia cannot be eliminated. Because the CaR is expressed in tissues beyond the parathyroid gland, including the kidney, C cells of the thyroid, chondrocytes, the intestine, lung, bone, nervous system, and bone marrow, the long-term effects of calcilytics on other tissue will need to be evaluated carefully. It is reassuring that extra-target effects of CaR antagonism have not been observed in animal studies, which may reflect differences in CaR sensitivity across cell types.

5.5.3. Dickkopf-1 (DKK-1) Inhibitors

5.5.3.1. What Is Known about the Target?

Among the various osteoanabolic targets that hold promise for treating osteoporosis, the canonical Wnt signaling pathway in bone may offer a high probability of success. Canonical Wnts signal through two co-receptors: frizzled and the low-density lipoprotein (LDL) receptor–related proteins (LRPs) 5 and 6. Loss-of-function mutations in LRP5 are associated with low BMD and increased fracture occurrence, whereas gain-of-function mutations result in significant increases in BMD in comparison with age-matched controls. The finding of these mutations in humans with their respective skeletal phenotypes further reaffirms the attractiveness of the Wnt signaling pathway as a target for developing agents to treat osteoporosis and other bone-related disorders.

Loss-of-function mutations in LRP5 are characterized by low BMD and skeletal fragility, resulting in an autosomal recessive disorder – osteoporosis-pseudoglioma syndrome (OPPG).[119] Although children with OPPG have low bone mass and are fracture prone, there is no evidence of a defect in collagen synthesis, mineral homeostasis, endochondral growth, or bone turnover.[119,120] In fact, bone biopsies from affected patients reveal decreased trabecular BV values but normal surface density as well as normal appearance of osteoclasts and osteoblasts on bone surfaces.[119] It appears that carriers of the OPPG mutation have an increased incidence of osteoporosis-related fractures. Patients with OPPG also have eye involvement varying from disruption of ocular structure, phthisis bulbi, to persistent hyperplasia of the primary vitreous (PHPV). LRP5 is expressed in osteoblasts in situ, and its expression changes with time as pluripotent mesenchymal cells differentiate along the osteoblastic lineage.[119] LRP5 mediates Wnt signaling in vitro via the canonical pathway and dominant-negative forms of LRP5 interfere with the process. Furthermore, it has been shown that dominant-negative forms of LRP5 affect bone thickness in mouse calvarial explant cultures. These data support LRP5 affecting the accrual of bone mass during Wnt-mediated osteoblastic proliferation and differentiation.

Patients with activating or gain-of-function mutations of the LRP5 gene manifest with a high bone mass phenotype.[121,122] In addition to the high bone mass phenotype, craniofacial abnormalities have been observed. These dysmorphisms include torus palatinus, which is an exostosis in the midline of the hard palate that can be found in up to 20% to 25% of the general population. Although the phenotype varies in different families, they all show a striking absence of fracture occurrence.[123,124]

Thus Wnt signaling plays an important role in the development and maintenance of a number of organs,[125,126] and the Wnt/β–catenin or canonical pathway is particularly important in bone biology.[127,128] Activation of Wnt/β–catenin signaling occurs on binding of Wnt to the 7-transmembrane domain-spanning frizzled receptor and LRP5 and LRP6 coreceptors.[126] Wnt signaling is highly regulated by members of secreted antagonists. Interactions between Wnt and frizzled receptors are inhibited by members of the secreted frizzled-related protein (sFRP-1) family and Wnt inhibitory factor 1 (WIF-1). LRP5/6 coreceptor activity is inhibited by members of the sclerostin (SOST gene product) and Dickoppf (DKK) families, which all bind LRP5 and LRP6.[126] DKK-1, -2, and -4 bind with different affinities to LRP5 and LRP6.

Dickkopf-1 (DKK-1) is a secreted glycoprotein member of the Dickkopf family of proteins. This family is made up of negative regulators of the canonical *Wnt* signaling pathway, which play a crucial role in bone formation.[129,130] DKK-1 inhibits Wnt signaling through an interaction with the Wnt coreceptors LRP5 or LRP6 as well as the Kremen proteins. LRP5 is the critical protein in regulating bone mass and is expressed in osteoblasts. Mice lacking LRP5 develop a low-bone-mass phenotype identical to that seen in patients with OPPG. By contrast, a single-amino-acid substitution in the β-propeller module of LRP5 results in an autosomal dominant high-bone-mass phenotype – a finding reproduced precisely in the LRPG171V mouse model.

A recent publication by Bodine et al. demonstrated the feasibility of developing small molecules that inhibit sFRP-1 and stimulate the canonical Wnt signaling to increase bone formation. High-throughput screening yielded a diaryl sulfone sulfonamide that bound to the sFRP-1 with a K_D of 0.35 μM and selectively inhibited sFRP-1 with an EC_{50} of 3.9 μM in the cell-based functional assay.[131] Further optimization yielded WAY-316606, which bound to sFRP-1 with a K_D of 0.08 μM and an EC_{50} of 0.65 μM. WAY-316606 was shown to increase total bone area in an ex vivo murine calvarial organ culture assay at concentrations as low as 0.01 nM.[131]

The piperidinyl diphenylsulfonyl sulfonamide scaffold has been further optimized to generate more selective and potent inhibitors of sFRP-1, including WAY-362692, which demonstrated binding affinity ($IC_{50} = 20$ nM) to sFRP-1 as well as potent functional activity both in the cell-based functional assay ($EC_{50} = 30$ nM) and in the ex vivo mouse calvarial tissue culture.[132] Further modifications have generated compounds with potent binding affinity ($IC_{50} \leq 100$ nM) as well as potent functional activity ($EC_{50} = 70–150$ nM). Profiling these sFRP-1 inhibitors in preclinical assays demonstrated increases in total bone area (47%–135%) when compared with vehicle in the ex vivo mouse calvarial assay with activation of osteoblasts.[132] The finding of increases in bone area as well as in osteoblasts holds promise for further translation in vivo.

5.5.3.2. Animal Models

Although the relevance of mouse models for probing the intricate physiology of the human skeleton remains unclear, genetically modified mice with gain- and loss-of-function LRP5 mutations have been generated, and these animals closely replicate the naturally occurring human findings. Transgenic mice were also created expressing the human LRP5 G171V substitution, the mutation responsible for the high-bone-mass phenotype in two human kindreds.[133] The mouse bearing the human G171V activating mutation demonstrates increases in vBMD by pQCT with increases in total vBMD (30%–55%) and trabecular vBMD (105%–250%) of the DFM.[133] Notable increases in the cortical size of the femoral diaphyses are also appreciated in these mutant mice. High-resolution μCT analysis of the distal femurs and lumbar vertebrae reveals significant increases (110%–232%) in the trabecular BV fraction in G171V mutant mice. These findings relate to both an increase in trabecular number (41%–74%) and an increase in trabecular thickness (34%–46%, $P < .01$ for all). The observed increases in bone mass also correlate with increases in bone strength. Increases in lumbar vertebrae volumes and cortical size correlate with increases in vertebral compression strength (80%–140%) and femoral bending strength (50%–130%), respectively. The mutant G171V transgenic mice showed an increase in actively mineralizing bone surface along with enhanced alkaline phosphatase staining in osteoblasts. It is believed that the bone phenotype (increases in trabecular vBMD and cortical size) seen in the $LRP5_{G171V}$ mice are caused by increased osteoblast activity and survival.[134]

The LRP5 knockout mouse generated by disruption of the extracellular domain of LRP5 yields a phenotype that is identical to OPPG.[119,135] The mice characteristically display two phenotypes: low bone mass due to decreased bone formation and persistent embryonic eye vascularization resulting from a failure in macrophage-mediated apoptosis.[135] The LRP5-deficient mice are characterized by early-onset osteoporosis with delayed ossification as well as multiple fragility fractures. Histological analysis of the skeleton of 2-month-old LRP5$^{-/-}$ mice reveals a significant decrease in BV compared with WT littermates. In particular, there is a marked reduction in the quantity of mineralized bone in the primary spongiosa of LRP5$^{-/-}$ mice.[135] Serum and urine levels of calcium and phosphorus are normal in the knockout mice, suggesting that the low-bone-mass phenotype cannot be ascribed to metabolic disturbances.

Histomorphometric analyses demonstrated a 2-fold decrease in BFR, an indicator of osteoblast activity, after double calcein labeling in 6-month-old LRP5$^{-/-}$ mice when compared with WT littermates.[135] The decreased BFR was ascribed to a decrease in matrix apposition rate (0.75 ± 0.05 vs. 0.45 ± 0.06 µm/d; $P < .05$) for WT and LRP5$^{-/-}$ mice, respectively. Urinary DPD cross-links, biochemical markers of bone resorption, were identical between both WT and knockout mice (urinary DPD/Cr ratio was 10.3 ± 2.1 in WT vs. 11.0 ± 6.2 in LRP5$^{-/-}$ mice).[135]

The LRP5 knockout mice generated by using a targeting vector that disrupts exon 18, which encodes the ligand-binding repeat, result in a low-bone-mass phenotype that is not apparent before 6 months of age.[136] The thickness of cortical bones (femur, tibia, and parietal bones) of LRP5$^{-/-}$ mice >6 months of age is 50% to 70% of that seen in the WT setting.

The two mouse models concur in demonstrating the central role for LRP5 in bone-mass determination[134] but differ in phenotypic expression. Kato's model exhibits reduced BMD evident at early onset as well as multiple fractures. In contrast, Fujino's mice were more mildly affected and of late onset. The differences between these models remain perplexing.

LRP5 encodes a co-receptor for ligands of the Wnt pathway that interact with serpentine receptors of the Frizzled (Fzd) family, which are necessary for intracellular signaling pathways. Using Affymetrix (Santa Clara, CA) GeneChip hybridization, it was shown that Fzd9 is the one gene that is differentially regulated together with known osteoblast marker genes in primary mouse osteoblasts.[137] A follow-up study was performed in vivo to ascertain whether Fzd9 in osteoblasts was necessary to regulate bone formation. Fzd9-deficient mice were found by histomorphometry to show a phenotype characterized by a >40% decrease in trabecular BV when compared with WT littermates.[137] Interestingly, it took time for the findings to become apparent. Nothing was seen at 6 weeks, but was certainly evident at 24 and 72 weeks of age. Dynamic histomorphometry further revealed that osteopenia could be attributed to a 50% reduction in BFR, whereas bone resorption was not affected. Similarly, *Fzd9*-deficient calvarial osteoblasts revealed a decreased rate of proliferation and a delayed matrix mineralization when compared with WT cultures. On the basis of these data, it was concluded that *Fzd9*, at least in mice, is a relevant Wnt receptor in osteoblasts.

The administration of DKK-1 to 6-month-old female adult C57BL/6 mice results in a decrease in BMD. Mice given a single i.v. dose of DKK-1 ($n = 12$/group) using an adeno-associated virus (AAV) delivery system resulted in a 14% decrease in L1–5 BMD at Week 2 and a 22% decrease at Week 8 compared with baseline BMD.[138] A significant decrease in whole-leg BMD was also seen. The osteoclast marker, TRAPC5b was significantly increased at Week 2 and remained significantly higher at Week 8 in the adenovirus-associated vector (AAV-DKK-1) group. Histomorphometric analysis revealed a decrease in trabecular BV (bone volume/tissue volume [BV/TV]) in the AAV-DKK-1 group by 73% compared with the control animals.[138] The decrease in BV/TV was associated with a decrease (-75%) in trabecular number but no significant change in trabecular thickness. Osteoclast surface as a percentage of bone surface was increased by 54%, whereas BFR/TV was significantly decreased by 72% in the AVV-DKK-1 mice. These findings are consistent with DKK-1 delivery's stimulating bone resorption and decreasing bone formation at the tissue level.

The effects of DKK-1 inhibition on bone do not appear to relate to skeletal maturity. Both young (6-week-old) and old (34-week-old) mice treated with an anti-DKK-1 antibody for 3 weeks demonstrated significant increases in BMD as assessed by pQCT at the LS. In addition, μCT analysis revealed significant increases in BMD, trabecular BV fraction, and trabecular number in distal femurs.

When intact female rats were treated with a neutralizing antibody to DKK-1 (anti-DKK-1; 30 mg/kg; 2x/week) for 3 weeks, significant increases in lumbar and whole-leg BMD were seen when compared with control animals.[139] Histomorphometry of the distal femur demonstrated increases in trabecular BV/TV of 39% in treated versus control rats ($P < .01$). Osteoblast surface per bone surface increased 377% versus control ($P < .001$), whereas a nonsignificant increase ($\sim38\%$) in osteoclast surface per bone surface was seen. In addition, BFR/TV was significantly increased by 89% versus controls ($P < .001$) in anti-DKK-1–treated animals.[139] Furthermore, cortical area and thickness of the midshaft femur were significantly greater ($\sim20\%$) in treated rats when compared to controls ($P < .01$).

The observed increases in trabecular and cortical bone mass and density in rodents further highlight the promise of inhibiting DKK-1 activity as a therapeutic target for the treatment of osteoporosis.

Proof of pharmacology for a small-molecule antagonist of sFRP-1 to increase BFR has been established in the OVX rat with WAY-262611,[140] which exhibited high potency ($EC_{50} = 0.63$ μM) as well as good solubility. Rats were allocated to 7 treatment groups: sham, vehicle, WAY-262611 (0.3, 1.0, 3.0., or 10.0 mg/kg/day), or hPTH (0.01 mg/kg/day s.c.) and treated for 28 days. The oral administration of WAY-262611 resulted in a clear dose response with increases in trabecular BFR in the tibia, including the low dose (0.3 mg/kg/day). WAY-262611 demonstrated good oral bioavailability ($F = 78\%$) and a plasma $t_{1/2}$ (5.6 hours) when dosed to OVX rodents as 0.5% methylcellulose/2% Tween-80. These data provide promise for the further assessment of a novel osteoanabolic mechanism that should be assessed in larger preclinical species as well as in the clinic.

5.5.3.3. Human Data

Although we are unaware of any Phase 1 clinical trials using small-molecule drugs to inhibit DKK-1 function, patents have been published claiming the development of antibodies and immunological functional fragments that neutralize DKK-1 function.[130] Significantly, patients with gain-of-function mutations in the LRP5 gene are characterized by a high-bone-mass phenotype. Affected individuals typically present with cortical thickening of long bones[123] and age- and sex-adjusted bone density of the LS ~5 standard deviations above the population mean.[122] Mineral homeostasis parameters are typically unaffected. Mean serum calcium and phosphate levels are normal, whereas urinary calcium tends to be at the high end of the normal range.[122] Both serum levels of PTH and vitamin D metabolites are normal. Markers of bone resorption, including levels of uNTx, and TRACP5b were within the normal range.[122] This is not the case for sOC, a marker of bone formation, which is elevated more than 3 times that of controls. In a report of 4 affected adults, sOC measured 32.3 ± 7.4 versus 9.8 ± 1.8 ng/mL in 9 controls, $P < .001$.[122] BSAP, another bone formation marker, was not elevated, however, in these individuals (mean value $= 25 \pm 6$ U/L; normal range 15–41).[122] The finding of increased markers of bone formation without changes in markers of bone resorption may be consistent with uncoupling of bone turnover and account for the increase in bone mass observed.

5.5.4. Sclerostin Inhibitors

5.5.4.1. What Is Known about the Target?

Sclerostin as a target was briefly discussed in the DKK-1 Inhibitor section earlier in the text, and the sclerostin pathway is also a promising osteoanabolic approach (supported by human genetic evidence) for treating osteoporosis. Two bone disorders, sclerosteosis and Van Buchem disease, are rare bone dysplasias caused by loss-of-function mutations of SOST[141] and are inherited in an autosomal recessive manner.[142]

Sclerosteosis is a progressive, sclerosing bone dysplasia characterized radiologically by increased generalized hyperostosis and sclerosis, resulting in a markedly thickened and sclerotic skull and also affecting the mandible, ribs, clavicles, and long bones.[141] Due to bone overgrowth and narrowing of foramina, these patients present with cranial nerve deficits, including facial nerve palsy, hearing loss, and optic nerve atrophy. Van Buchem disease manifests with a phenotype similar to that of sclerosteosis, although hand malformations and a large stature are characteristic of sclerosteosis.[141] Positional cloning efforts for both conditions indicated that the high-bone-mass phenotype is a consequence of a complete loss of function of sclerostin protein.[141,143–145] Importantly, it is reported that heterozygotic carriers of loss-of-function mutations in the SOST gene exhibit increased BMD.[146] The almost exclusive skeletal manifestations in patients with sclerosteosis and Van Buchem disease suggest a restricted expression of SOST in bone, although SOST transcripts have also been reported in nonskeletal tissue, including cartilage and multiple soft tissues (kidney and the vessel wall of the great arteries).[147] Patients with Van Buchem disease have elevated markers of bone formation, higher bone density, and greater polar moment of inertia.[148] When BMD and biochemical markers of bone turnover in Van Buchem patients were compared with those in Van Buchem carriers, significant differences were observed. In addition to the higher BMD in patients compared with carriers (153 ± 6 vs. 111 ± 4, $P < .01$), higher levels of markers of bone formation, serum P1NP (75.6 ± 13.7 vs. 29.4 ± 5.0, $P < .01$), and sOC (25.1 ± 3.8 vs. 13.6 ± 2.0, $P < .05$) were observed. It is interesting to note that the bone resorption marker, uNTx, was also higher in the patients (73.0 ± 19.6 vs. 36.9 ± 2.8, $P < .05$). It is also noteworthy that, when BMD was evaluated in patients with sclerosteosis, marked increases were observed at all skeletal sites.[146] Z-score ranges at the anatomical sites were LS ($+7.73$ to $+14.43$), total hip ($+7.84$ to $+11.51$), and forearm ($+4.44$ to $+9.53$) (Figure 5.9).

In adult bone, sclerostin protein and SOST mRNA are exclusively expressed in osteocytes,[147] which are nonproliferative, terminally differentiated cells of the osteoblast lineage. Osteocytes reside both in the mineralized bone matrix as well as in newly formed osteoid locked inside the lacuna spaces in the hard substance of bone and are considered nonmigratory.[149] Osteocytes have mechanosensory properties, and mechanical loading triggers them to modulate bone homeostasis.[150] It has been recently shown that in vivo mechanical loading of bone reduces sclerostin expression, thus providing a potential mechanism whereby mechanical loading increases bone formation.[151] Because sclerostin is located within osteocytes, it is optimally situated to signal rapidly to surface cells to limit their bone formation.[142] Inhibition of sclerostin production or signaling is predicted to increase bone mass. The exact mechanism by which sclerostin inhibits bone formation is not known. It was originally believed

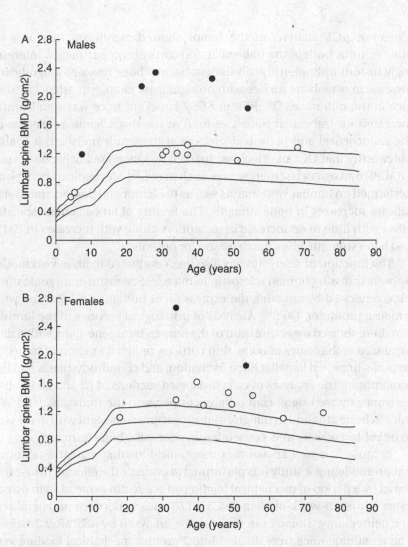

Fig. 5.9
Lumbar spine BMD in male and female homozygous (•) and heterozygous (○) individuals with sclerosteosis. Lines depict normal ranges. Reprinted with permission from Gardner JC, van Bezooijen RL, Mervis B, et al. (2005). Bone mineral density in sclerosteosis; affected individuals and gene carriers. J. Clin. Endocrinol. Metab. 90, 6392–6395. Copyright 2010, The Endocrine Society.

that sclerostin inhibited bone formation by antagonizing bone morphogenetic protein (BMP) activity.[143] It has been reported, however, that sclerostin behaves as a circulating inhibitor of the Wnt signaling pathway, which it accomplishes by binding to LRP5 and LRP6.[152] Furthermore, sclerostin inhibits BMP-stimulated bone formation but does not affect BMP signaling.[153]

5.5.4.2. Animal Models

A number of mouse models have been used to further explore the role of sclerostin in bone biology. These models include mice with targeted deletion of the sclerostin gene as well as transgenic mice overexpressing *SOST*. Male and female *SOST*-null mice display a similar phenotype with increased radiodensity throughout the skeleton but with general skeletal morphology appearing normal.[154] BMD evaluation using DXA revealed a >50% increase in BMD both at the lumbar vertebrae and whole leg.

Moreover, μCT analysis of the femur showed significant increases in bone volume, both in the trabecular and cortical compartments. Interestingly, histomorphometric analysis of trabecular bone revealed a significant increase in osteoblast surface with no significant change in osteoclast surface in the null mice. The BFR in *SOST* knockout mice was significantly increased for trabecular bone (>9-fold) at the distal femur as well as at the endocortical and periosteal surfaces of the femur midshaft. It is also noteworthy that OC, an osteoblast marker, was increased, whereas serum TRACP5b, an osteoclast marker, was unchanged.[154] Mechanical testing was performed on lumbar vertebrae as well as the femur and demonstrated significant increases in bone strength. The finding of an osteoblast-specific effect with little to no increase in resorption, along with increases in BMD and bone strength, gives much reason for optimism.

The function of sclerostin has also been evaluated in an in vivo model by overexpressing human sclerostin in mice.[155] Sclerostin-transgenic mice were generated by targeting the expression of human *SOST* to bone with a mouse promoter, *OGT*.[156] Analysis of histological sections of the lumbar vertebrae showed overexpression of the human transgene along with a disorganized architecture of bone, thin cortices, reduced amount of trabecular bone, impaired lamellar bone formation, and chondrodysplasia.[155] Histomorphometric analyses of calcein-labeled sections of L3 and L5 lumbar vertebrae showed significant differences between the transgenic and WT mice in bone area and in mineral apposition rate consistent with decreases in osteoblast activity and, consequently, decreased bone formation.

Because it is well known that mechanical loading regulates adaptive bone remodeling, a study was performed to evaluate the effect of disuse followed by a period of mechanical loading on sclerostin expression in osteocytes. Nineteen-week-old female C57BL/6 mice underwent unilateral sciatic neurectomy. Tibiae from 6 mice were analyzed by μCT after 3 weeks. The remaining mice were divided into 2 groups: mechanical loading versus no loading. The results confirmed that sclerostin expression in trabecular and cortical bone osteocytes is increased by disuse and reversed by mechanical loading with a distribution related to new bone formation.[157] It has previously been reported that loading decreases sclerostin protein expression in cortical bone, whereas unloading increases *SOST* mRNA expression.[158,159]

A sclerostin-neutralizing monoclonal antibody (Scl-AbII) was administered to 6-month-old female Sprague–Dawley OVX rats that were left untreated for a 1-year period to ensure significant estrogen deficiency–induced bone loss.[160] At the age of 19 months, OVX rats were divided into 2 groups and treated with either phosphate-buffered saline (PBS) or murine Scl-AbII for 5 weeks. A group of sham-operated rats were also treated with PBS. An evaluation of aBMD by DXA confirmed a significant decrease in BMD at the lumbar vertebrae and femur–tibia in the OVX animals when compared with sham-operated controls. Following Scl-AbII administration, robust BMD increases in lumbar vertebrae and femur–tibia were

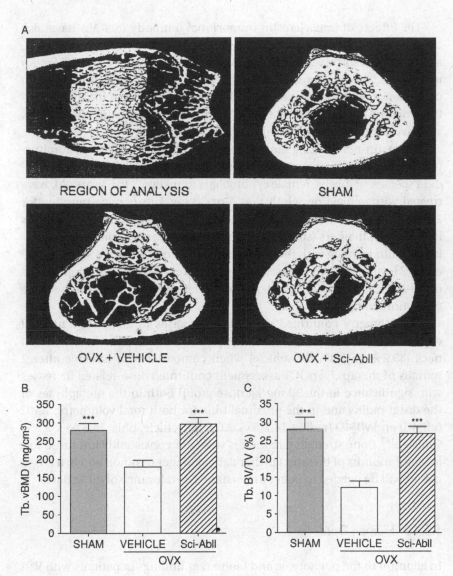

A
REGION OF ANALYSIS   SHAM

OVX + VEHICLE   OVX + Scl-AbII

B
Tb. vBMD (mg/cm³)

350
300 ***
250
200
150   ***
100
50
0
    SHAM VEHICLE Sci-AbII
            OVX

C
Tb. BV/TV (%)

35
30 ***
25
20
15
10   ***
5
0
    SHAM VEHICLE Sci-AbII
            OVX

Fig. 5.10
Scl-AbII treatment in osteopenic rats restores trabecular BMD and BV back to sham levels at distal femur. A, Distal femur region of analysis (top left) and representative 3-dimensional (3D) μCT images of a 1-mm central section (with attached cortices) from each of the three groups. Representative 3D images were selected based on the median trabecular BV of each group. B, Values for trabecular vBMD. C, Values for trabecular BV. Data represent mean ± standard error (SE) for 11 to 12 rats/group. ***$P < .001$ vs. OVX+vehicle. From LI X, Ominsky MS, Warmington KS, Morony S, Gong J, Cao J, et al. (2009). Sclerostin antibody treatment increases bone formation, bone mass, and bone strength in a rat model of postmenopausal osteoporosis. J. Bone Miner. Res. 24, 578–588. Reprinted with permission of John Wiley & Sons, Inc.

observed. In contrast, BMD in the sham OVX controls remained at pretreatment levels. In keeping with the robust increase in BMD, sOC was significantly increased following 5 weeks of therapy with Scl-AbII versus vehicle.

μCT analysis of the metaphyseal region of the distal femur confirmed significant bone loss in the vehicle-treated OVX rats compared with sham controls, and, within 5 weeks of Scl-AbII therapy, vBMD and BV/TV were restored to pre-OVX levels with a significant increase in trabecular number.[160] Histomorphometric analysis of trabecular bone in the proximal tibia confirmed the decrease in trabecular BV (BV/TV) for vehicle-treated OVX rats with restoration of trabecular BV to sham control levels following Scl-AbII treatment (Figure 5.10). Moreover, mechanical testing confirmed increases in bone strength to levels greater than those found in non-OVX controls.

The effects of antisclerostin monoclonal antibody (Scl-Ab) have also been assessed in the presence of ALN in OVX rats. It is noteworthy that ALN, a potent antiresorptive, did not blunt the bone restorative effects of Scl-Ab in OVX rats.[161] As confirmed by histomorphometry, Scl-Ab given alone or in combination with ALN was equally effective at increasing mineralizing surface, mineral apposition rate, and BFR.[161] Consistent with this observation, sOC levels were increased equally with both therapies.

Sclerostin-neutralizing monoclonal antibody (Scl-AbIV) was administered to hormonally intact monkeys to explore the bone effects in nonrodent species.[162] Twelve female cynomolgus monkeys, 3 to 5 years old, were treated with vehicle or Scl-AbIV at 3 or 30 mg/kg s.c. once-monthly for 2 months. Consistent with findings observed in rats, significant increases in formation markers (sOC and serum P1NP) were seen following administration. In keeping with the observed clearance of Scl-AbIV, serum P1NP and OC levels returned to baseline 4 weeks after the first and second doses of Scl-AbIV. Interestingly, again no clear effect was observed on the bone resorption marker, sCTx.

Densitometry confirmed significant increases in areal bone mineral content (aBMC) for the whole body (24% vs. 6.4% for vehicle) and femoral neck (35.2% vs. 5.4% for vehicle) when compared with baseline after 2 months of therapy.[162] pQCT assessment confirmed dose-related increases with significance in the 30 mg/kg dose group both in the metaphyses of the distal radius and in the proximal tibia for both total volumetric BMC (vBMC) and vBMD (radius, 14.2% vs. 2.6% for vehicle; tibia, 18.8% vs. 2.9%, vehicle).[162] Bone strength parameters were not consistently improved following 2 months of therapy. Further data of longer duration and in a larger cohort will be needed to better understand the relevance of these data.

5.5.4.3. Human Data

In addition to the phenotypic and biomarker findings in patients with Van Buchem disease and heterozygotic carriers described earlier in the text, proof-of-pharmacological principle has been obtained with antisclerostin monoclonal antibody administration in the clinic. In a blinded, placebo-controlled, rising single-dose study, 48 postmenopausal women were randomized (3:1) to receive a single s.c. dose (0.1, 0.3, 1.0, 3.0, 5.0, or 10 mg/kg) of a sclerostin-neutralizing monoclonal antibody (Scl-mAb) or placebo.[163] Dose-related increases in bone formation makers, P1NP, OC, and BSAP were observed (relative to placebo). The mean percent change from baseline for these markers was approximately 60% to 100% at the 3 mg/kg dose by 21 days.[163] A dose-related trend toward decreasing sCTx was also observed. The antibody was generally well tolerated.

Sclerostin levels have recently been evaluated in postmenopausal women immobilized after a single episode of stroke and compared with healthy postmenopausal counterparts. Immobilized patients had higher

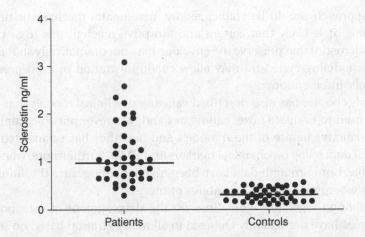

Fig. 5.11
Sclerostin serum levels (ng/ml) are higher in immobilized patients vs. healthy, free-living subjects (*P* < .001). Data are presented as medians. Reprinted with permission from Mirza FS, Padhi IS, Raisz LG, & Lorenzo JA. (2010). Serum sclerostin levels negatively correlate with parathyroid hormone levels and free estrogen index in postmenopausal women. J. Clin. Endocrinol. Metab. 95, 1991–1997. Copyright 1995, The Endocrine Society.

serum sclerostin levels (1.164 ± 0.654 vs. 0.298 ± 0.135 ng/mL, *P* < .0001).[164] In keeping with immobilization, sCTx was elevated in the patients compared with the controls (1.05 ± 0.57 vs. 0.46 ± 0.18 ng/mL, *P* < .001) as was serum BSAP (38.33 ± 25.21 vs. 14.68 ± 8.75 µg/L, *P* < .001).[164] These provocative data suggest that sclerostin may be at the center of increased bone turnover due to mechanical unloading in the setting of disuse osteoporosis.

Given the key role that sclerostin may play in bone metabolism, there are emerging data suggesting that it may regulate bone mass as an endocrine hormone. In a cross-sectional observational study comparing healthy pre- and postmenopausal women, the postmenopausal women had significantly higher serum sclerostin levels (1.16 ± 0.38 vs. 0.48 ± 0.15 ng/mL, *P* < .001) compared with their premenopausal counterparts (Figure 5.11).[165] Significant negative correlations between sclerostin and free estrogen index (β = −0.629, *P* = .002) and PTH (β = −0.554, *P* = .004) were found, further suggesting that sclerostin levels are regulated both by estrogen and PTH levels in postmenopausal women.

5.6. Conclusions

Osteoporosis presents unique translational challenges depending on the biomolecular mechanism. In this chapter, bone biology and several potentially exciting therapies have been reviewed as they relate to antiresorptive and anabolic properties. The usefulness and rationale for combination therapy in the context of understanding bone biology has also been presented. Optimal combination therapeutic regimens need to be informed by intrinsic bone biology (i.e., the temporal sequence of the remodeling cycle). Perhaps the most successful approach will be to introduce an anabolic and "consolidate" with an antiresorptive (e.g., bisphosphonates). Although this approach should be challenged by incremental mechanistic understanding, it is likely that certain antiresorptive mechanisms (e.g., Cat K and sclerostin) that preserve the envelope may not dramatically shut down the remodeling cycle and may allow coadministration or even preempt anabolic intervention.

This chapter has also described valuable preclinical models that have been used to evaluate novel candidates and, wherever possible, captured the predictive nature of these models and how they have translated into clinical data using biochemical markers and BMD. Furthermore, wherever possible, bone strength data have been highlighted because this information is essential to inform probability of success.

Although regulatory guidelines for the development of osteoporosis therapies have not recently changed to allow registration based on surrogate endpoints prior to outcome data demonstrating fracture risk reduction, it is a widely held view in the field that the constellation of predictive biomarker data, increased BMD, and positive bone strength data portends success. It is appropriate to envision that the field of bone biology will continue to mature and that we will see further inclusion of modeling and simulation strategies, including disease modeling. It is noteworthy that a number of the new targets have already challenged the prevailing dogma in the field, and we will therefore need to use iterative strategies, including predictive preclinical models along with appropriate clinical data. Whether successful or not, the pursuit of novel targets also enhances the mechanistic understanding of bone biology, as has been observed with sclerostin, which may now be viewed an a endocrine hormone regulating bone mass.

The selection of therapeutic targets remains a central tenet in drug development. Given the incremental cost of bringing new medications to patients, it is important to reflect on what determines success. Although animal models have been important in prosecuting novel targets, many have been discovered through "accidents of nature" (Cat K, $\alpha_v\beta_3$ integrin, calcilytic, DKK-1, and sclerostin). Human genetic mutations of potential drug targets and their related pathway molecules are resource sparing and help to predict the effects of target modulation through careful study of their phenotypic and biochemical consequences. Although rational drug development will and should prevail, we need to continue to take note of what is around us. It should not be forgotten that bisphosphonates, the most widely prescribed class of antiosteoporotic agents, were discovered by serendipity. Therefore, at least in osteoporosis, translational science will also continue to be shaped by the bedside-to-bench approach as a valuable and affordable strategy.

Although there are many principles that can be generalized across different mechanisms in bone biology, one needs to make appropriate adjustments at different stages to ensure effective and successful translation in the clinic. The predictive value of preclinical models has been particularly highlighted, including the use of biomarkers, both soluble (markers of bone turnover) and imaging (BMD), along with bone strength parameters to enhance probability of success as novel mechanisms enter the clinic. When tackling novel targets, one needs to challenge assumptions proactively and at times dispense with prevailing dogma based on those mechanisms already prosecuted with approved drugs. In the examples highlighted in this chapter, some of those assumptions have already been challenged. In the case of Cat K, a number of modifications needed to take place to better translate this mechanism. Preclinically, the rabbit OVX model needed to be established because the sequence homology of the enzyme is not conserved across species, calling into question the predictive value of rat and murine models.

Biochemical marker data have been highlighted in all of the case studies described and were particularly useful for Cat K inhibitors. They also confirmed more modest effects on bone formation than is evident with other antiresorptives, including bisphosphonates, estrogens, and the receptor activator of nuclear factor kappa B ligand (RANKL) antibody. The effects of RANK ligand inhibition were hypothesized preclinically based on knockout mice data, which exhibited increased fluorescein labeling, but longer studies in late development were necessary to confirm this activity. The required duration in part reflects the temporal nature of bone turnover and the relative length of time required to understand the clinical correlations of suppression of bone formation markers and, more importantly, the challenge of showing a relative lack of suppression. Other hypotheses based on preclinical data and an understanding of bone biology remain to be validated in the clinic. For example, the relative sparing of the bone formation envelope observed in the nonhuman primate (NHP) model requires human clinical confirmation with coadministered anabolic agents.

The calcilytic mechanism could pose an extraordinary challenge on two fronts. First, because this mechanism takes advantage of regulating in situ physiology, unless the PK profile is optimal this will result in a hyperparathyroid phenotype and paradoxically yield bone loss (in addition to hypercalcemia) rather than achieve bone formation. Taking advantage of validated biomarkers of bone turnover (resorption and formation) along with mineral homeostatic parameters (e.g., serum and urine calcium), one could try to "thread the needle" for this mechanism. Second, one needs to establish the ideal PK/PD relationship with BMD, which can be used to confirm bone gain rather than potential bone loss. This particular mechanism, almost more so than any other, underscores the governing principle of drug development – get the dose right. The calcilytic represents a narrow therapeutic index relationship in a way not seen with exogenous PTH administration. It is far more challenging to recapitulate this with an oral agent taking advantage of pulsatile PTH secretion. Exogenous PTH administration results in increases in both bone formation and resorption markers as well as increases in serum and urine calcium. Manipulating endogenous PTH is like fine tuning a precision instrument – any overshoot may not result in a neutral effect, but, in fact, a deleterious one. Under these constraints, a particular molecule's being subject to drug–drug interaction potential can further limit viability in this instance. Taking advantage of modeling and simulation and looking at the profile in aggregate would be the way to proceed.

We are poised to enter a new health care environment in which the justification of intervention based not only on clinical evidence but on sensitivity to economic considerations, along with appropriate medical justification, will be required. A better and more in-depth understanding of bone physiology will be required to sequence therapy rationally. We need to continue to pursue creative basic research and elegant clinical investigation to bring forward therapies for this important indication that, despite available therapies, remains inadequately treated. Osteoporosis numbers will continue to burgeon with the aging of the population, and future therapies will need to distinguish themselves to gain prescribing access.

5.7. References

1. MacLaughlin EJ. (2010). Improving osteoporosis screening, risk assessment, diagnosis, and treatment initiation: Role of the health-system pharmacist in closing the gap. Am. J. Health Syst. Pharm. 67, S4–S8.
2. Seibel MJ, Eastell R, Gundber CM, Hannon R, & Pols HAP. (2002). Biochemical markers of bone metabolism (pp. 1543–1571). In: Principles of Bone Biology, edited by Bilezikian JP, Raisz LG, & Rodan GA. San Diego: Academic.
3. Tesch G, Amur S, Schousboe JT, Siegel J, Lesko L, & Bai J. (2010). Success achieved and challenges ahead of translating biomarkers into clinical applications. AAPS J. 12(3), 243–253.
4. Cremers S, & Garnero P. (2006). Biochemical markers of bone turnover in the clinical development of drugs for osteoporosis and metastatic bone disease. Drugs. 66, 2031–2058.
5. Delaissé JM, Engsig MT, Everts V, del Carmen Ovejero M, Ferreras M, Lund L, et al. (2000). Proteinases in bone resorption: Obvious and less obvious roles. Clin. Chem. Acta. 291, 223–234.
6. Everts V, Delaissé JM, Korper W, Jansen DC, Tigchelaar-Gutter W, Saftig P, et al. (2002). The bone lining cell: Its role in cleaning Howship's lacunae and initiating bone formation. J. Bone Miner. Res. 17, 77–90.
7. Garnero P, Borel O, Byrjalsen I, Ferreras M, Drake F, McQueney MS, et al. (1998). The collagenolytic activity of cathepsin K is unique among mammalian proteinases. J. Biol. Chem. 273, 32347–32352.
8. Sassi ML, Eriksen H, Risteli L, Niemi S, Mansell J, Gowen M, et al. (2000). Immunochemical characterization of assay for carboxyterminal telopeptide of human type I collagen: Loss of antigenicity by treatment with cathepsin K. Bone. 26, 367–373.
9. Eyre D. (1992). New biomarkers of bone resorption. J. Clin. Endocrinol. Metab. 74, 470A–470C.
10. Halleen JM, Titinen SL, Ylipahkala H, Fagerlund KM, & Väänänen HK. (2006). Tartrate-resistant acid phosphatase 5b (TRACP 5b) as a marker of bone resorption. Clin. Lab. 52, 499–509.

11. Wichers M, Schmidt E, Bidlingmaier F, & Klingmüller D. (1999). Diurnal rhythm of CrossLaps in human serum. Clin. Chem. 45, 1858–1860.

12. Greenspan SL, Parker RA, Ferguson L, Rosen HN, Maitland-Ramsey L, Karpf DB. (1998). Early changes in biochemical markers of bone turnover predict the long-term response to alendronate therapy in representative elderly women: A randomized clinical trial. J. Bone Miner. Res. 13, 1431–1438.

13. Ravn P, Hosking D, Thompson D, Cizza G, Wasnich RD, McClung M, et al. (1999). Monitoring of alendronate treatment and prediction of effect on bone mass by biochemical markers in the Early Postmenopausal Intervention Cohort Study. J. Clin. Endocrinol. Metab. 84, 2363–2368.

14. Bauer DC, Garnero P, Bilezikian JP, Greenspan SL, Ensrud KE, Rosen CJ, et al. (2006). Short-term changes in bone turnover markers and bone mineral density response to parathyroid hormone in postmenopausal women with osteoporosis. J. Clin. Endocrinol. Metab. 91, 1370–1375.

15. Lathia CD, Amakye D, Dai W, Girman C, Madani S, Mayne J, et al. (2009). The value, qualification, and regulatory use of surrogate end points in drug development. Clin. Pharmacol. Ther. 86, 32–43.

16. U.S. Food and Drug Administration. (1985). Guidelines for clinical evaluation of agents used in the treatment and prevention of osteoporosis. Rockville, MD: U.S. Food and Drug Administration.

17. U.S. Food and Drug Administration. (1994). Guidelines for preclinical and clinical evaluation of agents in the prevention or treatment of postmenopausal osteoporosis. Rockville, MD: U.S. Food and Drug Administration.

18. Binkley N, Kimmel DB, & Bruner J. (1998). Zoledronate prevents the development of absolute osteopenia following ovariectomy in adult rhesus monkeys. J. Bone Miner. Res. 13, 1775–1782.

19. Lazner F, Gowen M, & Kola I. (1999). An animal model of pycnodysostosis: The role of cathepsin K in bone remodeling. Mol. Med. Today. 5, 413–414.

20. Stoch SA, & Wagner JA. (2008). Cathepsin K inhibitors: A novel target for osteoporosis therapy. Clin. Pharmacol. Ther. 83, 172–176.

21. Bossard M, Tomazek TA, & Thompson S. (1996). Proteolytic activity of human osteoclast cathepsin K. J. Biol. Chem. 271, 12517–12524.

22. Troen BR. (2004). The role of cathepsin K in normal bone resorption. Drug News Perspect. 70, 19–28.

23. Gelb BD, Shi GP, Chapman HA, & Desnick PJ. (1996). Pycnodysostosis, a lysosomal disease caused by cathepsin K deficiency. Science. 273, 1236–1238.

24. Marquis RW. (2004). Inhibition of the cysteine protease cathepsin K. Ann. Rev. Med. Chem. 39, 79–98.

25. Gauthier JY, Chauret N, Cromlish W, Desmarais S, Duong LT, Falgueyret JP, et al. (2008). The discovery of odanacatib (MK-0822), a selective inhibitor of cathepsin K. Bioorg. Med. Chem. Lett. 18, 923–928.

26. Saftig P, Hunziker E, Wehmeyer O, Jones S, Boyde A, Rommerskirch W, et al. (1998). Impaired osteoclastic bone resorption leads to osteopetrosis in cathepsin-K-deficient mice. Proc. Natl. Acad. Sci. U. S. A. 95, 13453–13458.

27. Pennypacker B, Shea M, Liu Q, Masarachia P, Saftig P, Rodan S, et al. (2009). Bone density, strength, and formation in adult cathepsin K (–/–) mice. Bone. 44, 199–207.

28. Marquis RW, Ru Y, LoCastro SM, Zeng J, Yamashita DS, Oh H-J, et al. (2001). Azapernone-based inhibitors of human and rat cathepsin K. J. Med. Chem. 44, 1380–1395.

29. Yasuma, T, Oi S, Choh N, Nomura T, Furuyama N, Nishimura A, et al. (1998). Synthesis of peptide aldehyde derivatives as selective inhibitors of human cathepsin L, and their inhibitory effect on bone resorption. J. Med. Chem. 41, 4301–4308.

30. Yamane H, Sakai A, Mori T, Tanaka S, Moridera K, & Nakamura T. (2009). The anabolic action of intermittent PTH in combination with cathepsin K inhibitor or alendronate differs depending on the remodeling status in bone in ovariectomized mice. Bone. 44, 1055–1062.

31. Pennypacker B, Duong LT, Cusick TE, Masarachia P, Gentile MA, Gauthier J-Y, et al. (2010). Cathepsin K inhibitors prevent bone loss in estrogen-deficient rabbits. J. Bone Miner. Res. Epub ahead of print..

32. Fisher JE, Caulfield MP, Sato M, Quartuccio HA, Gould RJ, Garsky VM, et al. (2002). Inhibition of osteoclastic bone resorption in vivo by echistatin, and "arginyl-glycyl-aspartyl" (RGD)-containing protein. Endocrinology. 30, 746–753.

33. Lark MW, Stroup GB, James IE, Dodds RA, Hwang SM, Blake SM, et al. (2002). A potent small molecule, nonpeptide inhibitor of cathepsin K (SB 331750) prevents bone matrix resorption in the ovariectomized rat. Bone. 30, 746–753.

34. Pennypacker B, Rodan S, Black C, Oballa R, Masarachia P, Rodan G, & Kimmel DB. (2006). Bone effects of cathepsin K inhibitors in the growing rabbit. J. Bone Miner. Res. 21, S304.

35. Guay J, Riendeau D, & Mancini JA. (1999). Cloning and expression of rhesus monkey cathepsin K. Bone. 25, 205–209.

36. Palmer JT, Bryant C, Wang DX, Davis DE, Setti EL, Rydzewski RM, et al. (2005). Design and synthesis of tri-ring P3 benzamide-containing aminonitriles as potent, selective, orally effective inhibitors of cathepsin K. J. Med. Chem. 48, 7520–7534.

37. Kumar S, Dare L, Vasko-Moser J, James IE, Blake SM, Rickard DJ, et al. (2007). A highly potent inhibitor of cathepsin K (relacatib) reduces biomarkers of bone resorption both in vitro and in an acute model of elevated bone turnover in vivo in monkeys. Bone. 40, 122–131.

38. Masarachia P, Pun S, & Kimmel D. (2007). Bone effects of a cathepsin K inhibitor in ovariectomized rhesus monkeys. J. Bone Miner. Res. 22, S126.

39. Pennypacker B, Wesolowski G, Heo J, & Duong LT. (2009). Effects of odanacatib on central femur cortical bone in estrogen-deficient adult rhesus monkeys. J. Bone Miner. Res. 24, S52.

40. Nishi Y, Atley L, Eyre DE, Edelson JG, Superti-Furga A, Yasuda T, et al. (1999). Determination of bone markers in pycnodysostosis: Effects of cathepsin K deficiency on bone matrix degradation. J. Bone Miner. Res. 14, 1902–1908.

41. Fratzl-Zelman N, Valenta A, Roschger P, Nader A, Gelb BD, Fratzl P, et al. (2004). Decreased bone turnover in deterioration of bone structure in two cases of pycnodysostosis. J. Clin. Endocrinol. Metab. 89, 1538–1547.

42. Stoch SA, Zajic S, Stone J, Miller DL, Van Dyck K, Gutierrez MJ, et al. (2009). Effect of the cathepsin K inhibitor odanacatib on bone resorption biomarkers in healthy postmenopausal women: Two double-blind, randomized, placebo-controlled phase I studies. Clin. Pharmacol. Ther. 86, 175–182.

43. Bone HG, McClung MR, Roux C, Recker RR, Eisman JA, Verbruggen N, et al. (2010). Odanacatib, a cathepsin-K inhibitor for osteoporosis: A two-year study in postmenopausal women with low bone density. J. Bone Miner. Res. 25, 937–949.

44. Peroni A, Zini A, Braga V, Colato C, Adami S, & Girolomoni G. (2008). Drug-induced morphea: Report of a case induced by balicatib and review of the literature. J. Am. Acad. Dermatol. 59, 125–129.

45. Desmarais S, Black WC, Oballa R, Lamontagne S, Riendeau D, Tawa P, et al. (2007). Effect of cathepsin K inhibitor basicity on in vivo off-target activities. Mol. Pharmacol. 72, 147–156.

46. Khalfan HA. (1991). Study of thiol proteases of normal human skin fibroblasts. Cell Biochem. Funct. 9, 55–62.

47. Bromme D, & Lecaille F. (2009). Cathepsin K inhibitors for osteoporosis and potential off-target effects. Expert Opin. Invest. Drugs. 18, 585–600.

48. Bühling F, Röcken C, Brasch F, Hartig R, Yasuda Y, Saftig P, et al. (2004). Pivotal role of cathepsin K in lung fibrosis. Am. J. Pathol. 164, 125–129.

49. Hou WS, Li Z, Gordon RE, Chan K, Klein MJ, Levy R, et al. (2001). Cathepsin K is a critical protease in synovial fibroblast-mediated collagen degradation. Am. J. Pathol. 159, 2167–2177.

50. Tepel C, Bromme D, Herzog V, & Brix K. (2000). Cathepsin K in thyroid epithelial cells: Sequence, localization and possible function in extracellular proteolysis of thyroglobulin. J. Cell Sci. 113, 4487–4498.

51. Friedrichs B, Tepel C, Reinheckel T, Deussing J, von Figura K, Herzog V, et al. (2003). Thyroid function of mouse cathepsins B, K, and L. J. Clin. Invest. 111, 1733–1745.

52. Leu C-T, Wesolowski G, & Nagy R. (1997). Osteoclasts have over 107 high affinity echistatin binding sites (RGD-Integrins). J. Bone Miner. Res. 12, S416.

53. Ruoslahti E. (1991). Integrins. J. Clin. Invest. 87, 1–5.

54. Wang N, Butler JP, & Ingber DE. (1995). Mechanotransduction across the cell surface and through the cytoskeleton. Science. 260, 1124–1127.

55. Clark EA, & Brugge JS. (1995). Integrins and signal transduction pathways: The road taken. Science. 268, 233–239.

56. Ruoslahti E, Noble NA, Kagami S, & Border WA. (1994). Integrins. Kidney Int. Suppl. 44, S17–S22.

57. Giancotti FG, & Mainiero F. (1994). Integrin-mediated adhesion and signaling in tumorigenesis. Biochem. Biophys. 1198, 47–64.

58. Cox D, Aoki T, Seki J, Motoyama Y, & Yoshida K. (1994). The pharmacology of the integrins. Med. Res. Rev. 14, 195–228.

59. Sato M, Sardana MK, Grasser WA, Garsky VM, Murray JM, & Gould RJ. (1990). Echistatin is a potent inhibitor of bone resorption in culture. J. Cell Biol. 111, 1713–1723.

60. Horton MA, Dorey EL, Nesbitt SA, Samamen J, Ali FE, Stadel JM et al. (1993). Modulation of vitronectin-receptor mediated osteoclast adhesion by the Arg-Gly-Asp peptide analogs: A structure-function analysis. J. Bone Miner. Res. 8, 239–247.

61. Sato M, Garsky V, Majeska RJ, Einhorn TA, Murray J, Tashjian AH, et al. (1994). Structure-activity studies of the s-echistatin inhibition of bone resorption. J. Bone Miner. Res. 9, 1441–1449.

62. Yamamoto M, Fisher JE, Gentile M, Seedor JG, Len CT, Rodan SB, et al. (1998). The integrin ligand echistatin prevents bone loss in ovariectomized mice and rats. Endocrinol. 139, 1411–1419.

63. Masarachia P, Yamomoto M, Lee C-T, Rodan G, & Duong L. (1998). Histomorphometric evidence for echistatin inhibition of bone resorption in mice with secondary hyperparathyroidism. Endocrinology. 139, 1401–1410.

64. Scarborough RM, Rose JW, Naughton MA, Phillips DR, Nannizzi L, Arfsten A, et al. (1993). Characterization of the integrin specificities of disintegrins isolated from American pit viper venoms. J. Biol. Chem. 268, 1058–1063.

65. McHugh KP, Hodivala-Dilke K, Zheng M-H, Namba N, Lam J, Novack D, et al. (2000). Mice lacking β3 integrins are osteosclerotic because of dysfunctional osteoclasts. J. Clin. Invest. 105, 433–440.

66. Teitelbaum SL. (2006). Osteoclasts and integrins. Ann. N. Y. Acad. Sci. 1068, 95–99.

67. McHugh KP, Kitazawa S, Teitelbaum SL, & Ross FP. (2001). Cloning and characterization of the murine β3 integrin gene promoter: Identification of an interleukin-4 responsive element and regulation by Stat-6. J. Cell. Biochem. 81, 320–325.

68. Teitelbaum SL. (2005). Editorial: Osteoporosis and integrins. J. Clin. Endocrinol. Metab. 90, 2466–2468.

69. Hutchinson JH, Halczenko W, Brashear KM, Breslin MJ, Coleman PJ, Duong LT, et al. (2003). Nonpeptide $\alpha v\beta 3$ antagonists. 8. In vitro and in vivo evaluation of a potent $\alpha v\beta 3$ antagonist for the prevention and treatment of osteoporosis. J. Med. Chem. 46, 4790–4798.

70. Hoffman SJ, Vasko-Moser J, Miller WH, Lark MW, Gown M, & Stroup S. (2002). Rapid inhibition of thyroxine-induced bone resorption in the rat by an orally active vitronectin receptor antagonist. J. Pharmacol. Exp. Ther. 302, 201–211.

71. Murphy GM, Cerchio K, Stoch SA, Gottesdiener K, Wu M, & Recker R, for the L-000845704 Study Group. (2005). Effect of L-000845704, an $\alpha v\beta 3$ integrin antagonist, on markers of bone turnover and bone mineral density in postmenopausal osteoporotic women. J. Clin. Endocrinol. Metab. 90, 2022–2028.

72. Yamani MH, Tuzcu RC, Starling NB, Ratliff Y, Yu D, Vince G, et al. (2002). Myocardial ischemic injury after heart transplantation is associated with upregulation of vitronectin receptor $(\alpha_v\beta_3)$, activation of the matrix metalloproteinase induction system, and subsequent development of coronary vasculopathy. Circulation. 105b, 1955–1961.

73. Gao W, Kim J, & Dalton JT. (2006). Pharmacokinetics and pharmacodynamics of nonsteroidal androgen receptor ligands. Pharm. Res. 23, 1641–1658.

74. Kawano H, Sato T, Takashi Y, Matsumoto T, Sekine K, Watanabe T, et al. (2003). Suppressive function of androgen receptor in bone resorption. Proc. Natl. Acad. Sci. U. S. A. 100, 9416–9421.

75. Sato T, Matsumoto T, Yamada T, Watanabe T, Kawano H, & Kato S. (2003). Late onset of obesity in male androgen receptor-deficient (ARKO) mice. Biochem. Biophys. Res. Commun. 300, 161–171.

76. Montero M, Quiroga I, Rubert M, Diaz-Curiel M, Bauss F, & De La Piedra C. (2008). PINP, a new available rat bone formation marker. Usefulness in osteopenia studies due to androgen lack and ibandronate treatment. J. Bone Miner. Res. 23(Suppl), S190.

77. Morko J, Peng Z, Rissanen J, Suominen M, Fagerlund K, Ravanti L, et al. (2009). A novel selective androgen receptor modulator (SARM) as monotherapy and combination therapy with alendronate in the treatment of established osteopenia in orchidectomized rats. J. Bone Miner. Res. 24(Suppl), S226.

78. Rissanen J, Peng Z, Morko J, Suominen M, Ravanti L, Kallio P, & Halleen J. (2009). The effects of a novel selective androgen receptor modulator (SARM) ORM-11984 on prevention of osteopenia in ovariectomized rats. J. Bone Miner. Res. 24(Suppl), S354.

79. Peng Z, Morko J, Rissanen J, Suominen M, Ravanti L, Kallio & Halleen J. (2009). The effects of a selective androgen receptor modulator (SARM) ORM-11984 on prevention of osteoporosis in rat immobilization model. J. Bone Miner. Res. 24(Suppl), S483.

80. Stoch SA, Tanaka WK, Hilliard DA, Chappell DL, Modur VR, Phillips RL, et al. (2006). Identification of skin biomarkers following testosterone administration in postmenopausal women. Clin. Pharmacol. Ther. 79, P84.

81. Colvard DS, Eriksen EF, Keeting PE, Wilson EM, Lubahn DB, French FS, et al. (1989). Identification of androgen receptors in normal human osteoblast-like cells. Proc. Natl. Acad. Sci. U. S. A. 86, 854–857.

82. Orwoll ES, Stibrska I, Ramsey EE, & Keenan EJ. (1991). Androgen receptors in osteoblast-like cell lines. Calcif. Tiss. Int. 49, 183–187.

83. Raisz LG, Wiita B, Artis A, Bowen A, Schwartz S, Trahiotis M, et al. (1996). Comparison of the effects of estrogen alone and estrogen plus androgen on biochemical markers of bone formation and resorption in postmenopausal women. J. Clin. Endocrinol. Metab. 81, 37–43.

84. Awdishu S, West SL, Scheid JL, & De Souza MJ. (2008). Elevated androgens associated with increased bone formation in premenopausal exercising oligomenorrheic women. J. Bone Miner. Res. 23(Suppl), S287.

85. Hassager C, Jensen LT, Podenphant J, Riis BJ, & Christiansen C. (1990). Collagen synthesis in postmenopausal women during therapy with anabolic steroid or female sex hormones. Metabolism. 39, 1167–1169.

86. Stoch SA, Friedman EJ, Zhu H, Xu Y, Wong P, Chappell DL, et al. (2008). A 12-week pharmacokinetic and pharmacodynamic (PD) study of MK-0773 in healthy postmenopausal (PMP) subjects. The Endocrine Society 90th Annual Meeting, June 12–15, San Francisco, CA.

87. Brown EM, Gamba G, Riccardi D, Lombardi M, Butters R, Kifor O, et al.(1993). Cloning and characterization of an extracellular Ca2+-sensing receptor from bovine parathyroid. Nature. 366, 575–580.

88. Wuthrich RP, Martin D, & Bilezikian JP. (2008). The role of calcimimetics in the treatment of hyperparathyroidism. Eur. J. Clin. Invest. 37, 915–922.

89. Silverberg SJ, Rubin MR, Faiman C, Peacock M, Shoback DM, Smallridge RC, et al. (2007). Cinacalcet HCl reduces the serum calcium concentration in inoperable parathyroid carcinoma. J. Clin. Endocrinol. Metab. 92, 3803–3808.

90. Peacock M, Bilezikian JP, Klassen PS, Guo MD, Turner SA, & Shoback D. (2005). Cinacalcet hydrochloride maintains long-term normocalcemia in patients with primary hyperparathyroidism. J. Clin. Endocrinol. Metab. 90, 135–141.

91. Bilezikian JP, Matsumoto T, Bellido T, Khosla S, Martin J, Recker RR, et al. (2009). Targeting bone remodeling for the treatment of osteoporosis: Summary of the proceedings of an ASBMR workshop. J. Bone Miner. Res. 24, 373–385.

92. Nemeth EF. (2002). Receptor antagonists. The search for calcium receptor antagonists (calcilytics). J. Mol. Endocrinol. 29, 15–21.

93. Brown EM. (2007). The calcium-sensing receptor: Physiology, pathophysiology and CarR-based therapeutics. Subcell. Biochem. 45, 139–167.

94. Brown EM, & Macleod RJ. (2001). Extracellular calcium sensing and extracellular calcium signaling. Physiol. Rev. 81, 239–297.

95. Bai M, Trivedi S, Lane CR, Yang Y, Quinn SJ, & Brown EM. (1998). Protein kinase C phosphorylation of threonine position 888 in Ca2+ sensing receptor (CaR) inhibits coupling to Ca2+ store release. J. Biol. Chem. 273, 21267–21275.

96. Nemeth EF, & Scarpa A. (1986). Cytosolic Ca2+ and the regulation of secretion of parathyroid cells. FEBS. Lett. 203, 15–19.

97. Nemeth EF, Steffey ME, Hammerland L, Hung BCP, Van Wagenen BC, DelMar EG, et al. (1998). Calcimimetics with potent and selective activity on the parathyroid calcium receptor. Proc. Natl. Acad. Sci. U. S. A. 95, 4040–4045.

98. Nemeth EF, DelMar EG, Heaton WL, Miller MA, Lambert LD, Conklin RL, et al. (2001). Calcilytic compounds: Potent and selective Ca2+ receptor antagonists that stimulate secretion of parathyroid hormone. J. Pharmacol. Exp. Ther. 299, 323–331.

99. Gowen M, Stroup GB, Dodds RA, James IE, Votta BJ, Smith BR, et al. (2000). Antagonizing the parathyroid calcium receptor stimulates parathyroid hormone secretion and bone formation in osteopenic rats. J. Clin. Invest. 105, 1595–1604.

100. Kessler A, Faure H, Petrel C, Rognan D, Césario M, Ruat M, et al. (2006). N1-benzoyl-N2-[1-(1-naphthyl)ethyl]-trans-1,2-diaminocyclohexanes: Development of 4-chlorophenylcarboxamide (Calhex 231) as a new calcium sensing receptor ligand demonstrating potent calcilytic activity. J. Med. Chem. 46, 5119–5128.

101. Arey BJ, Seethala R, Ma Z, Fura A, Morin J, Swartz J, et al. (2005). A novel calcium receptor antagonist transiently stimulates parathyroid hormone secretion in vivo. Endocrinology. 146, 2015–2022.

102. Yang W, Wang Y, Roberge JY, Ma Z, Liu Y, Lawrence RM, et al. (2005). Discovery and structure-activity relationships of 2-benzylpyrrolidine-situated aryloxypropanols as calcium-sensing receptor antagonists. Bioorg. Med. Chem. Lett. 15, 1225–1228.

103. Shcherbakova I, Balandrin MF, Fox J, Ghatak A, Heaton WL, & Conklin RL. (2005). 3H-Quinazolin-4-ones as a new calcilytic template for the potential treatment of osteoporosis. Bioorg. Med. Chem. Lett. 15, 1557–1560.

104. Petrel C, Kessler A, Maslah F, Dauban P, Dodd RH, Rognan D, et al. (2003). Modeling and mutagenesis of the binding site of Calhex 231, a novel negative allosteric modulator of the extracellular Ca2+-sensing receptor. J. Biol. Chem. 278, 49487–49494.

105. Petrel C, Kessler A, Dauban P, Dodd RH, Rognan D, & Ruat M. (2004). Positive and negative allosteric modulators of the Ca2+-sensing receptor interact within the overlapping but not identical binding sites in the transmembrane domain. J. Biol. Chem. 279, 18990–18997.

106. Silverberg SJ, Gartenberg F, Jacobs TP, Shane E, Siris E, Staron RB, et al. (1995). Increased bone mineral density after parathyroidectomy in primary hyperparathyroidism. J. Clin. Endocrinol. Metab. 80, 729–734.

107. Dobnig H, & Turner RT. (1997). The effects of programmed administration of human parathyroid hormone fragment (1–34) on bone histomorphometry and serum chemistry in rats. Endocrinology. 138, 4607–4612.

108. Fox J, Miller MA, Stroup GB, Nemeth EF, & Miller SC. (1997). Plasma levels of parathyroid hormone that induce anabolic effects in bone of ovariectomized rats can be achieved by stimulation of endogenous hormone secretion. Bone. 21, 163–169.

109. Ham AW, Littner BA, Drake TGH, Robertson EC, & Tisdall FF. (1940). Physiological hypertrophy of the parathyroids, its cause and its relation to rickets. Am. J. Pathol. 16, 277–286.

110. Wernerson A, Widholm SM, Svensson O, Reinholt FP. (1991). Parathyroid cell number and size in hypocalcemic young rats. APMIS. 99, 1096–1102.

111. Naveh-Many T, Rahamimov R, Livni N, & Silver J. (1995). Parathyroid cell proliferation in normal and chronic renal failure rats. The effects of calcium, phosphate, and vitamin D. J. Clin. Invest. 96, 1786–1793.

112. Gasser JA, Ingold P, Venturiere A, & Markus J. (2009). Splitting the daily dose of parathyroid hormone PTH (1–34) results in a faster bone anabolic response in rats. J. Bone Miner. Res. 24, S144.

113. Fukumoto S, Nakamura T, Nishizawa Y, Hayashi M, & Matsumoto T. (2009). Randomized, single-blinded placebo-controlled study of a novel calcilytic, JTT-305, in patients with postmenopausal osteoporosis. J. Bone Miner. Res. 24(Suppl), S40.

114. Fitzpatrick L, Dabrowski C, Cicconetti G, Papapoulos S, Bone H, & Bilezikian J. (2009). Roncaleret, a calcium-sensing receptor antagonist: Results of a 1 year double-blind, placebo-controlled, dose-ranging phase II study. J. Bone Miner. Res. 24(Suppl), S40.

115. Fitzpatrick L, Dabrowski C, Cicconetti G, Fuerst T, Engelke K, & Genant H. (2009). The calcium-sensing receptor antagonist, ronacaleret (SB-751689), causes modest increases in trabecular but not cortical BMD by QCT in postmenopausal women. J. Bone Miner. Res. 24(Suppl), S39.

116. Caltabiano S, Desjardins J, Hossain M, Kurtineez M, & Fitzpatrick L. (2009). Characterization of the effect of ronacaleret, a calcium-sensing receptor antagonist on renal calcium excretion. J. Bone Miner. Res. 24(Suppl), S16.

117. Fitzpatrick L, Smith PL, McBride TA, Fries MA, Hossain M, & Dabrowski C. (2009). Ronacaleret (SB-751689), a calcium-sensing receptor antagonist, has

no significant effect on radial fracture healing time: Results from a random-ized, double-blinded, placebo-controlled phase II clinical trial. J. Bone Miner. Res. 24(Suppl), S214.

118. Cosman F, Lane NE, Bolognese MA, Zanchetta JR, Garcia-Hernandez PA, Sees K, et al. (2010). Effect of transdermal teriparatide administration on bone min-eral density in postmenopausal women. J. Clin. Endocrinol. Metab. 95, 151–158.

119. Gong Y, Slee RB, Fukai N, Rawadi G, Roman-Roman S, Reginator AM, et al. (2001). LDL receptor-related protein 5 (LRP5) affects bone accrual and eye development. Cell. 107, 513–523.

120. Gong Y, Vikkula M, Boon L, Liu J, Beighton P, Ramesar R, et al. (1996). Osteoporosis-pseudoglioma syndrome, a disorder affecting skeletal strength and vision, is assigned to chromosome region 11q12–13. Am. J. Hum. Genet. 59, 146–151.

121. Little RD, Carulli JP, Del Mastro RG, Dupuis J, Osborne M, Folz C, et al. (2002). A mutation in the LDL receptor-related protein 5 gene results in the autosomal dominant high-bone-mass trait. Am. J. Hum. Genet. 70, 11–19.

122. Boyden LM, Mao J, Belsky J, Mitzner L, Farhi A, Mitnick MA, et al. (2002). High bone density due to a mutation in LDL-receptor-related protein 5. N. Engl. J. Med. 346, 1513–1521.

123. Van Wesenbeeck L, Cleiren E, Gram J, Beals RK, Bénichou O, Scopelliti D, et al. (2003). Six novel missense mutations in the LDL receptor-related pro-tein 5 (LRP5) gene in different conditions with an increased bone density. Am. J. Hum. Genet. 72, 763–771.

124. Raisz LG. (2005). Pathogenesis of osteoporosis: Concepts, conflicts, and prospects. J. Clin. Invest. 115, 3318–3325.

125. Cadigan KM, & Nusse R. (1997). Wnt signaling: A common theme in animal development. Genes Dev. 11, 3286–3305.

126. Krishnan A, Bryant HU, & MacDonald OA. (2006). Regulation of bone mass by Wnt signaling. J. Clin. Invest. 116, 1202–1209.

127. Westendorf JJ, Kahler RA, & Schroeder TM. (2004). Wnt signaling in osteoblasts and bone diseases. Gene. 341, 19–39.

128. Rawadi G, & Roman-Roman S. (2005). Wnt signalling pathway: A new tar-get for the treatment of osteoporosis. Expert Opin. Ther. Targets. 9, 1063–1077.

129. Glinka A, Wu W, Delius H, Monaghan AP, Blumenstock C, & Niehrs C. (1998). Dickkopf-1 is a member of a new family of secreted proteins and functions in head induction. Nature. 391, 357–362.

130. Terpos E. (2006). Antibodies to dickkopf-1 protein. Expert Opin. Ther. Patents. 16, 1453–1458.

131. Bodine PVN, Stauffer B, Ponce-de-Leon H, Bhat RA, Mangine A, Seestaller-Wehr LM, et al. (2009). A small molecule inhibitor of the Wnt antagonist secreted fizzled-related potein-1 stimulates bone formation. Bone. 44, 1063–1068.

132. Moore WJ, Kern JC, Bhat R, Bodine PV, Fukyama S, Krishnamurthy G, et al. (2010). Modulation of Wnt signaling through inhibition of secreted frizzled-related protein (sFRP-1) with N-substituted piperidinyl diphenylsulfonyl sul-fonamides. Bioorg. Med. Chem. 18, 190–201.

133. Babij P, Zhao W, Small C, Kharode Y, Yaworsky PJ, Bouxsein ML, et al. (2003). High bone mass in mice expressing a mutant LRP5 gene. J. Bone Miner. Res. 18, 960–974.

134. Koay MA, & Brown MA. (2005). Genetic disorders of the LRP5-Wnt signalling pathway affecting the skeleton. Trends. Molec. Med. 11, 129–137.

135. Kato M, Patel MS, Levasseur R, Lobov I, Chang BH-J, Glass DA 2nd, et al. (2002). Cbfa1-independent decrease in osteoblast proliferation, osteopenia, and persistent embryonic eye vascularization in mice-deficient in Lrp5 a Wnt coreceptor. J. Cell Biol. 157, 303–314.

136. Fujino T, Asaba H, Kang MJ, Ikeda Y, Sone H, Takada S, et al. (2003). Low-density lipoprotein receptor-related protein 5 (LRP5) is essential for normal cholesterol metabolism and glucose-induced insulin secretion. Proc. Natl. Acad. Sci. U. S. A. 100, 229–234.

137. Albers J, Gebauer M, Friedrich F, Schulze J, Priemel M, Francke U, et al. (2008). Mice lacking the Wnt receptor frizzled-9 display osteopenia caused by decreased bone formation. J. Bone Miner. Res. 23(Suppl), S3.

138. Li X, Grisanti M, Geng Z, Niu Q, Fan W, Daris M, et al. (2006). Dickkopf-1 delivery by adeno-associated virus caused bone loss in adult mice. J. Bone Miner. Res. 21(Suppl), S8.

139. Grisanti M, Niu QT, Fan W, Asuncion F, Lee J, Steavenson S, et al. (2006). Dkk-1 inhibition increases bone mineral density in rodents. J. Bone Miner. Res. 21(Suppl), S25.

140. Pelletier JC, Lundquist JT 4th, Gilbert AM, Alon N, Bex FJ, Bhat BM, et al. (2009). (1-(4-(Naphthalen-2-yl)pyrimidin-2-yl)piperidin-4-yl)methanamine: A Aingless β-catenin agonist that increases bone formation rate. J. Med. Chem. 52, 6962–6965.

141. Balemans W, Ebeling M, Patel N, Van Hul E, Olson P, Dioszegi M, et al. (2001). Increased bone density in sclerostosis is due to deficiency of a novel secreted protein (SOST). Hum. Mol. Genet. 10, 537–543.

142. Martin TJ, Sims NA, & Ng KW. (2008). Regulatory pathways revealing new approaches to the development of anabolic drugs for osteoporosis. Osteoporos. Int. 19, 1125–1138.

143. Brunkow ME, Gardner JC, Van Ness J, Paeper BW, Kovacevich BR, Proll S, et al. (2001). Bone dysplasia sclerosteosis results from loss of the SOST gene product, a novel cystine-knot containing protein. Am. J. Hum. Genet. 68, 577–589.

144. Balemans W, Patel N, Eberling M, Van Hul E, Wuyts W, Lacza C, et al. (2002). Identification of a 52 kb deletion downstream of the SOST gene in patients with Van Buchem disease. J. Med. Genet. 39, 91–97.

145. Staehling-Hampton K, Proll S, Paeper BW, Zhao L, Charmley P, Brown A, et al. (2002). A 52-kb deletion in the SOST-MEOX1 intergenic region on 17q12-q21 is associated with Van Buchem disease in the Dutch population. Am. J. Med. Genet. 110, 144–152.

146. Gardner JC, van Bezooijen RL, Mervis B, Hamdy NA, Löwik CW, Hamersma H, et al. (2005). Bone mineral density in sclerosteosis; affected individuals and gene carriers. J. Clin. Endocrinol. Metab. 90, 6392–6395.

147. ten Dijke P, Krause C, de Gorter DJ, Löwik CW, & van Bezooijen RL. (2008). Osteocyte-derived sclerostin inhibits bone formation: Its role in bone morphogenetic protein and Wnt signaling. J. Bone Joint Surg. Am. 90(Suppl 1), 31–35.

148. Wergedal JE, Veskovic K, Hellan M, Nyght C, Balemans W, Libanati C, et al. (2003). Patients with Van Buchem disease, an osteosclerotic genetic disease, have elevated bone formation markers, higher bone density, and greater derived polar moment of inertia than normal. J. Clin. Endocrinol. Metab. 88, 5778–5783.

149. Noble BS. (2008). The osteocyte lineage. Arch. Biochem. Biophys. 473, 106–111.

150. Suva LJ. (2009). Sclerostin and the unloading of bone. J. Bone Miner. Res. 24, 1649–1650.

151. Robling AG, Bellido T, & Turner CH. (2006). Mechanical stimulation in vivo reduces osteocyte expression of sclerostin. J. Musculoskelet. Neuronal Interact. 6, 354.

152. Li X, Zhang Y, Kang H, Liu W, Liu P, Zhang J, et al. (2005). Sclerostin binds to LRP5/6 and antagonizes canonical Wnt signaling. J. Biol. Chem. 280, 19883–19887.

153. van Bezooijen RL, Svensson JP, Eefting D, Visser A, van der Horst G, Karperien M, et al. (2007). Wnt but not BMP signaling is involved in the inhibitory action of sclerostin on BMP-stimulated bone formation. J. Bone Miner. Res. 21, 19–28.

154. Li X, Ominsky MS, Niu QT, Sun N, Daugherty B, D'Agostin D, et al. (2008). Targeted disruption of the sclerostin gene in mice results in increased bone formation and bone strength. J. Bone Miner. Res. 23, 860–869.

155. Winkler DG, Sutherland MK, Geoghegan JC, Yu C, Hayes T, Skonier JE, et al. (2003). Osteocyte control of bone formation via sclerostin, a novel BMP antagonist. EMBO J. 22, 6267–6276.

156. Desbois C, Hogue DA, & Karsenty G. (1994). The mouse osteocalcin gene cluster contains three genes with two separate spatial and temporal patterns of expression. J. Biol. Chem. 269, 1183–1190.

157. Moustafa A, Sugiyama T, Zaman G, Lanyon L, & Price J. (2009). Sclerostin expression in trabecular and cortical bone osteocytes is increased by disuse and reversed by loading with a distribution related to new bone formation. J. Bone Miner. Res. 24(Suppl), S310.

158. Robing AG, Niziolek PJ, Baldridge LA, Condon KW, Allen MR, Alam I, et al. (2008). Mechanical stimulation of bone in vivo reduces osteocyte expression of SOST/sclerostin. J. Biol. Chem. 283, 5866–5875.

159. Moustafa A, Sugiyama T, Saxon LK, Zaman G, Sunters A, Armstrong VJ, et al. (2009). The mouse fibula as a suitable bone for the study of functional adaptation to mechanical loading. Bone. 44, 930–935.

160. Li X, Ominsky MS, Warmington KS, Morony S, Gong J, Cao J, et al. (2009). Sclerostin antibody treatment increases bone formation, bone mass, and bone strength in a rat model of postmenopausal osteoporosis. J. Bone Miner. Res. 24, 578–588.

161. Li X, Warmington K, Niu QT, Asuncion F, Grisanti M, Dwyer D, et al. (2008). Effects of co-treatment with an anti-sclerostin monoclonal antibody and alendronate in ovariectomized rats. J. Bone Miner. Res. 23, S60.

162. Ominsky MS, Vlasseros F, Jolette J, Smith SY, Stouch B, Doellgast G, et al. (2010). Two doses of sclerostin antibody to cynomolgus monkeys increases bone formation, bone mineral density, and bone strength. J. Bone Miner. Res. 25, 948–959.

163. Padhi D, Stouch B, Jang G, Fang L, Darling M, Glise H, et al. (2007). Anti-sclerostin antibody increases markers of bone formation in healthy postmenopausal women. J. Bone Miner. Res. 22(Suppl), S37.

164. Gaudio A, Pennisi P, Bratengeier C, Torrisi V, Lindner B, Mangiafico RA, et al. (2010). Increased sclerostin serum levels associated with bone formation and resorption markers in patients with immobilization-induced bone loss. J. Clin. Endocrinol. Metab. 95, 2248–2253.

165. Mirza FS, Padhi IS, Raisz LG, & Lorenzo JA. (2010). Serum sclerostin levels negatively correlate with parathyroid hormone levels and free estrogen index in postmenopausal women. J. Clin. Endocrinol. Metab. 95, 1991–1997.

Case Studies in Neuroscience: Unique Challenges and Examples

Gerard J. Marek

6.1. Why Is Neuroscience Not Tractable?

The discovery of novel therapies for the treatment of psychiatric and neurological disease faces one major hurdle beyond other therapeutic areas. The blood–brain barrier requires that most central nervous system (CNS) active drugs be reasonably lipophilic to reach their molecular target in the brain. Thus, understanding in vivo receptor occupancy has become an important part of most development programs in making terminantion ("no-go") or continuation ("go") decisions on progressing to a Phase 2 proof-of-concept study, especially when the drug in question is an antagonist or inhibitor of a transporter, enzyme, receptor, or ion channel. In these cases, at least 50% to 80% receptor occupancy at given doses, exposures, or both is usually required to attain demonstrable clinical efficacy (Fig. 6.1).[1] When receptor occupancy studies are not available and maximally tolerated dose (MTD) strategies are executed, the success of this strategy is governed by the accuracy of defining the MTD.

The development of duloxetine provides an example of difficulties that may arise when an optimal biomarker is not available to define dose selection for initial efficacy studies. Initial efficacy testing for duloxetine in a Phase 1b/2 study of major depression was initiated in February 1993 using a 20-mg fixed dose. The completion date for the last patient enrolled in this study was November 1994. At that time no serotonin transporter (SERT) radiotracers were available that had been validated with the stringency needed for decision making. Unfortunately, this Phase 1b/2 study was negative with respect to the primary efficacy variable (change in the Hamilton Rating Scale for Depression [HAM-D] score from baseline). Selection of this single 20-mg dose level in this study was not based on its human pharmacodynamic (PD) activity or receptor occupancy studies. Additional Phase 2 studies started in 1999 at higher doses were positive, and Phase 3 studies using doses of 60 mg q.d. or ≥40 mg b.i.d. eventually began nearly 6 years later in October 2000. When multiple SERT radiotracers later

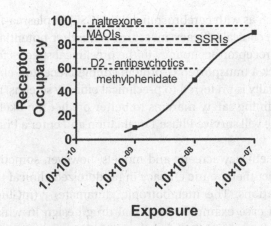

Fig. 6.1
Receptor occupancy
curve for CNS
therapeutics.
Generally, 60% to 95%
receptor occupancy is
required to observed
therapeutic effects for
CNS disease
indications.
Predictions of free
drug in the plasma
and CSF provide
improved predictions
for CNS occupancy/PK
relationships (x-axis).
Thus, for transporters,
therapeutic efficacy
for SSRIs
(depression/anxiety)
and methylphenidate
(ADHD) requires 80%
and 60% transporter
occupancy,
respectively. For
G-protein coupled
proteins, from 60%
(typical antipsychotics
at dopamine D_2
receptors) to 95%
occupancy (naltrexone
and alcoholism) is
required to observe
therapeutic effects.
For enzymes,
approximately 85%
inhibition of MAO-A
and B is required for
therapeutic effects by
nonselective MAOIs.
For ligand-gated ion
channels, 67% to 97%
occupancy of 5-HT$_3$
receptors needs to be
blocked to block
emesis. ADHD,
attention-
deficit/hyperactivity
disorder.

became available, receptor occupancy studies converged on the finding that doses resulting in at least 80% SERT occupancy are necessary to demonstrate efficacy of venlafaxine and selective serotonin reuptake inhibitors (SSRIs).[2,3] Thus, receptor occupancy studies improved the understanding of the basis for the efficacy dose-response relationship for duloxetine where the 40 mg/day dose has minimal effects and all doses between 60 mg and 120 mg are effective in the treatment of major depression.[4] Duloxetine doses at ≥60 mg/day are also associated with ≥80% SERT occupancy.[3] This retrospective case study highlights the necessity and urgency of using receptor occupancy when available to aid optimal dose selection for proof-of-concept Phase 2 studies.

6.2. Why Have New Mechanisms Failed?

There are several reasons why new mechanisms have failed in clinical testing. The first major problem is that preclinical disease models reflect a restricted range of biology underlying human diseases. These models have often been selected based on predictive validity when currently used therapeutics test positive and other drugs, which are not active in this indication, do not have a similar effect. Even when the directional prediction of the models does turn out to be true, the magnitude of the clinical effect size for the candidate drug may not be as good as, or better than, existing medications defined as the standard of care. The second major problem is that, for CNS drugs, often the margin between exposures that provide efficacious effects and those with either on-target or off-target interactions resulting in unacceptable adverse effects is small. This margin may result in significant safety issues that are not acceptable based on a limited advantage over the current standard of care. Failure to define margins from the toxicology studies by using truly translational endpoints to predict drug exposures (such as with cerebrospinal fluid [CSF] or plasma-free drug levels) for the preclinical efficacy measures is another potential pitfall. The use of in vivo receptor occupancy in the preclinical species for drugs that inhibit or block a transporter, G-protein coupled receptor, enzyme, or ion channel generally is preferred to preclinical efficacy screens/models as an anchor for defining safety margins to better predict the likelihood that a given molecule will survive Phase 1 evaluation and enter a Phase 2 efficacy study.

Preclinical efficacy screens and models, however, sometimes do successfully predict therapeutic efficacy in randomized clinical trials for CNS disease indications. The metabotropic glutamate$_{2/3}$ (mGlu$_{2/3}$) receptor agonists are a case example of rational drug design in which the rigid, glutamate-analogue LY354740 and the LY354740 prodrug, LY544344, were both found to be efficacious and well-tolerated in the treatment of generalized anxiety disorder (GAD).[5,6] Positive preclinical results in a range of models in rodents (fear-potentiated startle, elevated plus maze, and stress-induced hypothermia) originally validated with benzodiazepines led to clinical testing in translational, provocation-induced anxiety models in humans, and results were consistent with the lactate-induced panic model of rats.[7-9] The utility of these translational paradigms is limited by the relatively large sample size ($n = 15$/group) required if they are statistically powered for definitive go or no-go decision-making criteria. In addition to these translational paradigms, relatively small proof-of-concept clinical studies using LY354740 for patients with GAD had provided the initial confidence that supported both the preclinical profile and the translational, provocation-induced anxiety clinical studies. Despite the success with the translational studies and the confirmatory large multicenter, placebo- and comparator-controlled randomized Phase 3 clinical trials, convulsions were observed with these drugs in preclinical studies during late-stage clinical testing. Although no convulsions were observed in any patients on LY354740 for as long as 1 year, the benefit-to-risk ratio for GAD did not support further development in this indication. Nevertheless, this example does highlight that the currently used battery of preclinical efficacy screens and equivalent human models can predict that molecules targeting a novel mechanism of action will demonstrate efficacy in large, multicenter efficacy trials. This example also highlights the unpredictable occurrence of CNS safety issues in animals that may or may not translate to humans but the potential severity of which leads to discontinuation of the drug candidate.

A number of new mechanisms have failed in major depression trials. The list includes neurokinin-1 (NK1) receptor antagonists,[10] corticotrophin-releasing hormone-1 (CRH1) receptor antagonists,[11] glucocorticoid (GC) receptor antagonists, and 5-hydroxytryptamine$_{1B}$ (5-HT$_{1B}$) receptor antagonists. With the NK1 receptor antagonists, the presence of a radiotracer for this receptor has confirmed that the extensive set of depression trials conducted by Merck did truly test the hypothesis for this clinical target rather than simply test the mechanism.[12] Namely, Merck scientists used a dose of aprepitant at exposures saturating brain NK1 receptors. The positive comparator paroxetine in these studies was efficacious. Unfortunately, this proof-of-receptor engagement was not, and is not, available for CRH1 receptor antagonists or the GC receptor antagonists. For these two targets, the failure in clinical studies was due to either inadequate receptor occupancy or the lack of target relevance for these indications.

Almost all therapeutic drugs for CNS diseases have been found through serendipity. One of the most recent breakthroughs in therapeutics for depression, N-methyl-D-aspartate (NMDA) receptor antagonists, was discovered in this manner. Several years back, the channel-blocking NMDA receptor antagonist ketamine was being administered to depressed patients at Yale to explore the pathophysiology of depression.[13] The investigators were surprised that many of the patients experienced a temporary attenuation of their depressive symptoms for 1 to 2 weeks after a single ketamine infusion associated with known transient (minutes) psychotomimetic effects. Subsequently, a large, randomized clinical trial using a placebo condition confirmed that ketamine exerted a transitory antidepressant effect.[14] More recently, a selective antagonist binding to the NMDA NR2B subunit (NMDA GluN2B), CP-101,606, was found to augment the antidepressant action of an SSRI.[15] This approach is currently under investigation by AstraZeneca (see www.clinicaltrials.gov). AstraZeneca has completed a study of its NMDA NR2A/2B (NMDA GluN2A/2B) receptor antagonist AZD6765 for treatment-resistant depression. As of December 2009, it is recruiting patients for three additional major depression studies and another Phase 1 study testing the comparability of an oral formulation to their intravenous formulation.

The ongoing development of the $mGlu_{2/3}$ receptor agonist prodrug LY2140023 provides another example of successfully moving from preclinical efficacy models/screens to demonstrating efficacy in the clinic. The parent molecule of LY2140023, LY404039, and other orthosteric $mGlu_{2/3}$ receptor agonists have been found to (1) attenuate the increased locomotor activity induced by channel-blocking NMDA receptor antagonists, (2) suppress horizontal locomotor activity induced by amphetamine, (3) attenuate head shakes induced by the serotonergic phenethylamine hallucinogens, and (4) suppress avoidance responses without impairing escape responses in the conditioned avoidance response (CAR) model.[16–20] Activity of $mGlu_{2/3}$ receptor agonists in these models is not surprising in light of the CNS distribution of $mGlu_{2/3}$ receptors to cortical–subcortical macrocircuits implicated in the pathophysiology of schizophrenia. The second-generation atypical antipsychotic drugs also produce positive effects in these same preclinical screens/models. How this class of molecules will compare with the second-generation atypical antipsychotics with respect to positive and negative symptoms and cognition remains to be seen from additional studies.

In contrast to this successful translation of a robust preclinical efficacy package to a positive Phase 2 randomized clinical study for LY2140023, dopamine D_4 receptor antagonists represent an example of compounds that were brought forward in the absence of a package similar to the one supporting the $mGlu_{2/3}$ receptor agonists. In addition to a known affinity of clozapine for dopamine D_4 receptors, D_4 receptors have higher expression in the prefrontal cortex than striatum. Also, a number of reports suggested an up-regulation of D_4 receptor binding in postmortem brains from schizophrenic subjects. An additional rationale for testing D_4 receptor antagonists in the clinic is that these drugs were effective in blocking the behavioral sensitization of amphetamine. However, D_4 receptor antagonists do not reproduce this type of preclinical antipsychotic-like package shared between typical and atypical antipsychotics and $mGlu_{2/3}$ receptor agonists described in the previous paragraph. Not surprisingly, a large, multicenter, randomized, placebo-controlled, olanzapine-controlled clinical trial failed to demonstrate antipsychotic effects for the dopamine D_4 receptor antagonist sonepiprazole.[21] A 40-fold range of sonepiprazole was tested to minimize the likelihood that the highest dose did not engage the D_4 receptor. Given the absence of a selective D_4 receptor radiotracer, this possibility remains but is not likely given the robust range of doses tested in the clinical trial. The lack of efficacy for sonepiprazole was in contrast to the robust antipsychotic effects in the similarly powered olanzapine arm. This negative trial with the Pharmacia D_4 receptor antagonist essentially replicated the negative effects of a Merck dopamine D_4 receptor antagonist previously tested in a smaller study.[22] The $5-HT_3$ receptor is another example of a target that failed in the clinic after being brought forward in the absence of a robust preclinical package with systemic dosing of both the candidate molecule and psychotomimetic drugs.[23,24]

The $5-HT_{2A}$ receptor is an example of a target for which an intermediate preclinical antipsychotic package relative to the one predicting efficacy of $mGlu_{2/3}$ receptor agonists predicted equivocal clinical effects between those for the dopamine D_4 or $5-HT_3$ receptor antagonists cited earlier in text compared with the $mGlu_{2/3}$ receptor agonist prodrug LY2140023. Selective $5-HT_{2A}$ receptor antagonists such as M100907 (formerly known as MDL 100,907) suppress locomotor hyperactivity induced by NMDA receptor antagonists and head shakes induced by serotonergic hallucinogens.[25,26] $5-HT_{2A}$ receptor antagonists, however, generally do not suppress locomotor activity induced by amphetamine at doses selective for blocking $5-HT_{2A}$ receptors. Furthermore, $5-HT_{2A}$ receptor antagonists fail to suppress avoidance responding in the CAR model. $5-HT_{2A}$ receptor antagonists, however, do enhance the antipsychotic-like profile of known antipsychotic drugs in this paradigm. Two different $5-HT_{2A}$ receptor antagonists were tested in schizophrenic patients after verifying the doses needed to saturate brain $5-HT_{2A}$ receptors. M100907 was reported to decrease the symptoms of schizophrenia intermediate between placebo and the positive comparator haloperidol in two different, large, Phase 3 studies.[27] This drug was without effect in another large, multicenter, European study investigating schizophrenic patients primarily suffering from negative symptoms. Another $5\text{-}HT_{2A}$ receptor antagonist was found to produce a relatively modest but significant antipsychotic effect interme- diate between placebo and haloperidol.[28] Thus, one reason for a portion of failed Phase 2 studies relates to problems with preclinical target validation and selection and failure to demand an appropriately robust preclinical package. Although false positives undoubtedly will be seen using any particular battery of preclinical tests, these examples from antipsychotic drug development do emphasize that rigorous decision criteria from an appropriate preclinical battery should decrease the likelihood of failures in Phase 2 due to lack of efficacy. Improved decision making regarding compound advancement results will be made when these preclinical mod- els have human equivalents and the clinical results using these models confirm the animal model findings.

6.3. Can We Predict Efficacy in Short-Term Studies?

In some indications, preclinical models are not predictive for efficacy in humans. Cost-effective, short-term clinical trials in the target population may then be the best alternative. For antidepressants, the most useful kind of predictor would be the ability to predict an efficacious response to a novel drug after administration of only a single dose or after treatment for 1 to 2 weeks. Antidepressant drugs appear to normalize negative biases in information processing. A 2-week treatment duration with both the SSRI citalopram and the norepinephrine transporter (NET) inhibitor reboxetine has been found to increase the recognition accuracy of facial emotions like disgust, happiness, and surprise.[29] These effects correlated to clini- cal improvement observed during continued treatment for an additional 4 weeks. Thus, for some mechanisms, acute drug administration models may be predictive of antidepressant activity. For example, a 7-day treat- ment duration in healthy volunteers with either citalopram or reboxetine increased positive versus negative affective perceptions of facial recogni- tion and memory.[30] A single 4-mg dose of reboxetine, unlike placebo, also reversed a negative affective bias in depressed patients.[31] This result in patients similarly extended an earlier study in healthy volunteers showing that a single reboxetine dose resulted in an increase in emotional bias as measured by facial recognition, emotional categorization, and emotional memory.[32]

Three important questions are raised by these findings. The first is to understand the predictive validity of acute single-dose administration versus 1 or 2 weeks of drug administration. The second question is to understand the limitations of the predictive validity of these paradigms. The third question addresses whether there are other neurobiological measures providing convergent validity of these findings. Some limited evidence suggests that other mechanisms beyond monoamine reuptake inhibitors may possess these effects. A recent report has shown that the histamine $H_1/5\text{-}HT_{2/3}$ receptor antagonist mirtazapine improved emotional bias in healthy volunteers when administered as a single dose.[33] Conversely, a single dose of the NK1 receptor antagonist aprepitant in healthy volunteers produced a more restricted range of effects on emotional processing compared with monoamine reuptake inhibitors.[34] Further testing with drugs lacking any antidepressant efficacy is needed to better understand the predictive validity of this paradigm. A backdrop for these studies rests in the growing recognition of cognitive deficits in major depression.[35,36] Testing whether these neurocognitive deficits are consistent with the distributed neural circuits underlying the pathophysiology of mood disorders will be important in providing critical convergent validity of this paradigm.[37–39]

6.4. What Is the Role for Cognitive Biomarkers?

With an emphasis on CNS drug development for cognitive dysfunction in schizophrenia and Alzheimer's disease, the development of therapies that enhance cognition is at a premium. At least one example has defined a potential path toward developing cognitive enhancers. The stop-signal task model was designed to measure one aspect of response inhibition.[40] This model is based on inhibiting a prepotent response after it was already set in motion (e.g., action cancellation). The stop-signal task is one of the commonly used paradigms to measure the cardinal feature of attention-deficit/hyperactivity disorder (ADHD), response inhibition. The NET inhibitor atomoxetine was found to improve the performance of rats in the stop-signal task.[41] Translating from rats to humans, researchers found that a single 60-mg dose of atomoxetine also improved the performance of healthy volunteers on the stop-signal task.[42] Finally, patients with ADHD were tested. Like healthy volunteers, a single 60-mg dose of atomoxetine improved the stop-signal reaction time in adult patients with ADHD regardless of medication status.[43] These effects of atomoxetine are similar to past results obtained with methylphenidate, amphetamine, and modafinil.[40] Importantly, although SSRIs and serotonin depletions modulate response inhibition processes for go/no go tasks, SSRIs or depletion of brain 5-HT does not modify response inhibition assayed with the stop-signal task. Convergent validity of the translational rationale for this model for making predictions about therapeutic activity in ADHD is supported by the homologous frontostriatal circuits invoked by this task in both rats and humans.[40] This example provides two important teaching points. First, where homologous neural circuitry across species can be postulated for discrete cognitive tasks and verified, the translational use of cognitive models holds great promise for supporting the development of novel medications to improve different aspects of cognition. The Cambridge Neuropsychological Test Automated Battery (CANTAB) has been explicitly developed to provide these types of translational opportunities. Second, this work with atomoxetine on the stop-signal task is an additional example suggesting that a single dose of a potential therapeutic drug may provide a translational paradigm for early drug development.

6.5. What Translational Medicine Approaches Will Drive Innovation in Neuroscience Drug Development?

First and foremost, the development of optimal radiotracers to test target engagement during Phase 1 single or multiple dosing of compounds is critical to testing hypotheses concerning a mechanism of action or drug target rather than simply testing whether a given molecule may be active during Phase 2. The major limitation is that radiotracer development for positron emission tomography (PET) or single photon emission computed tomography (SPECT) neuroimaging is at least as difficult as developing new medications. Many targets are extremely difficult to address with these techniques, and significant questions exist for interpreting adequate occupancy for candidates that are agonists or positive allosteric modulators.

A second translational approach involves demonstrating that the drug is reaching the CSF in humans and attempting to bridge peripheral/CSF pharmacokinetic (PK)/PD data from animal models. This approach may be significantly strengthened if analytes modulated downstream from the drug target may also be altered and measured as a PD variable. The biomarker program leading to the Phase 3 study of the γ-secretase inhibitor semagacestat (LY450139) exemplifies such a PK/PD approach. Scientists at Washington University and Lilly first demonstrated an exposure-dependent decrease in amyloid-β (Aβ) production with single doses of semagacestat in healthy men.[44] The safety of semagacestat was then confirmed in a 14-week, Phase 2 safety and tolerability study.[45] Interestingly, although adequate CSF exposures were seen in this Phase 2 study, only a modest, nonsignificant reduction of Aβ in the CSF was observed. The apparent discordance between altering Aβ production in healthy volunteers and steady-state Aβ levels in the CSF of patients may imply differential CNS compartmentalization of drug, analytes, or both, which is a common problem complicating the interpretation of CSF studies. Additional proof of clinical activity for semagacestat in this Phase 2 study is that plasma $A\beta_{40}$ was also reduced by ~60% by doses of the γ-secretase inhibitor that decreased $A\beta$ formation in healthy volunteers by ~50%. On the basis of adequate Phase 2 safety/tolerability for semagacestat and the demonstration that it has engaged its molecular target, a Phase 3 program has begun.[46]

A third key translational approach revolves around demonstrating circuit engagement for molecules for which key nodal points both for the target and the disease pathophysiology have been identified. Here both fluorodeoxyglucose (FDG) PET and functional magnetic resonance imaging (fMRI) studies will need to be refined further. Recently, fMRI studies defining connectivity of different brain regions and how different drugs may alter the connectivity patterns have been gaining interest as a translational tool because the neurocircuits involved in the pathophysiology of neuropsychiatric disease appear to be better understood. Other techniques, such as magnetoencephalography (MEG), are being used to define the three-dimensional physiological connectivity of the brain on a more refined time dimension (ms) that is not possible with fMRI.[47] In addition to MEG, electroencephalography (EEG) time–frequency analysis is enjoying a resurgence of interest given a resonance between the basic neuroscientific understanding of γ-oscillations in cortical structures and disrupted local circuits in the cortex of schizophrenic patients that may play a role in their impaired cognition and negative symptoms.[48,49] These uses of EEG data go beyond previous graphical maps of electrical activity described by quantitative pharmaco-EEG studies.

A range of techniques can also define abnormalities of fiber pathways in macrocircuits involved in disease pathophysiology. Optical contrast tomography (OCT) is one specialized technique showing great promise as a novel biomarker for measuring the retinal nerve fiber layer in multiple sclerosis. Modifications of MRI such as diffusion tensor imaging (DTI) also help to define white matter tracts in the brain.

As these techniques are further refined and validated, they hold great promise for helping to speed up quality decision making in drug development and play a role supplementing relatively crude clinical outcome measures. The key feature of these approaches for CNS drug discovery is to ground these translational paradigms in shared homologous neurocircuitry across species. The examples described for $mGlu_{2/3}$ receptor agonists in GAD and schizophrenia, for duloxetine in depression, and for the NET inhibitor atomoxetine in ADHD highlight the potential for improving the quality of early drug development decision making by using these types of translational strategies. In contrast, the failure to bring all potential sources of translational data to the drug development process for CNS disease indications portends an even slower rate of making novel medications available to patients that is further limited by the current downsizing of the pharmaceutical industry, resulting in fewer clinical scientists able to pursue this type of translational research.

6.6. References

1. Grimwood S, & Hartig PR. (2009). Target site occupancy: Emerging generalizations from clinical and preclinical studies. Pharmacol. Ther. 122, 281–301.

2. Meyer JH, Wilson AA, Sagrati S, Hussey D, Carella A, Potter WZ, et al. (2004). Serotonin transporter occupancy of five selective serotonin reuptake inhibitors at different doses: An [11C]DASB positron emission tomography study. Am. J. Psychiatry. 161, 826–835.

3. Takano A, Suzuki K, Kosaka J, Ota M, Nozaki S, Ikoma Y, et al. (2006). A dose-finding study of duloxetine based on serotonin transporter occupancy. Psychopharmacol. 185, 395–399.

4. Pritchett YL, Marciniak MD, Corey-Lisle PK, Berzon RA, Desaiah D, & Detke MJ. (2007). Use of effect size to determine optimal dose of duloxetine in major depressive disorder. J. Psychiatr. Res. 41, 311–318.

5. Dunayevich E, Erickson J, Levine L, Landbloom R, Schoepp DD, & Tollefson GD. (2008). Efficacy and tolerability of an mGlu2/3 agonist in the treatment of generalized anxiety disorder. Neuropsychopharmacol. 33, 1603–1610.

6. Michelson D, Levine LR, Dellva MA, Mesters P, Schoepp DD, Dunayevich E, et al. (2005). Clinical studies with mGlu2/3 receptor agonists: LY354740 compared with placebo in patients with generalized anxiety disorder. Neuropharmacol. 49(Suppl 1), 257.

7. Kellner M, Muhtz C, Stark K, Yassouridis A, Arlt J, & Wiedemann K. (2005). Effects of a metabotropic glutamate(2/3) receptor agonist (LY544344/LY354740) on panic anxiety induced by cholecystokinin tetrapeptide in healthy humans: Preliminary results. Psychopharmacol. 179, 310–315.

8. Schoepp DD, Wright RA, Levine LR, Gaydos B, & Potter WZ. (2003). LY354740, an mGlu2/3 receptor agonist, as a novel approach to treat anxicty/stress. Stress. 6, 189–197.

9. Shekhar A, & Keim SR. (2000). LY354740, a potent group II metabotropic glutamate receptor agonist, prevents lactate-induced panic-like response in panic-prone rats. Neuropharmacol. 39, 1139–1146.

10. Keller M, Montgomery S, Ball W, Morrison M, Snavely D, Liu G, et al. (2006). Lack of efficacy of the substance P (neurokinin1 receptor) antagonist aprepitant in the treatment of major depressive disorder. Biol. Psychiatry. 59, 216–223.

11. Binneman B, Feltner D, Kolluri S, Shi Y, Qiu R, & Stiger T. (2008). A 6-week randomized, placebo-controlled trial of CP-316,311 (a selective CRH1 antagonist) in the treatment of major depression. Am. J. Psychiatry. 165, 617–620.

12. Bergstrom M, Hargreaves RJ, Burns HD, Goldberg MR, Sciberras D, Reines SA, et al. (2004). Human positron emission tomography studies of brain neurokinin 1 receptor occupancy by aprepitant. Biol. Psychiatry. 55, 1007–1012.

13. Berman RM, Capiello A, Anand A, Oren DA, Heninger GR, Charney DS, et al. (2000). Antidepressant effects of ketamine in depressed patients. Biol. Psychiatry. 47, 351–354.

14. Zarate CA, Singh JB, Carlson PJ, Brutsche NE, Ameli R, Luckenbaugh MA, et al. (2006). A randomized trial of an N-methyl-D-aspartate antagonist in treatment-resistant major depression. Arch. Gen. Psychiatry. 63, 856–864.

15. Preskorn SH, Baker B, Kolluri S, Menniti FS, Krams M, & Landen JW. (2008). An innovative design to establish proof of concept of the antidepressant effects of the NR2B subunit selective N-methyl-D-aspartate antagonist, CP-101,606, in patients with treatment-refractory major depressive disorder. J. Clin. Psychopharmacol. 28, 631–637.

16. Cartmell J, Monn JA, & Schoepp DD. (2000). Attenuation of specific PCP-evoked behaviors by the potent mGlu2/3 receptor agonist, LY379268, and comparison with the atypical antipsychotic, clozapine. Psychopharmacol. 148, 423–429.

17. Gewirtz JC, Chen AC-H, Duman RS, & Marek GJ. (1999). The group II metabotropic glutamate receptor agonist LY354740, suppresses behavioral and molecular effects of 5-HT2A receptor activation: Head shakes and neocortical neurotrophin expression. Soc. Neurosci. Abstr. 25, 449.

18. Klodzinska A, Bijak M, Tokarski K, & Pilc A. (2002). Group II mGlu receptor agonists inhibit behavioral and electrophysiological effects of DOI in mice. Pharmacol. Biochem. Behav. 73, 327–332.

19. Moghaddam B, & Adams BW. (1998). Reversal of phencyclidine effects by a group II metabotropic glutamate receptor agonist in rats. Science. 281, 1349–1352.

20. Rorick-Kehn LM, Johnson BG, Knitowski KM, Salhoff CR, Witkin JM, Perry KW, et al. (2007). In vivo pharmacological characterization of the structurally novel, potent, selective mGlu2/3 receptor agonist LY404039 in animal models of psychiatric disorders. Psychopharmacol. 193, 121–136.

21. Corrigan MH, Gallen CC, Bonura L, Mechant KM, & Sonepiprazole Study Group. (2004). Effectiveness of the selective D4 antagonist sonepiprazole in schizophrenia: A placebo-controlled trial. Biol. Psychiatry. 55, 445–451.

22. Kramer MS, Last B, Getson A, & Reines SA. (1997). The effects of a selective D4 dopamine receptor antagonist (L-745,870) in acutely psychotic inpatients with schizophrenia. Arch. Gen. Psychiatry. 54, 567–572.

23. Greenshaw AJ, & Silverstone PH. (1997). The non-antiemetic uses of serotonin 5-HT3 receptor antagonists. Drugs. 53, 20–39.

24. Newcomer JW, Faustman WO, Zipursky RB, & Csernansky JG. (1992). Zacopride in schizophrenia: A single-blind serotonin type 3 antagonist trial. Arch. Gen. Psychiatry. 49, 751–752.

25. Martin P, Waters N, Carlsson A, & Carlsson ML. (1997). The apparent antipsychotic action of the 5-HT2A receptor antagonist M100907 in a mouse model of schizophrenia is counteracted by ritanserin. J. Neural Transm. 104, 561–564.

26. Schreiber R, Brocco M, Audinot V, Gobert A, Veiga S, & Millan MJ. (1995). (1-(2,5-Dimethoxy-4 iodophenyl)-2-aminopropane)-induced head-twitches in the rat are mediated by 5-hydroxytryptamine(5-HT)2A receptors: Modulation by novel 5-HT2A/2C antagonists, D1 antagonists and 5-HT1A agonists. J. Pharmacol. Exp. Ther. 273, 101–112.

27. Marder SR. (1999). Limitations of dopamine-D2 antagonists and the search for novel antipsychotic strategies. Neuropsychopharmacol. 21(Suppl 6), S117–S121.

28. Meltzer HY, Arvanitis L, Bauer D, Rein W, & Meta-Trial Study Group. (2004). Placebo-controlled evaluation of four novel compounds for the treatment of schizophrenia and schizoaffective disorders. Am. J. Psychiatry. 161, 975–984.

29. Tranter R, Bell D, Gutting P, Harmer C, Healy D, & Anderson IM. (2009). The effect of serotonergic and noradrenergic antidepressants on face emotion processing in depressed patients. J. Affect. Dis. 118, 87–93.

30. Harmer CJ, Shelley NC, Cowen PJ, & Goodwin GM. (2004). Increased positive versus negative affective perception and memory in healthy volunteers following selective serotonin and norepinephrine reuptake inhibition. Am. J. Psychiatry. 161, 1256–1263.

31. Harmer C, O'Sullivan U, Favaron E, Massey-Chase R, Ayres R, Reinecke A, et al. (2009). Effect of acute antidepressant administration on negative affective bias in depressed patients. Am. J. Psychiatry. 166, 1178–1184.

32. Harmer CJ, Hill SA, Taylor MJ, Cowen PJ, & Goodwin GM. (2003). Toward a neuropsychological theory of antidepressant drug action: Increase in positive emotional bias after potentiation of norepinephrine activity. Am. J. Psychiatry. 160, 990–992.

33. Amone D, Horder J, Cowen PJ, & Harmer CJ. (2009). Early effects of mirtazapine on emotional processing. Psychopharmacol. 203, 685–691.

34. Chandra P, Hafizi S, Massey-Chase R, Goodwin GM, Cowen P, & Harmer C. (2010). NK1 receptor antagonism and emotional processing in healthy volunteers. J. Psychopharmacol. 24, 481–487.

35. Beck AT. (2005) The current state of cognitive therapy. Arch. Gen. Psychiatry. 62, 953–959.

36. Clark L, Chamberlain SR, & Sahakian BJ. (2009). Neurocognitive mechanisms in depression: Implications for treatment. Ann. Rev. Neurosci. 32, 57–74.

37. Drevets WC. (1998). Functional neuroimaging studies of depression: The anatomy of melancholia. Ann. Rev. Med. 49, 341–361.

38. Mayberg HS. (1997). Limbic-cortical dysregulation: A proposed model of depression. J. Neuropsychiatr. Clin. Neurosci. 9(3), 471–481.

39. Price JL. (1999). Prefrontal cortical networks related to visceral function and mood. Ann. N. Y. Acad. Sci. 29, 383–396.

40. Eagle DM, Bari A, & Robbins TW. (2008). The neuropsychopharmacology of action inhibition: Cross-species translation of the stop-signal and go/no-go tasks. Psychopharmacol. 199, 439–456.

41. Robinson ESJ, Eagle DM, Bannerjee G, & Robbins TW. (2006). Effects of atomoxetine on inhibitory control in the rat stop-signal task. J. Psychopharmacol. 20, A67.

42. Chamberlain SR, Muller U, Blackwell AD, Clark L, Robbins TW, & Sahakian BJ. (2006). Neurochemical modulation of response inhibition and probabilistic learning in humans. Science. 311, 861–863.

43. Chamberlain SR, del Campo N, Dowson J, Muller U, Clark L, Robbins TW, et al. (2007). Atomoxetine improved response inhibition in adults with attention deficit/hyperactivity disorder. Biol. Psychiatry. 62, 977–984.

44. Bateman RJ, Siemers ER, Mawuenyega KG, Wen G, Browning KR, Sigurdson WC, et al. (2009). A γ-secretase inhibitor decreases amyloid-β production in the central nervous system. Ann. Neurol. 66, 48–54.

45. Fleisher AS, Raman R, Siemers ER, Becerra L, Clark CM, Dean RA, et al. (2008). Phase 2 safety trial targeting amyloid β production with a γ-secretase inhibitor in Alzheimer disease. Arch. Neurol. 65, 1031–1038.

46. Henley DB, May PC, Dean RA, & Siemers ER. (2009). Development of semagacestat (LY450139), a functional γ-secretase inhibitor, for the treatment of Alzheimer's disease. Expert Opin. Pharmacother. 10, 1657–1664.

47. Bullmore E, & Sporns O. (2009). Complex brain networks: Graph theoretical analysis of structural and functional systems. Nat. Rev. 10, 186–198.

48. Ford JM, & Mathalon DH. (2008). Neural synchrony in schizophrenia. Schizophr. Bull. 34, 904–906.

49. Whittington MA, Faulkner HJ, Doheny HC, & Traub RD. (2000). Neuronal fast oscillations as a target site for psychoactive drugs. Pharmacol. Ther. 86, 171–190.

Translational Medicine in Oncology

Dominic G. Spinella

Translational medicine (TM) has many definitions in many settings, but a common theme is to take biomedical research from "bench-to- bedside" using various classes of biomarkers to speed drug-development decisions. For a variety of reasons that will be discussed in this chapter, TM and biomarkers have arguably had their greatest impact in the area of oncology. Cancer drug development differs in many ways from drug development in other therapeutic areas, and the use of biomarkers as surrogates for clinical benefit has had a long history in oncology. In this chapter, we will explore the use of various classes of biomarkers in oncologic drug development and establish some general principles and points to consider when using translational approaches to cancer therapeutics.

A biomarker is defined as "a characteristic that is measured and evaluated as an indicator of normal biological processes, pathogenic processes, or pharmacological responses to a therapeutic intervention."[1] For the purposes of this chapter, three major classes of biomarkers are defined based on how they are used in the development of cancer drugs: pharmacodynamic (PD) biomarkers, outcome biomarkers, and patient selection biomarkers.

7.1. Pharmacodynamic Biomarkers

PD biomarkers, sometimes called "target" or "mechanism" biomarkers, are largely concerned with direct biochemical or physiologic effects of drugs on their intended targets (e.g., enzyme inhibition, receptor antagonism) independent of any relationship to potential clinical benefit. PD biomarkers have two major uses in drug development: establishing dose (or dose range) and achieving "proof of mechanism" – the demonstration that a drug has hit and modulated its intended target at a tolerated dose.

Dose selection in oncology has historically been driven almost exclusively by toxicity and the concept of "maximum tolerated dose." A typical Phase 1 oncology study involves patients (only rarely healthy volunteers are included owing to the intrinsic toxicities of anticancer drugs) in what has come to be known as a "3+3 design." That is, a drug is initially given to cohorts of three patients. If no patient in a cohort experiences a dose-limiting toxicity (DLT), the dose is escalated according to a predefined schema, and a subsequent three-patient cohort is dosed at the next higher level. This escalation continues until a DLT is observed, at which time the cohort is expanded with an additional three patients. If at least one more DLT is observed in the expanded cohort, that dose is defined as the maximally administered dose, and the previous dose level is defined as the maximally tolerated dose (MTD). Otherwise, the escalation continues as before.

This process of establishing the MTD is related to several unique aspects of cancer drug development. First, Phase 2 clinical development in most other therapeutic areas is at least partly concerned with defining dose in patients. In oncology, dose is usually determined in Phase 1 in patients with any tumor type (i.e., "all-comers") – regardless of the type of cancer for which the drug is ultimately intended. Phase 2 development often uses a single dose level and regimen (most often the MTD) and is more concerned with defining the type of cancer in which the drug may be effective. Moreover, to be eligible for the trial, patients in Phase 1 trials are often among the sickest patients because they are typically first required to fail the standard therapeutic interventions and have no further approved therapeutic options. These considerations underscore another unique feature of cancer drug development: the ethical need to avoid foreclosing the possibility of clinical benefit to patients with a life-threatening disease. Patients who have other approved therapeutic options must first exhaust those options before embarking on an experimental regimen of uncertain clinical benefit. The motivation of cancer patients to participate in Phase 1 studies is largely driven by their hope for therapeutic benefit (although whether their hope is realistic is a complex and controversial issue).[2] As a consequence of these ethical constraints, placebos are virtually never used in Phase 1, and cohort sizes are relatively small compared with other therapeutic areas so as to minimize the number of patients exposed to low, and presumably subtherapeutic, drug doses. The net result, however, is that the dose of many cancer drugs is determined by the toxicity experienced by as few as two heavily pretreated patients, who are often extremely ill with metastatic or end-stage disease.

7.1.1. Traditional Phase 1 Dose Selection versus the Paradigm for Targeted Agents

The traditional Phase 1 approach is perhaps not unreasonable for the development of cytotoxic agents (which, until recently, constituted the vast majority of anticancer drugs) for a life-threatening disease. Dose selection, therefore, is largely a function of drug exposure, observed toxicity, and *projected efficacious exposure* (based on animal models of the intended tumor type and extrapolated human exposure using allometric scaling algorithms). Drugs can be terminated during the Phase 1 dose escalation studies if MTD is encountered before reaching the projected efficacious exposure; otherwise, the MTD often becomes the sole dose to explore in Phase 2. From this therapeutic perspective, more is always better: indeed, much of the practice of clinical oncology deals with mitigating the effects of high doses of cytotoxic drugs on healthy tissues such as bone marrow, gastrointestinal mucosa, and so forth. This approach, however, is clearly suboptimal for "targeted" anticancer agents. In some cases, the maximum pharmacologic (PD) effect of these drugs may be reached at doses much lower than MTD, resulting in unnecessary off-target toxicity for the patient. In addition, some drugs may produce nonlinear or even U-shaped exposure/response curves[3] in which maximal clinical benefit is achieved at some intermediate exposure beyond which clinical benefit actually decreases.

By using preclinical models, it is usually possible to determine the extent (and duration) of *PD modulation* of a drug target that is associated with efficacy and extrapolate this information for clinical studies, terminating drugs in which unacceptable toxicity is encountered at a dose lower than that necessary for sufficient modulation of the PD endpoint. Indeed, it may be that drug target modulation is a more appropriate metric than is mere drug exposure, and the relationship between PD and outcome may be better conserved between species than between drug exposure (PK) and outcome. In addition, if efficacy studies are negative and conducted at doses that do not have sufficient activity on the target, then there is still no information about the clinical validity of the drug target. The best approach is likely to incorporate both PK *and* PD data, which is why PK/PD modeling has assumed importance in early drug development. The use of PD markers both to define dose and "prove mechanism" is an important aspect of the TM approach.

In most therapeutic areas, the utility of proof of mechanism (POM) is at least debatable. Demonstration of POM has been embraced by many pharmaceutical companies in an effort to reduce the (~70%–80%) attrition rates of drugs in Phases 2 and 3)[4] and to help clinically validate novel drug targets. Most failures in Phase 2 are due to lack of clinical efficacy, the root cause of which can in principle be ascribed either to a failure of a drug to modulate its intended target or a failure of that modulation to have the intended impact on the disease in question. The latter cause may be the more important one, and, in the face of good preclinical data and reasonable clinical drug exposures, it will be relatively rare for a drug not to hit its intended target. For indications like cancers in which translational efficacy models are typically murine xenograft models with good negative but poor positive predictive value, demonstrating POM may do little to reduce attrition rates, and nothing substitutes for deep understanding of the disease and wise (or perhaps, lucky) choice of drug target.

Once again, however, oncology is a different beast because drug activity in the human tumor environment is influenced by factors difficult to predict with peripheral PK-PD models or animal models. In this context, the difference stems from the fact that many human tumors have a physiology that reduces their drug exposure. This physiology includes mechanisms such as high interstitial pressures,[5,6] expression of efflux pumps[7] and aberrant, leaky vasculature.[8] These mechanisms all conspire to reduce intratumoral drug exposure relative to that observed in normal tissues – or even the subcutaneous xenografted tumors in animal models. Moreover, the density of target expression in tumors may be much higher than that found in surrogate normal tissues, and exposures that completely agonize or antagonize a target in a surrogate tissue may have only marginal effect in tumor tissue. Hence, lack of sufficient target engagement/modulation *at the intended sites of action* (i.e., the tumor lesions themselves) may well be an important contributor to clinical failure. The implication here is that, although POM for drugs targeting abnormal pathways in tumor tissue may indeed be useful in reducing late-stage attrition of oncology agents, it cannot truly be established in surrogate tissues such as peripheral blood cells, hair follicles, or skin biopsies that are often used for this purpose. The only way to prove mechanism definitively for tumor targets in oncology is to analyze the PD effect of the drug in the tumor itself.

Unfortunately, the practical reality is that it is notoriously difficult to obtain posttreatment tumor biopsies consistently in clinical studies. For one thing, many patients do not present with readily biopsiable tumors, and patients who do are usually overrepresentative of the few tumor types (such as melanoma or head and neck cancers) in which superficial lesions are readily accessible. In any case, patients are often reluctant to participate in trials that require invasive or uncomfortable serial biopsies, and the inclusion of these biopsies as requirements of study protocols can dramatically slow enrollment. What, then, is the answer to this quandary? Certainly, one should obtain voluntary biopsies wherever possible and perform PD assays on these tissues. A more useful approach, however, may reside in the judicious use of outcome biomarkers.

7.2. Outcome Biomarkers

An outcome or mechanism-based biomarker with medium or high linkage to clinical outcomes can be used as a surrogate for clinical benefit – if not for registration purposes, then at least for internal program decisions and prioritization. In contrast to other therapeutic areas, oncology drug development has long relied on what is essentially such an outcome biomarker: Response Evaluation Criteria in Solid Tumors (RECIST) and its World Health Organization (WHO) antecedent. RECIST is simply a series of rules for the interpretation of radiographic images of changes in tumor size. Drug-induced reduction in tumor size is an imperfect surrogate for the true registration endpoint of survival, but it is widely used as a Phase 2 endpoint in a variety of guises, depending on the cancer under study, from response rate (the proportion of patients achieving at least a minimum regression in tumor size typically defined as >30% reduction in the sum of longest diameters of target lesions determined by computerized tomography [CT] or magnetic resonance imaging [MRI]) to progression-free survival (the length of time to radiographic progression usually defined as a >20% increase in the sum of the longest diameters, or death, whichever comes first). A full description of RECIST and its various iterations and uses is beyond the scope of this chapter,[9] but changes in tumor size (or stabilization of tumor size and prevention of growth) have long served as biomarkers to predict clinical outcome, substituting for the lengthy survival endpoints usually required for drug registration. In reality, the relationship between RECIST parameters and true survival benefit is quite variable by tumor type and may be more appropriate to the development of cytotoxic agents than to the current generation of targeted therapies. Certainly, there are many instances of clinical benefit without tumor regression and of tumor regression without concomitant prolongation of survival:[10] nevertheless, RECIST remains commonly used as a clinical endpoint.

Regardless of its relationship to survival, tumor regression or stabilization does not occur instantly upon drug exposure, and response rate or progression studies, although faster than survival studies, still take a good deal of time. This has led to efforts to develop or conscript other outcome biomarkers, especially imaging tools, that allow visualization of effects directly in tumor lesions and in which drug effects can be seen more quickly. From a purely theoretical perspective, and regardless of their proximate molecular etiology, virtually all cancer drugs ultimately work by one or more of five mechanisms: They inhibit tumor metabolism, inhibit tumor proliferation, induce tumor apoptosis/necrosis, enhance antitumor immunity, or – in the case of antiangiogenics – reduce intratumoral vascular density and permeability. A common thread among four of these mechanisms is that they are at least potentially measurable by noninvasive imaging techniques such as positron emission tomography with tracers like ^{18}F-fluorodeoxyglucose (^{18}F-FDG PET) or ^{18}F-3-fluoro-3-deoxy-L-thymidine (FLT), diffusion-weighted or dynamic contrast MRI scans, and a host of other imaging technologies in various stages of development. Antitumor immune effector mechanisms may also result in similar changes detectable by these imaging modalities.

These kinds of biomarkers essentially provide functional or biological images of a tumor as opposed to the anatomical images provided by traditional CT or MRI scans that form the basis of RECIST evaluations of objective response. Imaging modalities, such as FDG-PET, are already widely used clinically to evaluate patients and, in some tumors, may be more related to ultimate survival endpoints than are the traditional RECIST endpoints. More important, drug-induced changes in these biological imaging endpoints are often detectable far in advance of anatomical changes to the tumor – often soon after initial dosing of the therapeutic compound – and presage ultimate response to therapy in a variety of tumor types (see a review[11]).

Although there are clearly both technical and operational barriers to the immediate clinical application of some of these imaging modalities (e.g., low or extremely variable baseline uptake of tracer, poor availability of newer technology, intrinsic variation in the measures), in theory at least, it ought to be possible to use one or more of them as biomarkers to *infer* POM provided that these are first validated in preclinical models and that the methods are qualified in humans. These biological imaging methods are noninvasive, and they can be employed across all doses and even sometimes at multiple time points in the same patient. Preclinical biomarker development for imaging endpoints involves defining *which* of the imaging modalities is most appropriate for the drug in question, *when* is the optimal time after dosing to use it, and *what* the relationship is between the imaging endpoint and the actual target modulation in the tumor.

Circulating tumor cells (CTCs) and, to a lesser extent, circulating endothelial cells and circulating tumor deoxyribonucleic acid (DNA) are also emerging as potential substrates for PD and outcome biomarkers to assess drug effects in some tumor types. CTCs in particular are receiving a great deal of attention in many cancers. Although there is some question as to how representative CTCs are relative to intact tumor tissue, in some cases such cells may constitute an alternative to biopsy as a source of tissue for assessing PD biomarkers. At present, the use of CTCs for molecular studies (as opposed to merely enumerating them as a potential outcome biomarker) is limited by their low numbers and resultant difficulties in reproducibly isolating sufficient quantities of cells. Moreover, their utility in assessing drug pharmacodynamics is questionable because their presence in the peripheral circulation likely exposes them to far higher drug concentration than is achieved in the parent tumor. Nevertheless, new technologies[12] have the potential to increase the utility of CTCs as tumor biomarkers.

7.3. Patient Selection Biomarkers

The development of biomarkers to stratify patient populations into those who should or should not receive a given drug has received much attention in recent years and has probably had its most dramatic impact to date in oncology. Such a marker, or sometimes a composite or "signature" of multiple markers, is intended to identify those patients who are more or less likely to respond to (or experience adverse effects) from a drug, facilitating a "personalized medicine" approach to drug treatment. At the outset, it is perhaps useful to make two underappreciated points about personalized medicine. First, the idea that individual patients should have access to drugs that are especially likely to benefit their unique genotypic and disease characteristics is both attractive and almost diametrically opposed to another popular trend: Comparative Effectiveness Research, in which competing therapies are compared and only those with the highest *average* benefit across the patient population as a whole are made available (by placement on formularies if not outright approvals). It is not uncommon to hear health care pundits embrace both concepts without apparently recognizing this intrinsic contradiction.

Second, because it is possible to develop a biomarker predictor of efficacy does not mean that it is necessarily useful from either an economic or a drug development perspective. I argue that an empirical approach (give the drug blindly and see if it works) always trumps a biomarker-driven approach unless one of two conditions holds: (1) it takes a long time or is very expensive to know whether the drug has produced clinical benefit, or (2) the toxicity of the drug is such that patients should avoid exposure unless a priori probability of clinical benefit is reasonable. These conditions are typical for oncology drugs, which is why patient selection biomarker approaches have made the greatest inroads here.

To date, most of the examples of patient selection biomarkers in approved oncology drug labels, such as Her2/Neu levels for use of trastuzumab, estrogen receptor levels for use of tamoxifen or aromatase inhibitors in breast cancer, or UGT1A1 variants for use of irinotecan in colon cancer (from the U.S. Food and Drug Administration [FDA] Web site of validated genomic biomarkers: http://www.fda.gov/cder/genomics/genomic_biomarkers_table.htm), would seem to be relatively obvious from a pharmacologic perspective. A patient whose tumor does not express the presumed drug target is unlikely to respond to the drug, and a patient with low expression (or a poorly active variant) of a drug-metabolizing enzyme is more likely to be overexposed to drugs that are eliminated by that enzyme. These propositions are hardly surprising, although in the face of quantitative variation in target expression levels it is not always easy to know where to draw the treat/withhold line. Such biomarkers, however, typically account for only a fraction of the variability in drug responsiveness or toxicity. It is much more difficult to elucidate molecular factors that are not so directly related either to variations in target expression or structure or to polymorphisms in metabolizing enzymes involved in clearance. Nevertheless, apart from the obvious benefit of avoiding exposure to unhelpful or harmful drugs, the utility of such markers in oncology drug development is the increased probability of registrational success in studies of smaller subpopulations in which the average clinical benefit is higher and the trial costs are correspondingly lower.

The enthusiasm for developing biomarker approaches to patient selection is driven in part by the availability of new technologies that enable relatively rapid discovery of molecular markers that are at least correlated with drug response phenotypes. These hypothesis-independent approaches to biomarker discovery are widely used. Many clinical studies in oncology collect tumor or blood samples from as many subjects as possible for gene expression, mutation/polymorphism analysis, proteomic analysis, and so forth, to establish correlations with eventual clinical outcome. Putative biomarkers or predictive signatures resulting from such analyses in small numbers of patients must be considered, however, as no more than *hypotheses* that need to be tested in appropriately designed follow-up studies. This, in turn, often results in the process of biomarker qualification and validation lagging behind the drug development program it is intended to support. Often, the identification of a predictive biomarker is only made by retrospective analysis of postmarket studies (e.g., K-RAS for prediction of response to epidermal growth factor receptor [EGFR] inhibitors in colon cancer).[13,14] Of course, for drugs that fail pivotal studies despite achieving efficacy in a subset, that is a bit too late!

A key phrase in the previous paragraph is "appropriately designed," and, unfortunately, many biomarker hypotheses are never adequately tested because they are "grafted" onto other clinical studies that are not designed to test the biomarker hypothesis. A common mistake is to test the drug only in the subset of "marker+" patients in which efficacy is predicted, avoiding exposure of patients who are not expected to respond. Apart from the obvious fact that it is impossible to test a hypothesis by assuming it is true (what if the drug would have worked just as well in marker− patients?), such a design also gives rise to a common problem: failure to distinguish between a *predictive* and a *prognostic* marker. A predictive marker is one that is associated with response or lack of response to a particular therapy, whereas a prognostic marker is associated with clinical outcome regardless of therapy (i.e., it is a predictor of the natural history of the disease independent of treatment). It is not uncommon for molecular markers to have both prognostic and predictive effects (e.g., Her2 level is a positive predictive marker for trastuzumab treatment but has negative prognostic value, i.e., women with Her2+ breast cancer do somewhat worse than their negative sisters)[15], and the only way this distinction can be teased out is with a trial design that exposes both populations to drug plus standard of care versus standard of care alone.

7.4. Putting It All Together: The Translational Approach

7.4.1. Preclinical Work

The TM approach to drug development fundamentally involves asking three sets of questions.

- How do I know my drug has hit its intended target (and hit it hard enough)?
- What can I do to increase or decrease confidence quickly in the efficacy and safety of my drug early in clinical development?
- What patient population constitutes the best test of potential efficacy (i.e., if it doesn't "work" here, it is unlikely to work anywhere else)?

These questions need to be embedded in the drug discovery/development process well before the first patient is dosed. The last question is perhaps the first one that needs to be considered: given the chosen target, what cancer is most likely to respond? Answering this question will usually involve analysis of tumor cell lines, patient tumor samples, and so forth, to determine where the target is and is not in play. Here too is where the discovery of patient selection markers must begin. Of the tumors that appear to express the target, are there some *that* respond better than others? Poorly responsive tumors (either in vitro or in xenografts) are often ignored, but they can be informative in helping to generate a molecular hypothesis for nonresponsiveness. Are there polymorphisms or variations in the target or pathway that are associated with responsiveness or lack thereof? The time to begin the –omics work to establish molecular correlates of good and poor response that can be tested later in the clinic is during the preclinical phase and perhaps during Phase 1 by selecting different tumor types with needed molecular characteristics. Generating such hypotheses in Phase 2 is usually too late, although it may still be useful for backup programs.

Translation of in vitro and animal data to humans in an effort to establish how the drug will be evaluated in the clinic should also be conducted prior to Phase 1 evaluation. What level of target modulation is associated with efficacy in the models? How much drug exposure do I need to achieve it? How will I know I have attained this level of target modulation in patients? Are biopsies feasible for the intended tumor type? Have I worked out the reagents and operating characteristics of the assays that will be needed in the clinic? Are there alternative modalities (imaging, CTCs, etc.), and how are those endpoints quantitatively affected by my drug in the models? These translational questions will profoundly affect the design of the clinical studies to come, and they need to be addressed years before the human studies begin. All of these types of questions should be answered as part of the biomarker qualification program for a new cancer drug.

7.4.2. The Phase 1 Study

As always, the primary goal of a Phase 1 study is to ascertain safety and tolerability and to define MTD. An "all-comers" patient study (i.e., enrolling patients with any tumor type) is standard here, but of course not all tumors may be appropriate for assessing PD/target modulation. It is useful then to consider an expanded cohort Phase 1b study of perhaps 10 to 20 patients with the appropriate tumor type, molecular profile, or both (as defined in the preclinical work) in which to assess target modulation at the MTD. A good example of such a study was the evaluation of PF-02341066, a dual inhibitor of mesenchymal epithelial transition growth factor (c-Met) and anaplastic lymphoma kinase (ALK), which induced tumor shrinkage in 10 of 19 patients with non-small cell lung carcinoma (NSCLC) bearing the ALK translocation[16] in a Phase 1b study and was used as the basis for initiating a pivotal Phase 3 study of the drug for this indication. If a biopsy is necessary to establish the presence and primacy of the drug target, one can often employ archival biopsy samples (by and large, no one receives a diagnosis of cancer without an initial biopsy, and these biopsies are often archived – at least as paraffin-embedded, formalin-fixed samples). These archival samples can be used to assess mutational status, transcriptional overexpression, or, in some cases, protein expression level of the intended drug target.

The size of this Phase 1b study will depend on the intrinsic variation of the PD endpoint and its assay, but it need not be powered for traditional statistical significance. Depending on individual risk tolerance, one might assert that the target has been sufficiently modulated (POM achieved) if the defined preclinical level is reached with a P value of, say, 0.2. In the absence of either overt clinical benefit (as with PF-02341066) or evidence of sufficient target modulation in the expanded cohort, serious thought needs to be given about whether to continue the clinical program. This decision requires a surprising degree of discipline, for most projects that reach this stage of development have a "constituency," and terminating a drug development project this early is not easy. If Phase 2 or 3 drug failures can be considered type 1 errors (false positives), then abandoning a potentially effective drug in Phase 1 constitutes a type 2 error (false negative). Most project teams have nearly infinite tolerance for type 1 error but near zero tolerance for type 2 – despite the demonstrable frequency (~80%) of type 1 errors in late-stage clinical development. As any statistician will attest, however, type 1 and type 2 errors are inversely related, and, if one is serious about reducing the occurrence of the former, one must accept an increased probability of the latter!

7.4.3. The Phase 2 Study

Numerous articles have been written about Phase 2 study design in oncology and about the relative merits of historically controlled versus randomized trials, stage migration, appropriate endpoints, and so forth (for review[17]). From the perspective of this chapter, Phase 2 is the place to formally test any patient selection biomarker hypotheses that have emerged. Such testing will usually require that a putative predictive marker or signature be used to stratify patients into treatment and control arms, ensuring appropriate numbers of marker[+] and marker[−] patients in each arm. The primary endpoint of such a study may involve RECIST, other outcome biomarkers to predict efficacy, or both, but at least part of its goal is to verify or refute the biomarker hypothesis; to establish whether the marker is predictive, prognostic, or both (or neither); and to elucidate the magnitude of any predictive effect, either positive or negative. If the outcome of such a Phase 2 study points to clinical qualification or evidence of high linkage of the biomarker to clinical outcome, it becomes important to consider whether and how the biomarker will be further qualified for incorporation into a potential drug label and to continue working toward technical validation of the biomarker assay in preparation for development of a companion diagnostic, if required.

A second item to consider in the Phase 2 study is whether dose ranging is potentially useful or whether MTD will dictate the Phase 3 dose. In part, this determination will depend on the nature and clinical manageability of the dose-limiting toxicities. If MTD is much higher than the projected efficacious exposure, or if PD modulation at MTD is on a plateau of the dose-response curve and higher than required for efficacy in preclinical models, there is good rationale for at least exploring a lower dose range in subsequent studies – especially if toxicities are severe.

7.5. Conclusions

TM is more a way of thinking about drug development than it is a standalone discipline because it requires expertise and integration across several disciplines. Oncology drug development in particular has been among the most difficult of any therapeutic area with an estimated 50% attrition rate in Phase 3[4] – precisely the stage in which costs are highest. Cancer is a heterogeneous and complex disease, and it is no surprise that developing effective therapies is difficult, expensive, and often fraught with failure. The early adoption of translational thinking is really an effort to bring a level of scientific discipline and rigor to the process. We can no longer afford the time and expense involved in relying on standard clinical outcomes in Phase 2b and 3 clinical trials to make decisions. As drug discovery establishments, we are, quite simply, failing unsustainably. It is no longer enough to produce an experimental drug against a novel target and "throw it over the wall" to a standard clinical development paradigm. Along with the drug we need a way to evaluate it quickly in patients and a way to know which patients are most likely to derive benefit. This is what TM is trying to provide, and in no therapeutic area are the stakes higher than in oncology.

7.6. References

1. Biomarkers Definitions Working Group. (2001). Biomarkers and surrogate endpoints: Preferred definitions and conceptual framework. Clin. Pharmacol. Ther. 69, 89–95.
2. Horstmann E, McCabe MS, Grochow L, Yamamoto S, Rubinstein L, Budd T, et al. (2005). Risks and benefits of phase 1 oncology trials, 1991 through 2002. N. Engl. J. Med. 352, 895–904.
3. Calabrese EJ. (2005). Cancer biology and hormesis: Human tumor cell lines commonly display hormetic (biphasic) dose responses. Crit. Rev. Toxicol. 35(6), 463–582.
4. Kola I, & Landis J. (2004). Can the pharmaceutical industry reduce attrition rates? Nat. Rev. Drug Discovery. 3, 711–716.
5. Heldin C-H, Rubin K, Pietras K, & Östman A. (2004). High interstitial fluid pressure – an obstacle in cancer therapy. Nat. Rev. Cancer. 4, 806–813.
6. Jain RK. (1998). The next frontier of molecular medicine: Delivery of therapeutics. Nat. Med. 4, 655–657.
7. Fletcher JI, Haber M, Henderson MJ, & Norris MD. (2010). ABC transporters in cancer: More than just drug efflux pumps. Nat. Rev. Cancer. 10, 147–156.
8. Munn LL. (2003). Aberrant vascular architecture in tumors and its importance in drug-based therapies. DDT 8 (9), 396–403.
9. Therasse P, Arbuck SG, Eisenhauer EA, Wanders J, Kaplan RS, Rubinstein L, et al. (2000). New guidelines to evaluate the response to treatment in solid tumors: European Organization for Research and Treatment of Cancer, National Cancer Institute of the United States, National Cancer Institute of Canada. J. Natl. Cancer Inst. 92, 205–216.
10. Michaelis LC, & Ratain MJ. (2006). Measuring response in a post-RECIST world: From black and white to shades of grey. Nat. Rev. Cancer. 6, 409–414.
11. Hillner BE, Siegel BA, Shields AF, Liu D, Gareen IF, Hunt E, et al. (2008). Relationship between cancer type and impact of PET and PET/CT on intended management: Findings of the National Oncologic PET Registry. J. Nuclear Med. 49(12), 1928–1935.
12. Nagrath S, Sequist LV, Maheswaran S, Bell DW, Irimia D, Ulkus L, et al. (2007). Microchip-based isolation of rare circulating epithelial cells in cancer patients. Nature. 450, 1235–1239.
13. Amado RG, Wolf M, Peeters M, Van Cutsem E, Siena S, Freeman DJ, et al. (2008). Wild-type KRAS is required for panitumumab efficacy in patients with metastatic colorectal cancer. J. Clin. Oncol. 26, 1626–1634.
14. Khambata-Ford S, Garrett CR, Meropol NJ, Basik M, Harbison CT, Wu S, et al. (2007). Expression of epiregulin and amphiregulin and K-ras mutation status predict disease control in metastatic colorectal cancer patients treated with cetuximab. J. Clin. Oncol. 25, 3230–3237.

15. Ross JS, & Fletcher JA. (1999). The HER-2/Neu oncogene: Prognostic factor, predictive factor and target for therapy. Semin. Cancer Biol. 9(2), 125–138.
16. Kwak EL, Camidge DR, Clark J, Shapiro GI, Maki RG, Ratain MJ, et al. (2009). Clinical activity observed in a phase I dose escalation trial of an oral c-met and ALK inhibitor, PF-02341066. Journal of Clinical Oncology, ASCO Annual Meeting Proceedings. 27(15S), 3509.
17. Ratain MJ, & Sargent DJ. (2009). Optimising the design of phase II oncology trials: The importance of randomization. Eur. J. Cancer. 45, 275–280.

Biomarkers and Public–Private Partnerships

Discovery, development, and validation of biomarkers for use in early development to aid decision making are critical activities for translational medicine scientists. In the past, pharmaceutical companies attempted to create a competitive advantage for themselves by using biomarkers to reduce costs and improve productivity. Although these activities often must remain proprietary, biomarkers for some uses require external acceptance, and sponsors can benefit from sharing development costs. For these reasons, companies have recently come to the realization that much of this work can be done in the precompetitive space. This is especially true in the area of safety biomarkers and outcome biomarkers, where external acceptance of validity is critical to their value.

In this section, we describe the basic concepts involved in the process of biomarker validation within the proprietary space of early drug development and then provide three examples of organizational structures in which precompetitive partnerships for biomarker development projects can be created and executed.

Biomarker Validation and Application in Early Drug Development: Idea to Proof of Concept

Pfizer Global Research and Development 2004

Editors' Note: In 2004, Pfizer leadership sponsored the creation of a confidential "Biomarker Best Practices" document by a cross-discipline and cross-development team of experts that we would today call a "translational research team" or "advisory group." This work was completed, and Pfizer decided also to produce a public version with the goal of establishing a common view of biomarker definitions, development, validation, and application in drug development. The following chapter was extracted from this public version of Pfizer's "Biomarker Best Practices" document. The editors are grateful for Pfizer's permission to publish it in this book.

The contributors to this document were Michael Bleavins, John Castledine, Joseph C. Fleishaker, Scott Fountain, Frank Hermann, David Lester, Bruce H. Littman, Frank Marcoux, Patrice M. Milos, Damian O'Connell, David Slavin, and Stephen A. Williams.

The Pfizer leadership sponsors of this work were Jim Bristol, Kelvin Cooper, Jeffrey Ives, Diane Jorkasky, Martin Mackay, and Jack Reynolds.

8.1. Definitions and Summary of Overarching Principles

Before beginning a discussion of best practices, we establish a consistent language and new ways of classifying biomarkers so that there is less room for confusion: the "biomarker lexicon." Key definitions and issues include the following:

- Definition of a biomarker as "a characteristic that is measured and evaluated as an indicator of normal biologic processes, pathogenic processes, or pharmacological responses to a therapeutic intervention." [agreement with NIH definition]
- New definition of validation as "characterization of the biomarker that demonstrates to the user, its fitness for a specific purpose."

- New description of three types of biomarkers: Target, Mechanism, or Outcome and new qualitative assessment of the linkage of each of the three types of biomarker with a Clinical Outcome measure (high/medium/low) [Editors' note: See definitions in Chapter 1 (Section 1.1) of this book].
- Description of four phases of the biomarker lifecycle: pathfinding, research, development, and application

We do not reiterate in depth the original business case for biomarkers – to reduce the cost and increase the value of decisions – but we do discuss business.

The following latent assumptions are exposed:

- Any uncertainty from using a biomarker earlier does not lead to an intolerable increase in probability of a wrong decision.
- The expense of developing the biomarker does not erase the financial advantage.

We also establish some principles that maximize the value of biomarkers:

- Optimize biomarker investment choices based on return on investment (ROI) and team demand.
- Focus biomarker R&D on making biomarkers fit for purpose in the areas with best return on investment.
- Use biomarkers in every instance they can deliver better (or equivalent) decisions at lower cost.
- Do not use new biomarkers when there is no economic benefit versus existing measures or the risk is intolerable.
- Define, monitor, and achieve acceptable biomarker quality during application in drug development.
- Consider additional benefits as a potential product diagnostic or quid for licensing candidates and other biomarkers.

We define an optimal approach to biomarker validation as follows:

- Define the specific purpose(s) of the biomarker and create the plan to evaluate fitness for that purpose.
- Examine the hypothetical impact of making a false decision (business impact if false = BIIF). A high BIIF drives intolerance to uncertainty and increased rigor of validation. If the BIIF is not high, there is a greater tolerance for uncertainty about the biomarker, and it can be used at a more immature stage of its lifecycle.
- Select the appropriate technical validation attributes that should be evaluated to understand all sources of technical noise, biological variation, and biological signal – to the degree of rigor appropriate to the BIIF.

- Create "minimally acceptable criteria" (biomarker "MAC") and decision rules in advance as a part of the biomarker validation plan for each purpose and evaluate the biomarker against them.

We explain how the new validation principles can be applied to optimize planning for decision points in drug development – for exploratory development candidate selection, for confirmation of pharmacodynamics, decisions to proceed to

Phase 1 and utility within Phase 2.

Finally, we provide principles that will enable biomarker developers to optimize selection of biomarker investments, taking into account return on investment, team demand, technical opportunism, and portfolio balance. We also provide guidance on optimization of strategic planning for biomarkers.

8.2. Biomarker Validation Terminology

Additional teminnology includes the following:

- *Validation:* Characterization of the biomarker that demonstrates to the user its fitness for a specific purpose.
- *Technical validation:* The process of selecting all technical attributes that are required for the demonstration of fitness for the purpose, setting appropriate performance requirements for each attribute, and evaluating the biomarker against these requirements. Examples of some of the elements of the technical evaluation process that may be required are demonstrations of selectivity/specificity, accuracy, precision, responsiveness to pharmacology or disease, and robustness of all necessary procedures and assay steps under conditions similar to those that will be encountered in use (e. g., in a clinical methods study, sample storage stability and matrix effects are considered).
- *Biomarker Translation:* The activities needed to ensure that the biomarker (assay and underlying biology) is valid between different preclinical species, between preclinical species and humans, or between all of them.
- *Validity:* This is the existence of a technical validation package and a perception by the user that the biomarker is sufficiently competent to be fit for the intended purpose and there is a perceived understanding by the customer of how it should be used for making a decision.

Note: the term *clinical validation* is considered misleading and is discouraged. The term is nonspecific and can confuse clinical use of the biomarker with how the process of establishing the degree of linkage

Fig. 8.1
Elements of biomarker validation.

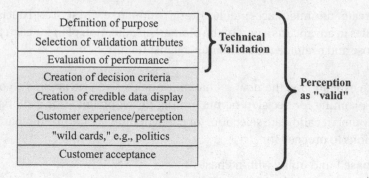

to clinical outcomes was undertaken. The process of clinical evaluation should lead to validation of the biomarker for use in humans and an accurate classification of the biomarker using the Linkage to Outcome (Human Efficacy/Safety) Scale (low, medium, or high).

8.3. Stages of Biomarker Lifecycle

Just as it is convenient to have stage definitions for drugs, this is also true for biomarkers to facilitate understanding of how far a biomarker has to go to become applicable to its purpose and as a framework to describe the most appropriate types of activities that should be taking place. To move from one stage of biomarker development to the next requires satisfying "stage-gate" criteria.

Pathfinding is the earliest stage of technical development, but not all biomarkers start in it. A biomarker starts life in this stage if it is invented as a technique but an appropriate purpose is not yet clear and objectives are not defined. The objective of experimentation in this stage is to evaluate multiple opportunities and learn what the technique would be good for. At this stage, if an invention has been made it must be discussed with the therapeutic area (TA) leaders and intellectual property attorney to review if a patent should be applied for. Once the objectives are defined and hypotheses stated, the stage-gate criteria are satisfied and the biomarker project can move into the next phase of development.

Research is the second stage of biomarker development in which objectives can be defined, including requirements for proof of concept and an outline of the biomarker minimal acceptable criteria (MAC). Biomarkers invented for a specific purpose start their life here. The aim is to reach a basic proof of concept for the biomarker in the species of application or to terminate efficiently. Uncertainty may be high. The biomarker should be reviewed for "freedom to operate" (FTO) and a decision made if any possible third-party infringements are identified. This may be accomplished by seeking a license or developing a work around. Once the proof of concept criteria are satisfied in the species in which the biomarker will be used, the biomarker project satisfies the stage-gate criteria for next phase of development.

Development is the third stage in which proof of concept has been reached and issues of practicality, cost, and performance are evaluated. At this stage, the MAC document becomes much more detailed and the biomarker is prospectively evaluated against it. Any intellectual property (IP) aspects should be included in the overall risk/benefit analysis and any potential license payments included in the project costs. Once the minimally acceptable criteria for the biomarker are fulfilled, the project meets requirements to move into the final stage.

Application is the stage after the minimally acceptable criteria have been fulfilled and the biomarker is used for its purpose. The emphasis is on incremental improvements in performance, cost reduction, and management of quality. A biomarker that is in this stage for one purpose may still be in an earlier stage for a different purpose – with a different MAC.

Box 8.1. Key Points

- The objective of this document is to provide performance guidance for biomarkers that is consistent, straightforward, and applicable across sites, lines, and teams and that optimizes the biomarker value proposition. To achieve these objectives it is important that consistent language be used throughout Pfizer.

- A biomarker may be defined as "a characteristic that is measured and evaluated as an indicator of normal biologic processes, pathogenic processes, or pharmacological responses to a therapeutic intervention."

- For applications in drug development, all biomarkers should be classified in two dimensions, (1) the type of biomarker [target, mechanism, or outcome] and (2) the degree of linkage of the biomarker to efficacy or safety outcomes in humans. This new classification should be used when describing biomarkers being developed and deployed.

- Outcome biomarkers always require some degree of linkage to an efficacy or safety outcome to be useful. For target and mechanism biomarkers, the importance of linkage to clinical outcome depends on the purpose – linkage may be irrelevant or important. All biomarker development and use must be guided by the principle of being "fit-for-purpose" and linked to how the biomarker will be used strategically in the development plan.

- The term *clinical validation* is considered misleading and is discouraged. The term is nonspecific and can confuse clinical use of the biomarker with clinical experiments to establish validity.
- Four phases of the biomarker lifecycle can be consistently described: (1) "pathfinding" – seeking the objectives and purpose, (2) "research" – seeking proof of concept in the species of application, (3) "development" – seeking evaluation of the MAC, and (4) "application" – use of the biomarker for the purpose for which the MAC was developed.

8.4. Why Biomarkers?

Fig. 8.2
Tradeoffs that optimize biomarker value during the biomarker lifecycle from "Pathfinding" to "Application."

The business case has been discussed in many other documents and will not be reexamined in this chapter in detail. However, very few documents have examined how the business value can be optimized or what tradeoffs must be managed. (See Figure 8.2). This is the purpose of this section, and it is completed by a new set of high-level principles. (See also Box 8.2.)

The intent of developing and applying new biomarkers is to reduce the cost and increase the value of decisions, either by making such decisions earlier in drug development or by reducing study size or duration.

Tradeoffs that optimize biomarker value during the biomarker lifecycle from "Pathfinding" to "Application"

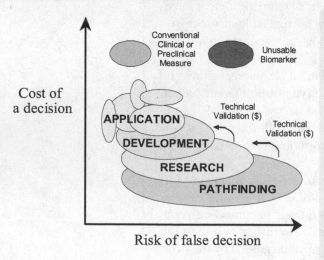

Explaining the Graph.

o The degree of uncertainty in true cost or risk is represented by the size of the oval.

o Conventional endpoints or existing biomarkers [represented by the top left-hand oval] carry a certain degree of risk and may have a high cost (usually in size and duration of trials).

o When biomarker investment starts [represented by the large "Pathfinding" oval], there is great uncertainty about the performance; thus, the oval is wide. The overall cost is low versus the conventional endpoint because little money has been invested.

o As research funds are spent on the biomarker, the cost of technical validation contributes to the decision cost and the ovals move upward.

o If technical validation is successful at reducing uncertainty and reducing the risk of a wrong decision, the ovals get smaller and are displaced to the left as biomarkers pass from "Research" into "Development."

o When sufficiently valid to be usable ["Application" biomarkers' ovals], a variety of risk/cost/uncertainty profiles are acceptable for various applications (multiple ovals).

o Thus, cost and risk are traded off against each other, and compared with the conventional endpoint or pre-existing biomarker

o A biomarker may be unusable (oval) if it does not reduce the cost of a decision but increases uncertainty.

A biomarker may serve multiple purposes as another source of value (e.g., one biomarker may reduce Phase 2 attrition, confirm confidence in rationale of a novel target for Discovery, and aid dose selection in Phase 2).

However, to be successful, this strategy has some latent assumptions that must be addressed:

- Any increased uncertainty from applying a biomarker does not lead to an intolerably increased probability of a wrong decision.
- The expense of developing the biomarker does not erase the financial advantage versus existing approaches.
- The biomarker must be available in time for the intended use in the program.

Box 8.2. Key Points That Guide Biomarker Best Practices

- Biomarker investment choices should be optimized to deliver the highest perceived business value per unit cost.
- The return on investment should be maximized by promoting acceptance of biomarker decisions, use multiple times across programs, and translation between clinical/preclinical lines.
- R&D of the biomarker should be balanced so that technical validation resources are not wasted and are focused on managing performance or uncertainty for the decision to which the biomarker is to be applied.
- Biomarkers should be used in every instance in which they can deliver decisions at lower cost, earlier timing, higher commercial value capture, or realize all of these advantages and when the level of uncertainty/risk is tolerable. Biomarkers should not be used when, there is no economic benefit or the level of uncertainty/risk is intolerable.
- Acceptable biomarker quality during application in drug development must be defined, measured, and achieved. This depends on all factors that can influence the acquisition, handling, and interpretation of data.

Practical implications of these points for early development leaders:

- Teams will need guidance on defining optimal investments.
- Teams will need guidance to optimize management of biomarker performance and uncertainty.
- Teams will need guidance to determine when they should or should not use biomarkers and how to define and manage risk.
- Teams will need guidance on how to determine what "acceptable" quality is for their application.

8.5. Biomarker Validation

The objective of developing and applying new biomarkers is to reduce the cost of decisions, either by making such decisions earlier in drug development or by reducing study size or duration. All biomarker development and use must be guided by the principle of being "fit-for-purpose" and linked to how the biomarker will be used strategically in the development plan.

When it has been determined that biomarker research should be carried out, the following activities should take place. These are discussed in sequential order in the subsections of this chapter.

[8.5.1] Define the specific purpose(s) of the biomarker:
- creates a foundation for all other questions

[8.5.2] Examine the business impact of making a wrong decision:
- sets the appropriate level of risk tolerance for all other questions

[8.5.3] Select appropriate technical validation attributes:
- defines what elements of performance must be assessed

[8.5.4] Create the biomarker MAC [minimally acceptable criteria] and appropriate decision criteria:
- sets the limits for minimum performance

8.5.1. Define the Specific Purpose(s) of the Biomarker

PRINCIPLE: Define a clear purpose or set of purposes prior to planning biomarker validation; purpose must relate the science to the decision being made.

There are two main reasons why purpose is particularly important:

- Purpose drives evidence gathering – specifying the very nature of biomarker research and defining proof of concept.
- Purpose drives performance – the "how good is good enough" question.

8.5.1.1. Relevance to Evidence Gathering

The purpose of a biomarker is directly analogous to a labeled "therapeutic indication" for a drug. Thus, a biomarker can have more than one purpose (just as a drug can have more than one indication), but just like drugs, the supporting evidence for each purpose/indication is often quite different, and a biomarker can be in different phases of its evolution for different purposes.

Table 8.1. Examining the Business Impact of Making a Wrong Decision: Examples Using Screening Diagnostic Biomarkers

Biomarker	Purpose	Consequences of False Positive	Consequences of False Negative	Message
Prostate Specific Antigen (PSA)	Screen for prostate cancer	Subject gets an unnecessary transrectal ultrasound and biopsy	Subject presents later with more advanced disease and greater risk of death	Moderate tolerance for false positives, but low tolerance for false negatives
Frozen section breast pathology	Intrasurgical verdict on malignancy	Subject gets an unnecessary mastectomy	Subject presents later with more advanced disease and greater risk of death	Low tolerance to any false result
Mammography	Screen for breast cancer	Subject gets an unnecessary breast biopsy	Subject presents later with more advanced disease and greater risk of death	Moderate tolerance for false positives but low tolerance for false negatives

8.5.1.2. Relevance to Performance

Diagnostics used as screening tools provide excellent illustrations of the point that different purposes underpin corresponding performance requirements (see Table 8.1).

8.5.2. Examine the Business Impact of Making a Wrong Decision

8.5.2.1. Key Principles

The following principles guide the rigor of biomarker validation:

- The key driver for biomarker performance is the *seriousness* of the business impact of making a false decision (BIIF).
- Teams should carefully evaluate the BIIF as a key part of planning biomarker validation.
- If the BIIF is high, the performance of a new biomarker (diligent estimate of false positive or false negative risk) must be no worse than the best available existing measure.

These principles will help drug development teams understand for themselves whether they could/should be "aggressive" [risk tolerant] or "conservative" [requiring more validation rigor and evidence] when developing and applying a biomarker for their situation. It is important to note the following:

8.5.2.1.1. Initiating New Biomarker Research Is Unlikely to Change the Consequence of a Wrong Decision but Will Reduce the Probability of Making a Wrong Decision

Individual circumstances will determine whether a BIIF is high. Making a false assertion that a drug is clinically safe could have a high BIIF, but equally it could be low if the safety issue is minor and would not harm subjects or affect commercialization. Similarly, termination of a viable candidate in the clinic will often have a high BIIF, but it could be moderate/low if there are multiple backups or if the portfolio is unusually rich so that application of resources to other projects would deliver a good return. The individual circumstances must be determined by the team and agreed to by the governing body.

For biomarkers that have application to multiple projects, a generic estimate of BIIF should be made to underwrite appropriate validation planning. When such biomarkers are to be applied for an individual project, the BIIF should be reevaluated for those specific circumstances. This is analogous to a physician's evaluations when prescribing a drug for an individual patient, although a label for the population already exists. If the individual circumstances are substantially different from the generic estimate, then more or less variability/risk can be allowed as appropriate (e.g., if the existence of a close backup reduces the impact of a false termination decision, the changing sample size could be reduced or decision criteria made less stringent).

8.5.2.1.2. Practical Implications of Applying These Principles

- The principles replace the supposition that the phase of drug development is the key driver for rigor of validation.
  - They explain why Phase 4 is accepting of innovative biomarker application and Phase 3 much less so.
  - They explain why candidate termination often requires rigor of validation and application (e.g., electrocardiogram Q-T interval change (QTc) in Phase 1) and how the BIIF of a go decision will often be different from that of a "no go" decision; they are not mirror images.
  - They explain why termination of a discovery approach requires more rigor of validation and application than termination of an individual candidate.

- The principles explain why certain decisions may or may not require more rigorous validation than others (see also Box 8.3):
  - Why a biomarker that is in the "research" or "development" phase for a decision with a high BIIF might meet the MAC and be in the "application" phase for a decision with a lesser BIIF – where there is more risk tolerance
  - That reluctance to accept a biomarker for a decision with a high BIIF when it is already accepted for a different decision with a low BIIF is not necessarily "bad team behavior" if it is determined in advance that the biomarker's performance is not sufficiently robust (i.e., does not meet the MAC) for the high-BIIF decision
  - That the existence of multiple backups (which reduce the BIIF for a "no go" decision for any candidate that is easily replaced) supports a more risk-tolerant approach to biomarker development/application
  - That, if there are many other attractive candidates in the portfolio and insufficient resources for all, the BIIF for any one candidate's no go is reduced and the appropriate risk tolerance is higher

---

Box 8.3.   Frequently Asked Question

Question: If termination decisions are often high BIIF, why not just use conventional endpoints for them so we can avoid having to validate a biomarker to high standards?

Answer: Conventional endpoints used in clinical trials routinely carry a substantial risk of false positive and false negative results. It is not necessarily difficult or expensive to equal or exceed this performance with a biomarker at substantially lower cost. Linkage to clinical outcome – possibly the most expensive part of validation – is not necessary for a nonviability decision based on the absence of pharmacology (negative proof of mechanism (POM)). A precise pharmacologic measure can do the job.

8.5.3. Select Appropriate Technical Validation Attributes

- All technical validation attributes relevant to the determination of fitness for purpose must be appropriately identified using the list in Figure 8.3 and the best available current information.
  - All probable sources of technical noise (any purpose)
  - All probable sources of biological variation (any purpose)
  - All relevant changes induced by drug or disease as relevant to the purpose
- If the cost of timely evaluation of the biomarker on all of the identified attributes is low, they should *all* be evaluated.

GUIDE FOR SELECTION OF APPROPRIATE TECHNICAL VALIDATION ATTRIBUTES FOR BIOMARKERS

	DISCOVERY		EXPLORATORY / FULL DEVELOPMENT	
	LEAD DISCOVERY	**CANDIDATE SUPPORTING**	**CLINICAL**	
CRITERIA COMMON TO ALL BIOMARKER TYPES_ INTERNALLY OR EXTERNALLY SOURCED (Target, Mechanism & Outcome Biomarker)	**Attributes relevant to technical noise that should be considered:** • Sample handling • Linearity (calibration model) • Instrument calibration • Calibration matrix • Reagents and reference materials • Draft procedure in place **Attributes relevant to biological signal and noise that should be considered:** • Sample stability • Specificity & sensitivity to effects of standard pharmacologic agents	**Attributes relevant to technical noise that should be considered:** All of the attributes listed under "Lead Discovery" plus: • Written procedure in place • Reagents, reference, and QC materials • Precision • Limit of quantitation • Accuracy **Attributes relevant to biological signal and noise that should be considered:** All the attributes under "lead discovery" plus: • Acceptance criteria defined • Acceptable specimens identified • Acceptability for translation evaluated	**Attributes relevant to technical noise that should be considered:** All of the attributes listed under "Candidate Supporting" plus: • Appropriate GCP / GLP • Recovery determined • Accreditation and compliance • Hardware and software 21CFR part11 compliance • Outliers defined and criteria for handling defined • Reference ranges calculated • Comparison with known/ reference method (if available) completed • Assay interferences examined • Matix effects characterized • Cross-site and within-site differences in laboratory or machine type/brand/calibration • Cross-site and within-site differences in signal processing, compression, data handling • Interreader and intra-reader differences if humans involved • Coding/blinding of samples	**Attributes relevant to biological signal and noise that should be considered:** All of the attributes listed under "Candidate Supporting" plus: • Linkage with established clinical disease endpoints and biomarkers • Appropriate and inappropriate populations • Healthy versus patient samples or measurements • Degree of biological effect change within and between human subjects • False positive and false negative rates in humans • Panic values • Temporal effects in humans • Critical review and assessment by stakeholders • Positive and negative control samples or pharmacologies in humans • Compatibility of measurement with clinical trial conditions

PRU   Produced for the Global Biomarker Taskforce by the Pfizer Research University

Fig. 8.3
Guide for selection of appropriate technical validation attributes for biomarkers based on purpose and stage of drug candidate development.

- The BIIF evaluation (Section 8.5.2) should be used to modify selection of attributes from the list in Figure 8.3 as follows:
  - If the cost or time required to evaluate all relevant attributes is high, but the BIIF is not high, some of the lower likelihood or magnitude evaluations can be appropriately left out (high risk tolerance).
  - If the drug candidate is in one of the early phases, but the BIIF evaluation for biomarker application to a decision is high, then attributes usually included only in the later stages should considered for addition (low risk tolerance).
- All relevant biological signals and noise should be sufficiently understood to enable them to be managed and for them to have an appropriate impact on experimental design and decision criteria.

The following three types of attributes are to be evaluated as a part of the technical validation process:

- Technical sources of variance ("Technical Noise") – intrinsic sources of variability in the assay or biomarker
- Biological variation – the real biological variability that is independent of drug or disease

■ Changes induced by drug or disease (the biomarker "signal") – the magnitude, variability, and linkage to an outcome.

First, contributions to these attributes must be identified or selected as described in this section and by using the guide table in Figure 8.3; then acceptable limits and decision criteria must be defined as described in Section 8.5.4.3– the biomarker MAC.

BOX 8.4. Guidance for Biomarker Development and Validation Activities for Translatable Biomarkers

---

OPTIMIZING TECHNICAL BIOMARKER VALIDATION FOR HUMANS WITH ACCEPTABLE QUANTITATIVE MEASUREMENTS

When translating a preclinical biomarker into humans,

■ Demonstrate that the preclinical biomarker has a human equivalent that has the same biological significance

■ Demonstrate that the preclinical biomarker assay or a specific human biomarker assay or test has performance characteristics similar to the previously validated preclinical assay or test.

OPTIMIZING CLINICAL METHODS STUDY TO CONFIRM THE APPLICABILITY OF THE BIOMARKER

To use a biomarker in Phase 1 or Phase 2 clinical trials for decision-making purposes, it is essential to

■ Confirm its technical performance in a clinical trial-like setting similar to one planned in the Phase 1 or 2 study

■ Consider implications of single-center versus multicenter requirements

■ Sample collection, storage, and shipment

■ Examine facilities and expertise at study site

■ Understand requirements for population selection

■ Obtain human results in the target population for sample sizing

■ Understand the degree of change that can practically be studied and/or the degree of change that may be expected such as the difference between biomarker results in a patient population compared with a normal population.

OPTIMIZING HUMAN PK/PD RELATIONSHIPS USING BIOMARKERS IN PHASE 1

■ The relationship between exposure and biomarker response in preclinical species must be understood. This will enable PK/PD modelers to evaluate the effect of time on response (delayed biomarker responses or responses to last longer than exposure) and will affect the protocol design of Phase 1 studies.

■ The relationship between biomarker response and efficacy in pre-clinical models must be understood to establish the degree of biomarker signal associated with the desired outcome.

■ The biomarker signal must be quantitative and reflect activity of the compound in the tissue of interest, which is relevant to the indication. For this reason, in some cases the study must be done in the target population.

■ The biomarker response should be evaluated over a wide range of doses and exposures in single and, if applicable multiple dose studies and also include sampling times that provide an understanding of the relationship between time of dosing (exposure) to biomarker response.

BOX 8.5. Guidance When Selecting a Minimal Acceptable Phase 1 Biomarker Signal that is Required (Proof of Mechanism) to Proceed to Phase 2

The use of biomarkers in Phase 1 to help compounds through Phase 2 is an important benefit, but selection of a threshold level of pharmacological activity that is required to initiate Phase 2 (Proof of Mechanism – POM) has the inherent risk of discontinuing development after Phase 1 if the amount of pharmacological activity at the maximum tolerated dose is less than an agreed upon threshold. A false negative decision at this stage is serious because it could lead to the loss of a good compound and possibly the discontinuation of a program due to an incorrect conclusion about the efficacy or safety of the mechanism.

Therefore, the following principles are important:

■ Setting biomarker criteria for the decision to advance to Phase 2 should be data driven.

  ■ Understand the relationship between biomarker signal and outcomes (efficacy) in preclinical animal models.

  ■ Understand the relationship between biomarker signal and disease activity from human data.

  ■ Understand the relationship between biomarker signal and disease activity from previous Phase 2 studies with similar compounds.

- The minimally acceptable signal must be defined before generating biomarker data in Phase 1. Waiting for the data and then deciding on acceptable criteria is poor practice.
- A high business impact for false termination (BIIF) leads to pressure to be reasonably conservative in setting decision criteria for proof of nonviability (PONV) decisions in Phase 2.

  - If there is clear precedence for the predictive power of the biomarker, then decision criteria may be more stringent and a higher biomarker signal threshold is appropriate.
  - If there is no clear precedence, then set a low biomarker threshold for PONV.
  - If there are backups at near-similar stage, then BIIF is reduced and the team can be more risk tolerant.
  - If the overall portfolio is unusually rich, then BIIF for termination is reduced (because resources can be applied to other good candidates) and the team can be more risk tolerant [but conversely, BIIF for a false go decision is increased, and so the team should be more conservative on go criteria].
  - Phase 2b false decisions have a higher BIIF than Phase 2a. Performance standards should therefore be higher because tolerability of risk is lower.

- Ideally, Phase 1 should have already have been a convincing test of the compound's mechanism for feedback to Discovery, but if this cannot be done it should be done in Phase 2a. This may mean not establishing a hair-trigger termination decision in Phase 1 for the first candidate with a new mechanism.

If the uncertainty for acceptable biomarker activity is large, then the PONV threshold, should be set low and the "proof of mechanism" thresholds should be set high. A "gray zone" for pharmacologic signal, above PONV threshold and below POM threshold, may be acceptable.

8.5.4. Create the Biomarker MAC and Appropriate Decision Criteria

8.5.4.1. Principles for Setting Performance Standards in the Biomarker MAC

- The MAC should be outlined when a biomarker reaches the "research" phase and finalized when it reaches proof of concept (POC) and enters the "development" phase.

Fig. 8.4
Schematic illustrating
the idealized
relationship between
signal and noise.

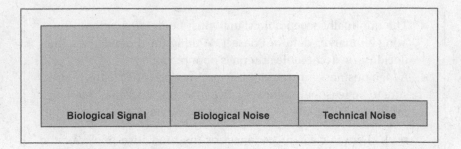

- The MAC should contain an evaluation of the minimally acceptable biological signal, the maximally acceptable biological noise and the maximally acceptable technical noise (see Figure 8.4).
- The degree of biomarker change from drug or disease is much greater than the degree of biological variability, which is much greater than the biomarker technical variability.
- All sources of variation should be sufficiently understood to enable their management and to have an impact on experimental design (e.g., issues as diverse as sample handling and software performance).

Having selected the appropriate attributes to evaluate, teams should set performance criteria for them that are appropriate to the purpose and the BIIF evaluation of risk tolerance. This will usually be done after proof of concept for the biomarker is reached.

8.5.4.2. Contents of the Biomarker MAC

- The MAC should contain all of the selected attributes grouped by their contribution to the three categories above.
- Wherever possible, a quantitative performance target should be set for each category (see Section 8.5.4.3).
- The MAC should identify key issues that must be solved to enable understanding of the meaning of the effect or linkage to outcome if needed, and, if the biomarker is being developed for more than one purpose, the MAC will need to contain attributes and standards for each purpose.

8.5.4.3. Guidance for Setting Quantitative Performance Targets Prior to Executing the Biomarker Validation Plan

It is recommended that a great effort be made to predefine a meaningful change in the biological signal because doing so greatly reduces the uncertainty around setting performance targets and improves acceptance of the decision. This is usually a fundamental part of the POC of a biomarker and thus will commonly be available here because the MAC is not generated in detail until biomarker POC.

Best practice: if the size of the biological signal resulting from the drug is known or a target has been set but the noise is unknown.

■ An upper limit on the sample size that is cost effective or practical should be defined. Using this and the known biological signal, the team should make a statistical calculation to define the highest variance that would be consistent with statistical significance if the biological signal is present. Achieving this variance (or less) becomes part of the biomarker MAC.

Fallback position: if the technical and biological noise is known but the required degree of change resulting from the drug is not.

1) An upper limit on the sample size that is cost-effective or practical should be defined by the team, and a statistical calculation should be made using this sample size and the known noise to define the smallest statistically significant change.
2) If we know that the smallest statistically significant degree of change in (1) is biologically or clinically insignificant, then absence of statistical significance would be a reasonable candidate no go decision.

   If we do not have agreement about where "meaningful" change starts, using statistical significance as a threshold for go or no go decision criterion is not best practice (see example in Section 8.5.4.5 for guidance on setting decision criteria in these circumstances). Nonetheless, the study might be worth doing to learn about the biomarker, to define meaningful change for the next relevant candidate, or to obtain other information.

8.5.4.4. When Is Linkage to Outcome a Part of the MAC?

Table 8.2 is a guide to when and why biomarker linkage to clinical outcome should be included as a part of the MAC for some purposes.

8.5.4.5. Example MAC (hypothetical)

Biomarker: serum rhubarb
Specific purpose: proof of nonviability in Phase 1 due to absence of pharmacology for drugs that block rhubarb absorption.
Business impact if false: High. This is the only drug with this important mechanism, and the rest of the portfolio represents more risky investment. Competitors have blocked ownership of all relevant alternative structures, and so this represents our last chance for this approach. A false termination would therefore be highly costly. Tolerance for risk is consequently low.

Table 8.2. Examining the Requirement for Biomarker Linkage to Clinical Outcomes

Scenario	Decision	Required Linkage	Why Biomarker Linkage Is/Is Not Needed	Overall Message
Pharmacology is absent	No Go	Low	The no go decision is based on absence of a signal. The meaning of a signal (if it had been present) is unnecessary.	Linkage is not needed in the MAC for proof of nonviability owing to absence of pharmacology/target.
Pharmacology is present	Go to Exploratory Development Go to FIH Go to P2a Go to P2b Go to Full Development (P3) Planning Go to P3	Low linkage Low linkage Low linkage Medium linkage Medium linkage High linkage	If there is no linkage, the biomarker may be an epiphenomenon (i.e. independent of the therapeutic benefit). To support forward clinical investment, some linkage is needed.	The greater the forward clinical investment, the greater linkage is needed as part of the MAC.
Safety issue	Go (absence of toxicity) No Go (presence of toxicity)	Usually medium Usually high	Absence of a signal is only reassuring if the biomarker is linked. Degree of linkage depends on seriousness of effect (risk). Presence is only a real danger signal if linked; termination is a serious decision	Safety biomarkers require linkage to outcome in the MAC in proportion to the forward investment, or in proportion to forward risk

Notes: Low linkage is where there is no information or animal model information only. FIH, First in human
Medium linkage between biomarker results and clinical outcome:

■ Requires association with efficacy, disease, or safety outcome data in humans but does *not* require a prospective (longitudinal data) demonstration in clinical studies

■ The study must be robustly designed with buy-in by key stakeholders, and the results must be carefully analyzed and hold up to scientific review and agreement by governing bodies

High linkage between biomarker results and clinical outcome

■ Requires *reproducible* demonstration of the relationship between biomarker change and clinical outcome in longitudinal prospective studies in the target population (two or more studies with similar findings)

■ Results of studies establishing linkage must stand up to independent review for scientific merit and validity because development decisions based on high linkage will result in large resource investments.

Selection of relevant technical attributes and setting performance standards:

The program is at the candidate-seeking stage but the biomarker's key use will be in Phase 1, and so the complete list for clinical biomarkers was considered. In setting performance standards, we know from natural history studies that a 20% reduction in serum rhubarb in humans is required for prevention of gout; the upper bound on our practical sample size was 50 subjects per group. That number was used to calculate the upper limit for technical noise.

- Total noise from all sources of technical variation must be less than a coefficient of variation (CV) of 3% to fulfill the sample size requirement.
- Sample handling: freeze thaw experiments. Storage of up to 3 weeks must show <1% difference versus fresh samples.
- Linearity: linearity to within 2%.
- Instrument calibration: rhubarb standards must be prepared and used throughout the study.
- A written procedure must be in place prior to clinical use that includes quality control (QC) procedures for the trial and assurance that the lab will be run to good laboratory practice (GLP) standards.
- The assay must be insensitive to serum raspberry (<1% change for a concentration of 2 punnets per litre).
- Within-subject variability on the same sample must be <1% between subject variability at baseline <1%.
- Subjects with congenital insensitivity to rhubarb represent <1% of the population and will be treated as statistical outliers.
- Linkage to clinical outcomes was not relevant to this purpose.
- Assay performance using serum from healthy volunteers should be equivalent to rat serum (within 2%).
- No other listed attributes were considered relevant to this purpose.

Decision criteria:

A candidate will be considered nonviable if the 95% confidence interval for reduction in serum rhubarb at 48 h at the maximum tolerated dose (MTD) in 12 healthy volunteers does not include 20% reduction and the variance is within 5% of that predicted.

The MAC should also contain the decision criteria that will be used for the decision(s) that form the biomarker purpose. When these are based on linkage with known pharmacology, they will specify how much the biomarker has to change to represent a meaningful change in pharmacology. When they are based on linkage with a clinical outcome, they will specify how much the biomarker has to change to represent a meaningful change in disease/toxicity.

Guidance on adjusting decision criteria to compensate for biomarker variability or uncertainty about the required degree of change so that an adequate MAC can be achieved:

- If failure to meet the MAC is for some reason other than variability or uncertainty about degree of change, changing decision criteria cannot compensate and is not appropriate.
- For go pharmacology decisions, the degree of change needed for a clear go decision can be increased to compensate for greater than expected biomarker variability so that there is still sufficient confidence that this change really means go.
- For no-go pharmacology decisions, the degree of change needed for a clear no-go decision can be decreased to compensate for greater than expected biomarker variability so that there is a high level of confidence that this really means no go.
- For safety decisions, the appropriate response to increased variability is to increase the required change in toxicity signal for no go and to decrease the required change for go decisions.
- A gray area of "insufficient information from biomarker" in between the go and no-go areas occurs in these cases. This may be acceptable to governing bodies and far preferable to the illusion of a binary decision. However, it should be recognized that there is a negative economic impact because there is a greater likelihood that a degree of change in the biomarker will deliver insufficient information to make a decision. This situation will usually spur further research to improve the biomarker's performance – or a search for a new biomarker!

8.5.5. Summary

Definition of adequate biomarker validation: Validation is "good enough" when

- There is a well-defined business-related scientific purpose.
- A full understanding of the business impact of making a false decision (BIIF) has been used to set the risk tolerance.
- Minimally acceptable criteria for performance have been defined in advance.
- Decision criteria have been defined in advance.
- All relevant technical validation attributes have been appropriately examined and limits set in the MAC achieved.
- All relevant biological signals and noise are sufficiently understood to enable the management of practical aspects of quality during application to drug development.

Box 8.6. Key Points

- Biomarker development and use must be guided by the principle of being "fit-for-purpose" and linked to how the biomarker will be used strategically in the development plan.

- The validation plan requires the definition of a specific purpose, understanding of the risk tolerance, selection of appropriate performance attributes, definition of minimally acceptable criteria, and specification of decision criteria.

- The key driver for rigor of biomarker performance is the business impact of making a false decision (BIIF).

- The "Selection of Technical Validation Attributes for Biomarkers" listed in Figure 8.3 can be used to select common potential sources of technical variance (i.e., noise) and biological variance for a given biomarker when applied at various stages of development. Teams should use it as a guide/checklist for completeness, but there will be issues that are irrelevant to a particular application, and there will be issues not on the list that are peculiar to a given biomarker. The key principle is that all attributes necessary to determine fitness for the intended purpose should be addressed, whether or not they are listed on Figure 8.3.

- The biomarker MAC should define all relevant minimally acceptable criteria, quantitative performance standards, and decision criteria.

- Manipulation of decision criteria based on the degree of change may be used to manage some of the uncertainty; for example, for go pharmacology decisions (or no-go safety decisions), selecting a larger degree of change in the biomarker compensates for greater than expected uncertainty or poorer performance.

8.6. When and How to Apply Biomarkers in Drug Development: Biomarker Development Is Described for Each Stage of Drug Development

8.6.1. Biomarker Development Must Occur So That Biomarkers Are Validated for their Purpose Prior to Application for Drug Development Decisions

Biomarkers are used in every instance in which they can deliver decisions at lower cost, and/or earlier timing and/or higher commercial value capture, and when the level of uncertainty/risk is tolerable.

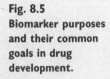

Fig. 8.5
Biomarker purposes and their common goals in drug development.

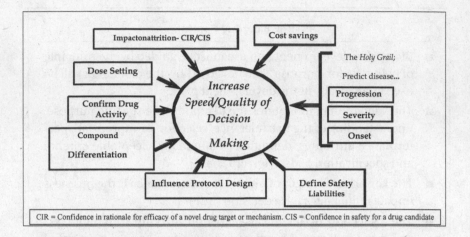

Biomarkers are not used when there is no economic benefit or the level of uncertainty/risk is intolerable.

(See Figure 8.5.)

8.6.2. Biomarker Selection and Development between "Target Idea" and Decision on Drug Candidate Selection

Goal: (1) Select and validate a target or mechanism biomarker for use in preclinical species that is translatable to humans and (2) develop a biomarker plan to define resources and responsibilities as well as an outline of the biomarker MAC.

Purpose: Generation of pharmacology data for drug candidate selection with *potential* for measuring pharmacodynamic activity in humans during Phase 2 – translatable biomarker.

Risk Assessment: A false negative biomarker-driven decision usually has moderate business impact because it could lead to discarding a potentially good candidate and trigger resources to find alternative candidates. A false positive biomarker-driven decision usually has a high business impact because it would trigger larger investments for candidate development. However, it is likely that conflicting data during validation would alert Discovery teams that the biomarker performance was not satisfactory long before any drug candidate decision would be made. The main risk at this stage, therefore, is related to whether the biomarker will actually be translatable to humans. (See Table 8.3).

8.6.3. Biomarker Best Practice between Drug Candidate Selection and First In-Human (FIH) Study

Goals: (1) Complete human biomarker translation validation activities for preclinical biomarkers and ensure human biomarkers are validated

Table 8.3. Biomarker Best Practice Between "Idea" and Decision on Drug Candidate Selection for Preclinical Use and Translation to Humans

Principle	Activity
The purpose(s) must be defined first in order to identify potential biomarkers and set criteria for performance based on the BIIF for the decisions under consideration. **Biomarker activities at this time are focused on use in preclinical species and human translation.**	More than one biomarker may be needed to satisfy multiple purposes. List specific purposes of biomarkers relevant to exploratory drug (ED) candidate selection such as (but not limited to) the following: ■ go from demonstration and understanding of pharmacologic mechanism/target in preclinical models ■ characterization of PK/PD if go in preclinical models ■ no go from demonstration of absence of pharmacologic mechanism/target in preclinical models ■ no go from demonstration of presence of toxicity in preclinical models ■ go from demonstration of the absence of toxicity in preclinical models ■ combination of safety and efficacy biomarkers to establish therapeutic index in efficacy models and toxicology species ■ translation of pharmacologic signals from preclinical models to humans.
Biomarker must reflect the pharmacology of the compound in tissues relevant to the site of pathology in animal models and human disease.	Identify animal species used for efficacy models, nature of the model, and tissues where mechanism of action is found and list potential/most appropriate target and mechanism biomarkers that might fulfill the purposes identified: ■ Need experts: project biology and clinical therapeutic area experts in disease biology and others as dictated by the nature of the project ■ Scientists from the Biomarker Technology groups ■ Pharmaceutical Sciences if development requires the use of challenge agents or other exogenous substances ■ Other experts, internal and external, as needed.
Biomarker selection is based on an evaluation of cost (including validation cost), benefit (including application to other projects and candidates), and likelihood of success compared with alternatives, including proceeding without a biomarker.	■ Using consensus from appropriate experts in the area and diligent review of all available internal/external information, select the appropriate biomarkers, taking into account whether the pathways are active in normal animals (and humans), and availability of challenge agents if required with the following "musts": 1) Biomarker(s) must deliver understanding of the mechanism of action. 2) Biomarker must be translatable to humans in a clinical trial setting or a plausible plan to translate it must be created ■ Using the list in Figure 8.3, and any other known sources of signal or noise, select the validation attributes that should be evaluated.

(continued)

Table 8.3 (*continued*)

Principle	Activity
	■ Using the options in Box 8.5, determine what the appropriate quantitative performance standard should be for the biomarker MAC and set decision criteria using the understanding of risk tolerance from considering the BIIF.
	■ Estimate the cost of validating each biomarker to the appropriate performance standard. If the cost is high, a formal ROI calculation may be needed.
	■ Determine which biomarkers (if any) are appropriate to pursue (e.g., having a significant return on investment versus executing the program without the biomarker).
Select biomarker for application to CAN selection and potential for human translation based on validation results compared with the MAC	■ Evaluate technical performance of selected biomarkers on sources of biological noise and biological variation versus MAC.
	■ Evaluate technical performance of selected biomarkers for demonstration of biological signal using reference compounds as positive and negative controls, including PK/PD relationships and, if required, evaluate appropriate linkage to outcome as described in Table 8.2 and Box 8.8.
	■ If the MAC is met and decision criteria have been produced, evaluate drug candidates by running appropriate experiments using the biomarker(s)

prior to use in the clinic. **(2)** Ensure that criteria for biomarker driven decisions in Phase 1 are appropriately defined and integrated into the clinical plan.

Purpose(s): Generation of pharmacology (pharmacodynamic) data in humans during Phase 1 that may be used for POM, Phase 2 dose selection, candidate discontinuation for insufficient pharmacology, or additional investments based on confirmed pharmacology at a well-tolerated dose (POM) and biomarker linkage to clinical outcomes if present.

Risk Assessment: A false negative biomarker-driven decision usually has high business impact because it could lead to discarding a potentially good candidate and trigger resources to develop alternative candidates. A false positive biomarker-driven decision usually has a very high business impact because it would trigger large Phase 2 investments and also incur opportunity costs. (See Table 8.4.)

8.6.4. Biomarker Best Practice between FIH and Phase 2 Start

Goals: Selection and validation of efficacy, safety, and differentiation biomarker(s) included in Phase 2A studies (confirm medium or high linkage to clinical outcome).

Table 8.4. Biomarker Best Practice between the Candidate Selection Decision and First In-Human Study (FIH) for Biomarker Use in Phase I

Principle	Activity
The purpose(s) must be defined first in order to set criteria for performance based on the BIIF for the decisions under consideration. **Biomarker activities at this time are focused on use in Phase I or both Phase 2A**	List specific purposes of biomarkers such as (but not limited to) the following: 1) "no go" at FIH based on toxicology findings at exposures lower than those needed for efficacious pharmacology in animal models. 2) go to Phase 2A from demonstration and understanding of pharmacological mechanism/target in FIH or multidose (MD) Phase I study 3) no go from demonstration of insufficient degree of pharmacologic mechanism/target binding in FIH/MD Phase I 4) dose selection for Phase 2 from characterization of PK/PD from FIH single and multidose studies or from trial simulation 5) differentiation through demonstration of presence or absence of a key pharmacologic/toxicity feature 6) no go from demonstration of presence of toxicity in FIH/MD Phase I 7) go from demonstration of the apparent absence of toxicity in FIH/MD Phase I 8) combination of safety and efficacy biomarkers to establish acceptable therapeutic index in FIH/MD Phase I 9) go to Phase 2B (high investment option) based on high biomarker linkage to clinical outcome 10) feedback to Discovery for termination of approach if mechanism does not translate to humans

Biomarker selection is based on an evaluation of cost (including validation cost), benefit (including application to other projects and candidates), and likelihood of success compared with alternatives, including proceeding without a biomarker.	1) Continue to pursue most appropriate target, mechanism, and outcome biomarkers that might fulfill the purposes at acceptable cost.
	  ■ favor those used preclinically having a translation plan that is being executed and biomarkers already under evaluation.
	2) Using the list on Figure 8.3, and any other known sources of signal or noise, select additional validation attributes for evaluation (if any)
	  ■ If the purpose requires linkage to clinical outcome, complete the plan for validation of linkage
	3) Using the options in Box 8.5 refine the biomarker MAC and set decision criteria using the understanding of risk tolerance.
	4) Estimate additional costs and benefits of validating each biomarker.
	5) Pursue validation for cost-effective biomarkers.

Select biomarker for application in Phase I based on validation results compared with the MAC.	Evaluate technical performance of selected biomarkers on sources of biological noise and biological variation versus MAC using appropriate laboratory and clinical methodology studies. Confirm technical performance in a clinical trial-like setting comparing across sites if necessary.

Table 8.5. Biomarker Best Practice between FIH and Phase 2 Start for Biomarker Use in Phase 2

Principle	Activity
The purpose(s) must be defined first in order to set criteria for performance based on the BIIF for the decisions under consideration. **Biomarker activities at this time are focused on use in Phase 2A**	Define what the biomarker data will be used for after stage-gate 2: ■ Setting the dose and regimen for Phase 2 (role of PK/PD modeling and simulation) ■ go to Phase 2b ■ Full-development strategic planning ■ Proof of nonviability in Phase 2a from insufficient biomarker signal ■ Proof of nonviability in Phase 2a from undesirable pharmacology or toxicity ■ Proof of nonviability in Phase 2a from inadequate differentiability. Define the BIIF for each purpose. In general this is very high for this stage of development.
The cost of biomarker validation for each purpose must be weighed against the benefit(s) of using biomarker data for development decisions compared with alternatives, including proceeding without a new biomarker.	Validation activities to consider may include the following: ■ Studies in patients and normal subjects to confirm linkage to clinical outcome or to define biomarker signal differences associated with disease activity ■ Studies in the target population to estimate sample size ■ Studies with marketed drugs for differentiation biomarkers ■ Studies with marketed drugs to set threshold for efficacy or safety decision ■ Studies across sites using actual types of equipment and data processing.
Select biomarker for application in Phase 2 based on validation results compared with the MAC.	Evaluate technical performance of selected biomarkers on sources of biological noise and biological variation versus MAC using appropriate methodology studies or existing data in humans. Confirm technical performance in a clinical trial-like setting if not already demonstrated. At this stage, this usually involves demonstration of medium or high linkage of biomarkers to clinical outcome, which may be related to efficacy, safety, or differentiation

Purpose(s): (1) Discontinuation of the candidate after Phase 2A, (2) go to Phase 2B, (3) go to Full Development planning, (4) trigger high investment strategy – straight to Phase 3.

Risk Assessment: A false negative biomarker-driven decision usually has very high business impact because it could lead to discarding a potentially good candidate and trigger resources to develop alternative candidates. A false positive biomarker-driven decision also has a very high business impact because it would trigger large Phase 2 or 3 investments and also incur opportunity costs. See Table 8.5 and Boxes 8.7 and 8.8.

Box 8.7. Guidance for Optimizing Selection of Phase 2 Dose and Regimen Using Biomarkers in Phase 1

Biomarker signals (desirable and undesirable pharmacological activity) that are safe and needed for efficacy must be established:

- This may come from preclinical models, from studies of the biomarker in patients with various levels of disease activity, and from comparison of the biomarker signal in patients and normal subjects.

- Detailed knowledge of biomarker responses associated with efficacy such as whether intermittent high levels of pharmacological activity or constant levels of pharmacological activity are preferred.

- Time relationships between biomarker signals and PK should be understood: the biomarker signal may not be synchronous with the pharmacokinetic exposure data (hysteresis). Some direct pharmacological effects may not be rapidly reversible or may have irreversible downstream effects on the disease.

- Doses selected should result in clearly separated levels of pharmacological activity based on biomarker data and exposure-response modeling.

Box 8.8. Guidance for Establishing Linkage to Clinical Outcome

- Literature or in-house generated data are required to establish relationships between biomarker change and disease activity or safety findings.

- The following sources of data should be considered based on cost and data quality;

  - Similar data from more than one study in peer-reviewed literature.
  - Significant data from a methods study in the target population.
  - Analyses of samples derived from completed or ongoing drug studies in the target population.
  - Significant data from external study samples analyzed in-house.
  - Cross-sectional data in a target population is often acceptable, but longitudinal biomarker data are generally more reliable because within-subject changes can be determined.

Imaging Biomarkers in Drug Development: Case Studies

Johannes T. Tauscher and Adam J. Schwarz

9.1. Introduction

The discovery and development of novel treatments is a lengthy and costly endeavor: for drug candidates entering clinical trials between 1989 and 2002, the estimated cost per new drug varied from approximately 500 million to more than 2 billion U.S. dollars.[1] Biomarkers – objective and measurable responses to a putative drug candidate – have been heralded as one potential solution to the ever-increasing expenditure of developing new medicines, and anatomical or functional medical imaging can be one tool in the armamentarium of biomarkers. Conceptually, the utility of imaging biomarkers for facilitating drug development, especially go/no go decisions in early development, includes the following:

- *confirming the presence of a drug target* in a (sub)population entering a clinical trial (e.g., accumulation of β-amyloid, as measured with positron emission tomography [PET] and a specific ligand for β-amyloid in the brain of patients entering a clinical trial for a novel Alzheimer's drug candidate[2]);
- *assessing target engagement* of a novel drug candidate (e.g., confirmation of dopamine-2 [D_2] receptor antagonism of antipsychotics using PET imaging of [^{11}C]-raclopride displacement[3]);
- *demonstrating a functional effect* of a drug on a mechanism- or disease-relevant biological parameter (e.g., blockade of ketamine-induced functional magnetic resonance imaging [fMRI] signal in the central nervous system [CNS] by antipsychotics or glutamate-normalizing compounds[4]);
- *informing dosing* for clinical trials (e.g., if the degree of desired target engagement is known from preclinical data, previous drug candidates aimed at the same target, or both, then a "receptor occupancy" study can inform dosing for subsequent clinical trials[5]); or using a functional dose-response relationship to establish a biologically effective

dose range or schedule to be explored in larger oncology clinical trials (rather than using the maximum tolerated dose)[6]; or

- *Becoming a surrogate* for clinical response (e.g., joint-space narrowing measured from x-rays in osteoarthritis,[7] or Response Evaluation Criteria in Solid Tumors (RECIST) measure of solid tumor burden in oncology).[8]

Biomarkers used for research purposes (i.e., "internal decision making") require a different, less stringent validation approach than those used in the context of applications to regulatory agencies. For the purpose of this chapter, we will mainly describe imaging biomarker methods that are "validated" or of substantial potential utility and in the process of validation, which refers to a characterization of their performance characteristics so they can be confidently used as analytical endpoints.[9] These thus represent imaging biomarker approaches that drive scientific decisions (e.g., go/no-go decisions), particularly in the early phases of drug development. At the other end of the spectrum are "qualified" biomarkers that are accepted as objective measures for a particular purpose by regulatory authorities.[9] In late-phase registration trials, MRI, X-rays, and computed tomography (CT) are widely used in an anatomical (radiological) mode as surrogate endpoints or well-established parameters of disease status. In translational research (the phase of preclinical through preregistration clinical phases of drug discovery and development), however, there is greater scope for the use of molecular, functional, and other emerging imaging techniques to increase understanding of a drug's biological mode of action and for internal decision making in the drug development process. Imaging methods present an array of appealing experimental constructs to obtain anatomical and, in particular, functional information about a drug's interaction with both on-target and off-target biology in an experimental medicine setting. In appropriate animal and human experimental models as well as in patient populations, imaging techniques can also provide a longitudinal, insitu window of drug effects on the biological and disease processes. As increasing emphasis is placed on novel mechanisms, the uncertainties inherent in bringing forward new candidate drugs aimed at new biological targets with unprecedented mechanisms of action are correspondingly greater. Imaging techniques present a powerful possibility to probe a molecule's interaction with the human organism. In many instances, these experiments can be informed by (and, in turn, inform) preclinical experiments.

In order to address the widening gap between scientific discoveries that have the potential to prevent and cure some of today's biggest killers, such as diabetes, cancer, and Alzheimer's disease, and their translation into innovative medical treatments, the U.S. Food and Drug Administration (FDA) in March 2004 launched the Critical Path Initiative with the release of a landmark report entitled "Innovation/Stagnation: Challenge and Opportunity on the Critical Path to New Medical Products."

In that report, advanced imaging technologies were listed as one biomarker modality, besides fields like genomics or bioinformatics, that "could be applied during [drug] development to improve the accuracy of the tests that predict the safety and efficacy of potential medical products" with the intent to modernize drug development.[10]

In this chapter, we attempt to provide examples illustrating the role of imaging biomarkers in modern drug development. Specifically, we will review how molecular imaging was initially introduced as a biomarker for brain penetration and target engagement and how this information can be used to inform dosing in clinical trials. Furthermore, we will list examples of how functional imaging can be used to interrogate downstream consequences of pharmacodynamic (PD) actions at specific targets and how this information can be used in the context of drug development. Last, but not least, we will review the existing scientific literature on the role of imaging as a tool to enrich patient populations, and – representing the Holy Grail for biomarkers – as a surrogate for treatment response.

9.2. Molecular Imaging: PET "Receptor Occupancy" as a Marker for Target Engagement

9.2.1. A Brief History of Dopamine Receptor Occupancy with Antipsychotics

The introduction of in vivo molecular neuroimaging modalities using radionuclides, such as PET or single photon emission tomography (SPECT) has greatly added to our knowledge about the molecular effects and the mechanisms of action of psychotropic medications. With these nuclear medicine techniques it is possible to quantitatively analyze the targets of drugs such as brain dopamine or serotonin neurotransmitter receptors.

Initial evidence that PET could serve as a biomarker for target engagement and guide dosing of psychotropic drugs emerged in the late 1980s with antipsychotics. Researchers at the Swedish Karolinska Institute showed that haloperidol, a first-generation antipsychotic drug, led to substantial blockade of D_2 receptors in the putamen[3] and that there was a relationship between dose, striatal D_2 receptor occupancy, and motor adverse events, such as extrapyramidal symptoms (EPS), that appear more likely in patients exceeding 80% D_2 receptor occupancy.[11,12] In this context, the term "receptor occupancy" refers to the proportion of neurotransmitter receptors that is occupied by a drug. The binding potential (BP) can be obtained using PET and a ligand that specifically binds to the receptor population under study, such as $[^{11}C]$raclopride to D_2 receptors, and is a measure of the number of available receptors to which a ligand can bind.[13]

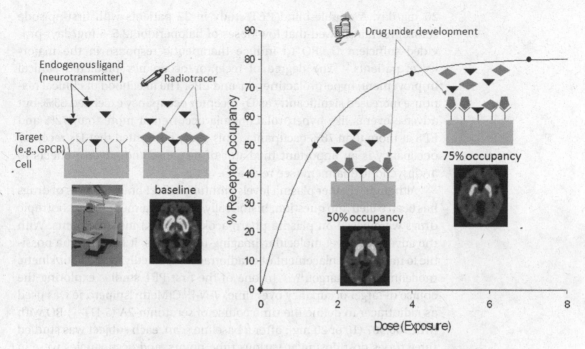

Fig. 9.1
Example of using a displacement paradigm with a radiolabeled PET tracer to determine receptor occupancy of a novel drug candidate. GPCR, G-protein coupled receptor.

The underlying principle for receptor occupancy studies is relatively simple and straightforward. First, a radiotracer specific to a particular target is needed, for instance [^{11}C]raclopride for D_2 receptors. After establishing that this radiotracer can be used reliably and safely in humans, its baseline (i.e., untreated) BP can be determined (Figure 9.1). In a next step, the degree of receptor occupancy can be measured by determining whether a novel drug candidate is able to displace the radiotracer from its target. If this is the case, it may serve as proof of target engagement.

Specifically, the BP after an individual has taken a medication is compared with an untreated baseline value, and the proportion of receptors blocked by a drug [receptor occupancy (RO)] can be calculated using the following equation:

$$\% \ receptor \ occupancy = [1 - \frac{BP \ during \ treatment}{baseline \ BP}] \times 100$$

In some instances, it is not possible to obtain a baseline BP value during untreated conditions. In these cases, an age-corrected estimate from a historical group of antipsychotic-naive patients with schizophrenia and healthy volunteers can be used.[14]

Molecular imaging provided a novel biomarker approach to determine more rational dosing schemes with psychotropic medications. In the case of the conventional neuroleptic haloperidol, PET data became instrumental for questioning the clinical practice of dosing in the range of 10 to

20 mg/day. A double-blind PET study in 22 patients with first-episode schizophrenia showed that low doses of haloperidol (2.5–5 mg/day) provided sufficient D_2 RO to induce therapeutic response in the majority of patients.[11] The degree of receptor occupancy predicted clinical improvement, hyperprolactinemia, and EPS. The likelihood of clinical response increased significantly as D_2 receptor occupancy exceeded 65%, but adverse events like hyperprolactinemia occurred at more than 72% and EPS at more than 78% occupancy. This study confirmed that D_2 receptor occupancy is an important mediator of response and adverse effects to antipsychotic treatment (see review[15]).

Although whether plasma levels faithfully reflect brain kinetics of drugs has been called into question, historically, dosing regimens of psychotropic drugs were based on plasma pharmacokinetic (PK) measurements. With the advent of novel molecular imaging techniques, it has become possible to measure displacement of a radiotracer repeatedly to allow for kinetic modeling at the target.[16,17] In one of the first PET studies exploring the course of target occupancy over time, 3-N-$[^{11}C]$Methylspiperone was used as radiotracer to define the time course of serotonin-2A (5-HT_{2A}) RO with MDL100,907 (10 or 20 mg): after a baseline scan, each subject was studied three times post dosing at various time points, and occupancies were in the range of 70% and 90% after each dose. Although RO remained in that range over 24 hours after 20 mg, it decreased by approximately 20% after 24 hours.[16]

In a more systematic study, the kinetics of plasma levels of two widely used antipsychotics, olanzapine and risperidone, were studied versus the time course of their effects in the brain.[17] PET and $[^{11}C]$-labeled ligands were used to quantify striatal and extrastriatal D_2 as well as cortical 5-HT_{2A} RO. The authors found a significant dissociation of brain and plasma kinetics: Mean terminal plasma elimination half-lives of olanzapine and risperidone were 24 and 10 hours, respectively, whereas it took much longer, on average 75 hours with olanzapine, and 67 hours with risperidone, to decline to 50% of their peak striatal and extra-striatal D_2, as well as 5-HT_{2A} RO. Those results question relying on plasma kinetics as the main basis for dosing regimens of psychotropic drugs and suggest that imaging biomarker studies of brain kinetics may provide a sounder basis for determining dosing schedules.

9.2.2. Serotonin Transporter Occupancy with Antidepressants

The first evidence that imaging biomarkers could be useful in the context of determining target engagement of antidepressants came from a SPECT serotonin transporter (SERT) occupancy case study with the selective serotonin reuptake inhibitor (SSRI) antidepressant fluoxetine.[18] More systematic research with citalopram, fluoxetine, sertraline, paroxetine, or extended-release venlafaxine revealed that all these antidepressants led to at least 80% SERT occupancy at clinically used doses.[19–21] In contrast, the tricyclic antidepressant clomipramine has been shown to occupy 80% of the SERT at doses as low as 10 mg,[22] which is a dose much lower than the clinically recommended range of 50 to 150 mg/day-in depression. Overall, results from PET and SPECT studies with antidepressants support the notion that sustained and considerable engagement of monoaminergic targets is necessary to exert the clinically desired antidepressant effects.

9.2.3. Case Study of a Translational PET Imaging Biomarker Strategy

The following example showcases the usefulness of an imaging biomarker in the clinical development of LY686017, a neurokinin-1 (NK1) receptor antagonist.[5] The translational imaging biomarker strategy was based on preclinical evidence showing LY686017's activity in a gerbil social stress model at doses exceeding 80% target occupancy. The clinical development of LY686017 included a human PET study and a clinical proof of concept (POC) trial in social anxiety disorder (SAD). The radioligand [11C]GR205171 and PET were used in healthy volunteers receiving LY686017 at 1 up to 100 mg/day for 28 days to determine brain RO. The mean NK1 RO ranged from 25% with 1 mg to 93% with 100 mg. Subsequently, a 12-week randomized clinical trial tested LY686017 versus paroxetine, or placebo in SAD. PK/RO modeling based on the PET results predicted that once-daily dosing of >30 mg of LY686017 led to sustained trough RO of more than 80%. On the basis of those PET results, a dose of 50 mg/day was selected to be brought forward to a clinical trial: 189 outpatients suffering from SAD were randomly assigned to 12 weeks of treatment with 50 mg/day LY686017, placebo, or 20 mg/day paroxetine. LY686018 showed no clinical activity in the Phase 2 clinical trial. The use of a biomarker for target engagement, in this case PET imaging of NK1 receptors with the specific NK1 antagonist ligand [11C]GR205171 enabled confident rejection of the hypothesis that NK1 antagonism plays a role in the treatment of SAD, for it was established in the noted PET study that the dose of 50 mg LY686018 once daily led to near-maximal target saturation in the human brain throughout the entire dosing interval.

Although LY686017 did not show efficacy in SAD, there was value in the reported biomarker strategy, and it may serve as an excellent example for a drug development program in which a biomarker – target engagement as measured with PET – simplified the development program to a point at which only one dose in one POC trial needed to be tested, thereby minimizing further, potentially equally futile exposures to a therapeutic candidate while helping to save costs. Traditional clinical plans may have comprised more than one Phase 2 trial in order to confidently reject the hypothesis of NK1 antagonism in anxiety. Conceivably, without a target-engagement biomarker and without the translational model of >80% NK1 antagonism targeted as biologically relevant for antianxiety effects, more patients could have been exposed to higher doses to allay concerns about "non-efficacy due to underdosing" the test drug. Thus, the reported development program underscores the importance of a seamless integration of a biomarker component into the overall development plan of a novel compound.

9.3. Functional Imaging: fMRI as a Probe of Drug Effects in the CNS

Although RO-PET can provide a sensitive measure of target engagement in the CNS, it provides no information on the functional effect of the drug candidate's engagement with the target receptor. Because CNS drugs are designed to counter aberrant brain function, functional imaging methods such as $[^{18}F]$-fluorodeoxyglucose $([^{18}F]FDG)$-PET) measuring glucose metabolism, $[^{15}O]H_2O$-PET measuring blood flow, and blood oxygenation level-dependent (BOLD) fMRI have begun to be evaluated as a noninvasive means of probing drug effects on brain function.[4,23–49] The fMRI technique is flexible and, in most standard implementations, allows measurements under a variety of functional conditions over the entire brain at a temporal scale of ~6 seconds (limited by the hemodynamic response) and a spatial scale of a few millimeters. Figure 9.2 illustrates how fMRI methods (and functional imaging, generally) can reflect engagement of a target brain system or region as an important bridge between molecular target engagement (e.g., receptor occupancy) and behavioral endpoints or clinical instruments.

Fig. 9.2 Functional imaging methods probe PD drug effects downstream of target engagement but provide a window on tissue function upstream of the final behavioral effect underlying the eventual clinical response (or lack thereof).

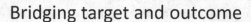

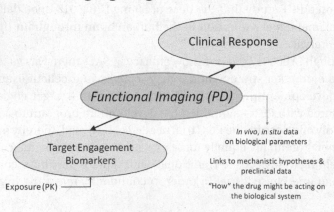

Bridging target and outcome

Clinical Response

Functional Imaging (PD)

Target Engagement Biomarkers

Exposure (PK)

In vivo, in situ data on biological parameters

Links to mechanistic hypotheses & preclinical data

"How" the drug might be acting on the biological system

Different variants of the fMRI approach can be used to detect drug effects on brain function. These can be summarized as follows:

- **Pharmacological MRI (phMRI)**: This approach entails direct detection of a compound's effect on baseline hemodynamic parameters, in the absence of applied stimulus or cognitive paradigm, reflecting the functional interaction between the drug candidate and its target in the task-free ("resting") state. If a drug can be injected intravenously, phMRI responses may be detected by infusing the drug during an image time series.[36,45,50–63] If not, perfusion imaging techniques such as arterial spin labeling (ASL)[64–66] allow the comparison of baseline brain perfusion between different scanning sessions and are hence amenable to oral drug administration or chronic dosing studies. The phMRI approach has a strong translational potential and has been widely implemented in animal models as well.[54–63,67,68]

- **Task-evoked fMRI:** The most common application of fMRI involves the use of a specific stimulus or neuropsychological paradigm chosen by the experimenter to modulate the hemodynamic response during the image time series. These might be sensory stimuli (e.g., peripheral somatosensory, visual, auditory), emotional challenge (e.g., facial affect, emotive picture libraries, emotional words), appetitive stimuli (e.g., monetary reward, food, addictive substances), or cognitive tasks (e.g., working memory, attentional control, episodic or spatial memory). Task-evoked fMRI allows brain circuits (more generally, a brain state) associated with a particular aspect of brain function to be selectively probed. The paradigm is thus typically chosen with a particular functional effect or therapeutic indication in mind; for example, a putative analgesic might be assayed against a painful somatosensory stimulus[31,43,47,69–73] or in a peripheral sensitization model,[74] whereas a compound hypothesized to modulate cognitive processes might be assayed in appropriate cognition paradigms.[35,40,46,75–78] A large number of studies have demonstrated that drug effects on evoked fMRI responses can be detected,[30–32,38,40,42,47,73,74,76,77] and task-evoked fMRI represents the most mature fMRI approach in terms of detecting both disease and drug effects.

- **Resting state functional connectivity:** As another means of probing pharmacological effects directly on baseline brain function, this approach examines temporal correlations in low-frequency fluctuations between different brain regions in the "resting state" (i.e., in the absence of any cognitive paradigm or stimulus).[79–82] This approach is also amenable to oral or chronic dosing studies, and data on disease state signatures and pharmacological modulation of functional connectivity endpoints are beginning to emerge.[41,66,83–86] For application to drug development, however, much remains to be elucidated, including the endpoints that are most robust and sensitive to drug effects.

9.3.1. fMRI Biomarkers and Mechanistic Models in Early Drug Development

Key questions in early clinical development center on evaluating the safety of the molecule in humans, confirming that the target at which the compound is designed to act is in fact engaged, and selecting a dose range for subsequent POC trials. In the case of molecules designed to act within the CNS, target engagement is preconditioned by whether the molecule is brain-penetrant. fMRI can provide a measure of central PD drug effect from which central penetration can usually be inferred, and, albeit with lower sensitivity than a good RO-PET ligand, it can potentially be applied to determine exposure-response and dose-response relationships. The relationship between drug dose, or both PK parameters (e.g., reflecting drug exposure) and the PD effect of the assay is an important consideration in the clinical pharmacology setting. To date, only a few pharmacological fMRI studies in the literature have reported dose-response or exposure-response relationships: In acute pain fMRI experiments, dose-dependent attenuation of evoked fMRI signals by opioid analgesics has been demonstrated[31,73]; in another study, plasma levels (area under the curve [AUC] from drug administration until end of the fMRI scanning session) of the DA/norepinephrine-enhancing psychostimulant methylphenidate were found to correlate positively with BOLD responses to a visuospatial attention task.[77] This latter study demonstrates that, even with a single dose cohort, the variability in exposure and in the central response can be leveraged to examine exposure-response relationships. Compared with other single-endpoint assays, PK/PD relationships in fMRI are likely to depend both on brain region and on the paradigm used. Because the ability to inform dose selection for later-phase clinical trials is of high value, further elucidation of these relationships will be an important area of focus as fMRI methods are increasingly applied to drug development. Thus, fMRI studies in healthy volunteers represent a plausible early-phase PD imaging biomarker to characterize the central functional effect of a novel compound.[87] Working with healthy volunteers generally allows for easier and more rapid subject recruitment than do patient studies and avoids some of the heterogeneity and confounds (e.g., prior or concomitant medication) that arise with many disease populations. Such studies can often be performed at a single imaging site, greatly simplifying the associated logistics and reducing data variability.

phMRI experiments can be designed to examine the direct CNS response to the drug of interest or its modulation of the response to a probe drug (e.g., an antagonist–agonist design) and are well suited to early-phase, mechanistic biomarker studies. A good example of the latter is a drug interaction paradigm based on N-methyl-D-aspartate (NMDA) receptor antagonists such as phencyclidine (PCP) or ketamine. In addition to being a widely used pharmacological model of schizophrenia – especially in preclinical pharmacology[88] – when administered acutely these drugs yield a robust and consistent phMRI response in rats and humans that

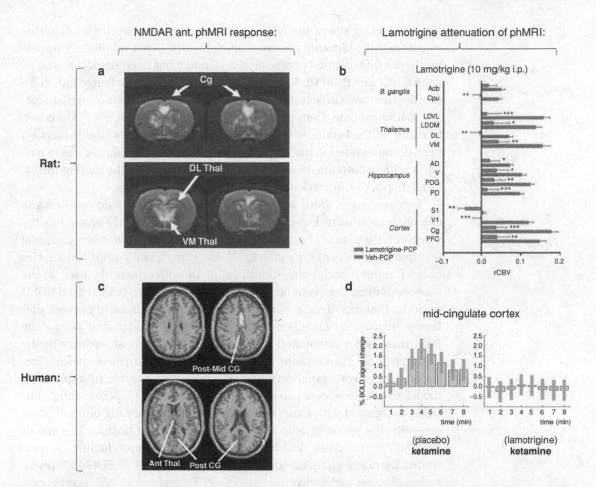

Fig. 9.3 NMDA receptor antagonist (NMDAR-ant.) challenge as a translational phMRI biomarker. Acute intravenous injection of NMDAR-ants., such as PCP or ketamine, induces regionally specific hemodynamic changes that are remarkably consistent across species. This phMRI signature serves as an imaging probe of glutamatergic dysregulation that can be modulated by pretreatment with compounds of interest. In the rat, relative cerebral blood volume (rCBV) increases in the brain following PCP challenge (a) can be attenuated by acute pretreatment with compounds such as lamotrigine (b). In humans, ketamine challenge evokes BOLD response in similar brain regions (c) that can also be blocked by pretreatment with lamotrigine (d). [Panels (a) and (b) first published in ref. 60. Panel (c) adapted from ref. 4 with permission from the American Medical Association (copyright © 2008 American Medical Association. All rights reserved.) Panel (d) courtesy of S. McKie and the authors of ref. 4.]

can serve as a CNS probe for the modulatory effect of other drugs (Figure 9.3).[60,89–92] Both drugs can be administered intravenously, facilitating the use of standard phMRI time series methods. In one such study in the rat, pretreatment with either the sodium channel blocker lamotrigine or the metabotropic glutamate$_{2/3}$ (mGlu$_{2/3}$) agonist LY354740 significantly attenuated the phMRI response to PCP (Figure 9.3, a and b).[60] In the same study, the atypical antipsychotic clozapine blocked the PCP response (most strongly in the thalamus), whereas it was not significantly attenuated by raclopride. Both the phMRI response to the NMDA receptor antagonist and its blockade by pretreatment with atypical antipsychotics are consistent with analogous, conscious 2-deoxyglucose (2-DG) studies.[93,94] In another phMRI study, the PCP signal was suppressed by activation of the allosteric glycine binding site of the NMDA receptor complex directly via D-serine or indirectly by blocking glycine reuptake with a GlyT1 inhibitor.[92] Importantly, the translational potential of this model has been demonstrated by several PET and fMRI studies in which acute ketamine challenge induced a positive hemodynamic response in brain regions (prefrontal/cingulate cortex, thalamus) consistent with those identified in the rat.[4,95–97] Moreover, blockade of the ketamine BOLD phMRI response by lamotrigine has also been demonstrated in healthy human volunteers,[4] providing a direct parallel to the lamotrigine blockade of the PCP response in the rat (Figure 9.3, c and d) and preclinical ketamine phMRI studies.[90]

Two reports of fMRI studies with the opioid analgesic remifentanil demonstrate how task-evoked fMRI can be used in early-phase healthy volunteer trials as a central PD biomarker to determine both temporal and spatial profiles of drug effect.[47,71] The experiment comprised a series of brief, painful peripheral stimuli using an MR-compatible laser. In the absence of drug, this paradigm evoked a central pattern of increased BOLD response that included primary and secondary somatosensory cortex, thalamus, insula, and cingulate cortex. Infusion of remifentanil during the fMRI time series attenuated this evoked response most strongly in the insula cortex.[47] Furthermore, because remifentanil is an intravenously formulated drug with rapid onset of action, it was possible to apply a PK model to the temporal profile of this modulation to derive time constants associated with onset and offset of this central drug effect.[71] More generally, the spatial profile observed in response to noxious thermal or mechanical stimuli in healthy subjects has been reproducibly demonstrated by many groups using modalities including $[^{18}F]$FDG-PET (measuring glucose metabolism), $[^{15}O]H_2O$-PET (perfusion), ASL (perfusion), and BOLD fMRI.[72,74,98–102] As such, it represents a particularly robust fMRI probe to modulate with drug candidates targeting pain indications.[31,37,48] Although opioid analgesics are effective in acute pain, there is a major unmet need in the treatment of pathological and chronic pain states,[72] and neuroimaging correlates of pain conditions (both baseline and evoked) are less well established than healthy volunteer acute pain models.[72,98,103,104] An intermediate role may be played by combining imaging with experimental pain models, for example, capsaicin-induced peripheral sensitization. In one study using such a model as a probe for drug modulation effects, the analgesic pregabalin was demonstrated to attenuate responses in the opercular cortex to evoked pain both in the normal and sensitized states (reflecting an antinociceptive effect of the drug) but also to attenuate positive responses in the brainstem and normalize aberrant and widespread deactivations that were observed only in the sensitized state (indicating an antihyperalgesic effect of the drug).[74]

Another approach is to directly probe differential CNS responses associated with specific genetic variants as a link to neural mechanisms underlying aspects of psychiatric disorders.[105–113] Studies to date have identified several genetic variants that alter BOLD responses to common neuropsychological paradigms implicated in depression and schizophrenia. An example is the Val[158/108] Met polymorphism in the gene coding for the catecholamine-O-methyltransferase (COMT) enzyme that plays an important role in breaking down DA in the prefrontal cortex (PFC), where few DA transporters are present.[114] A number of studies have shown that COMT genotype translates into differential BOLD activation in the PFC to working memory and executive function tasks,[114–118] implicating an optimal level of DA turnover for PFC-dependent tasks in an inverted-u relationship between DA signaling and function.[35,105,117] In this scenario, an ideal therapeutic would increase synaptic DA in individuals with suboptimal DA signaling but decrease it in subjects with supraoptimal DA levels. In reality, the picture is more complex with epistasis – interactions between different genes – playing an important role.[119–121] Nevertheless, in drug development such intermediate phenotypes may allow the interaction between target-relevant genetic variants and the effect of pharmacological treatment to be elucidated both in healthy populations[117] and in the disease state.[122] Ultimately, imaging genetics approaches may help, for example, to optimize dosing regimens for different subpopulations of patients.

9.3.2. Normalization of Brain Function: fMRI Studies in Patient Populations

fMRI studies in patient populations allow the functional effects of a putative therapeutic to be ascertained in the disease state and with respect to the aberrant functional responses associated with a particular pathology. Working in patient populations is relevant, for the manner in which a pharmacological agent modulates baseline or evoked responses in a pathological brain state may differ from its effects in control subjects; it is the disease state that represents the therapeutic target of the drug. For example, a meta-analysis of 12 published working-memory fMRI studies in schizophrenic patients[123] revealed a consistent hypoactivation in the dorsolateral PFC and a hyperactivation in the anterior cingulate cortex. In the context of mood disorders, exaggerated BOLD responses in limbic brain regions, including the amygdala, in emotional stimulus paradigms have been observed in depressed individuals compared with controls.[39,44,124–126] Importantly, a number of studies have documented "normalization" of this aberrant brain function following pharmacological treatment, with the increased amygdala response resolving toward levels observed in healthy controls following 8 weeks of treatment with different antidepressant medications (sertraline, venlafaxine, fluoxetine).[39,44,124] Moreover, an attenuated response in patients to positive affect (happy faces) in subcortical brain structures was found to be reversed by 8 weeks of fluoxetine treatment.[38] Interestingly, a study of facial affect in healthy volunteers also showed the amygdala response to fearful and disgusted faces to be attenuated by acute administration of citalopram, implying a pharmacological modulation of brain structures involved in basic processes underlying the disorder.[33] Note, however, that each of these studies examined a marketed drug of either the SSRI or serotonin–norepinephrine reuptake inhibitor (SNRI) class for which efficacious doses are already established; the extent to which these findings generalize to compounds with divergent mechanisms of action remains to be established.

Patient population fMRI studies are thus more typically associated with Phase 2 of the standard drug development paradigm, when clinical trials in patient populations are first carried out. The imaging study may be an addendum to a Phase 2 trial performed at a subset of the trial sites. In this situation, the geography and sites selected for the main trial can constrain options for the imaging study. This point is important for fMRI studies, which are complex in execution and typically rely on substantial expertise at specialist sites. Moreover, patient studies bring additional issues, including confounding effects of prior and current medication, heterogeneity across subjects, slower recruitment rates, and increased demands on scan-day logistics and clinical monitoring. Thus, to obtain sufficient sample sizes to be adequately powered, such imaging studies may need to be multisite, bringing requirements for the harmonization of acquisition protocols, appropriate and consistent quality assurance/quality control (QA/QC) procedures, well-defined and efficient analysis pipelines, and mechanisms for clear communication of progress and study diagnostics (e.g., summary results of acquisition and analysis QC steps). Given that fMRI remains a relatively specialized endeavor, an alternative to running the imaging study as a trial addendum is a stand-alone imaging study, which can allow more choice in site selection and protocol definition but may still need to be multicenter to reconcile expected recruitment rates and study timelines.[127,128]

9.3.3. Validation and Standardization of fMRI for Drug Development Applications

Despite many drug studies performed using fMRI, the technique has yet to become firmly established in the drug development process. In part, the technique is a victim of its own flexibility, for an extremely wide variety of paradigms and experimental designs have been used as fMRI methods have rapidly developed over the past two decades. Small differences in acquisition parameters, image reconstruction, and paradigm implementation, however, can result in subtle (or not so subtle) differences in the measured functional effect. To robustly detect a pharmacological effect – and confidently interpret the absence of an observed effect – with a novel compound, a stable, well-characterized paradigm is required in which the candidate drug is the primary experimental variable. Application to drug development thus requires precisely defined and well-characterized imaging protocols that can be reliably and reproducibly applied, appropriately powered, and for which clear numerical endpoints are established.

Although hemodynamic responses measured by fMRI methods can, under ideal circumstances, be considered a reasonable surrogate for underlying changes in metabolic demand and neuronal activity in the CNS, the fact that the hemodynamic response is downstream from these underlying changes means that potential confounds involving nonneurally mediated vasoaction and neurovascular coupling must be carefully considered when studying disease populations or pharmacological intervention.[49,129,130] In particular, a control task is often recommended[130] in which the lack of a significant pharmacological modulation provides evidence of functional specificity of the drug effect. For formal use in drug trials, powering considerations are mandatory, and these have begun to be addressed,[131–134] although data on actual pharmacological effect sizes have been less explicitly reported in the literature. Part of the complication is that the effect size can depend strongly on the statistical contrast reported and on brain region; significant drug effects may, for example, be detected in brain regions that do not strongly respond to the stimulus in the absence of drug. Moreover, in multisite studies, harmonization of the complex fMRI process and a rigorous statistical accounting for differences between sites are requisites.[127,128,131,135,136]

Several initiatives are under way to address the validation of fMRI for application in clinical trial and drug development contexts. The NIH-funded Biomedical Informatics Research Network (BIRN) has included an fMRI component ("fBIRN"), which has systematically addressed issues related to multicenter (and multivendor) fMRI[135,136] and has produced QA/QC protocols and analysis pipelines. These practices have also been applied to large trials of schizophrenic patients,[127,128] illustrating the utility of multicenter trials for both fast and large studies in patient populations. The Imaging Consortium for Drug Development (ICD) was recently established as a precompetitive collaboration between several pharmaceutical companies and Harvard University to characterize and validate fMRI systematically from the explicit viewpoint of application to drug development.[48] This initiative is evaluating both preclinical and clinical fMRI approaches, including phMRI, evoked fMRI, and resting-state functional connectivity in the particular context of pain and the development of analgesic compounds. It is hoped that efforts such as these will provide well-characterized fMRI protocols and associated procedures and help to establish de facto standards that will be greatly beneficial to the further application of fMRI methods to the drug development process.

9.4. Imaging as a Biomarker to Enrich Study Populations

In October 2004, academic researchers, the U.S. National Institutes of Health, and pharmaceutical companies launched the Alzheimer's Disease Neuroimaging Initiative (ADNI) with the goal of developing methods for improving Alzheimer's disease (AD) clinical trials.[137] Today, ADNI has enrolled more than 800 volunteers between the ages of 55 and 90, about a quarter of them healthy, another quarter clinically diagnosed with probable AD, and the rest diagnosed with mild cognitive impairment (MCI). They underwent testing every 6 to 12 months with a variety of methods, including volumetric MRI (vMRI), brain PET scans with [^{18}F]FDG or a ligand for β-amyloid, and lumbar punctures to collect cerebrospinal fluid with the goal of determining which biomarker(s) track the progression of AD more faithfully than the cognitive and clinical measures previously used in clinical trials.

Comparison of the imaging modalities used in ADNI – [^{18}F]FDG PET, [^{11}C]Pittsburgh compound B (PIB), and vMRI – has revealed that vMRI is the best powered to detect a given (e.g., 25%) reduction in the rate of progression of that endpoint.[138,139] β-amyloid imaging, however, appears to be an essential biomarker to enrich study populations; in other words, if, for instance, a novel amyloid-modifying treatment candidate is tested in an AD clinical trial, β-amyloid PET imaging is useful to ensure that only subjects with β-amyloid deposition in their brains are enrolled, for it is one of the hallmark features of AD. It needs to be remembered that, until relatively recently, the only way to determine whether a patient had β-amyloid plaques in the brain was during a postmortem using brain-staining techniques. Several PET amyloid imaging ligands have recently been developed and tested in AD patients, among them [^{11}C]PIB,[2] 3'[^{18}F]FPIB, [^{18}F]FDDNP,[140] [^{11}C]SB-13,[141] [^{18}F]F-SB-13, and most recently [^{18}F]AV45.[142] Although it is debatable which particular ligand may be best for a particular scientific question, it appears that there is a rich database documenting the usefulness of PET ligands to determine β-amyloid plaque deposition in AD patients and also in patients with amnestic MCI.[143] They represent an important clinical group because they are at increased risk of developing AD. It was found that PIB-positive subjects – those who had increased [^{11}C]PIB retention at baseline – with mild MCI were more likely to convert to AD than PIB-negative patients and that faster converters had higher PIB retention levels at baseline than slower converters.

9.5. Oncology

9.5.1. Anatomical Imaging in Cancer Drug Development

The primary application of imaging to drug development in oncology has been anatomical. As in standard-of-care clinical practice, MRI or CT scans are widely used in clinical trials to assess disease extent and solid tumor size. Typically, anatomical scans are performed before and after treatment to assess the effect of a drug or therapeutic regimen on the radiologically visible tumor burden. Using medical imaging to assess a potential change in tumor burden has become part of the clinical evaluation of cancer drug candidates: Tumor shrinkage and time to disease progression are important endpoints in clinical cancer trials. The use of tumor regression as an endpoint for Phase 2, POC clinical trials is supported by evidence suggesting that agents that produce solid tumor shrinkage have a reasonable chance of subsequently demonstrating an improvement in overall survival in larger, randomized Phase 3 cancer studies [reviewed in (144–147)]. At both, Phase 2 and 3 of clinical cancer drug development, clinical trials are using time to progression, or progression-free survival, based on anatomical measurement of tumor size, as an endpoint on which efficacy conclusions are drawn.

Since RECIST was published in 2000,[148] many investigators, cooperative groups, and industry and government authorities have adopted these criteria in the assessment of treatment outcomes. A number of questions and issues have arisen, which have led to the development of a revised RECIST guideline (version 1.1).[8] Major changes included a reduction in the number of lesions required to assess tumor burden for response determination. This number was reduced from a maximum of 10 to a maximum of 5 total (and from 5 to 2 per organ). Furthermore, assessing pathological lymph nodes is incorporated in the revised RECIST guidelines: Nodes with a short axis of 15 mm are considered measurable and assessable as target lesions. Nodes that shrink to a <10 mm short axis are to be considered normal. It has also been suggested that confirmation of response is required for trials with response as a primary endpoint but is no longer required in randomized, controlled studies. Disease progression is clarified in several aspects: In addition to the prior definition of progression in target disease of 20% increase in sum, a 5-mm absolute increase is now required to reduce false positives.

A key issue considered by the RECIST Working Group in developing RECIST 1.1 was whether it was appropriate to move from anatomic unidimensional assessment of tumor burden to either volumetric anatomical assessment or to functional assessment with PET or MRI. It was concluded that, at present, there is not sufficient standardization or evidence to abandon anatomical assessment of tumor burden. The only exception to this is in the use of [18F]FDG-PET imaging as an adjunct to determining of progression. In earlier phases of drug development, however, volumetric or functional imaging methods are more applicable and have the potential to assay the effects of a therapeutic candidate on a greater range of biological parameters.

9.5.2. Functional Imaging in Cancer Drug Development

The motivation for considering functional imaging methods is that changes in tumor biology may occur well before eventual clinical response and that imaging methods can detect drug effects on relevant parameters of tumor biology in a non- or minimally invasive manner within hours or days after the start of treatment.[6,149-154] More saliently, novel, targeted therapies may induce clinically meaningful changes in tumor status and function that do not necessarily translate into shrinkage amenable to RECIST classification of response.

The detection of drug effects on tumor biology can help to define a dose window between a biologically effective dose (BED) and the conventionally determined maximally tolerated dose (MTD).[6] The definition of an MTD-BED window allows a more flexible trade-off between efficacy and side effects to be explored. Such information could be gleaned by the incorporation of relevant imaging biomarkers in early-phase trials, for example, that provide an opportunity to obtain PD measurements over a range of doses, treatment regimens, and tumor types. The availability of such PD data in turn allows for an explicit assessment or modeling of PK/PD relationships – the relationship between the systemic exposure to the drug and macroscopic parameter(s) reflecting some aspect of the tumor's biological phenotype (e.g., vascular parameters, metabolism, cell density). Importantly, these methods are feasible in the translational space – often, the same method can be performed in both animal models and human subjects. At this juncture, the most advanced of the functional imaging methods are [18F]FDG-PET as a probe of tumor glucose metabolism and dynamic contrast-enhanced MRI (DCE-MRI) to report tumor vascular status.

Recently, the status and limitations of anatomic tumor response metrics, including the World Health Organization (WHO) criteria, RECIST, and RECIST 1.1, led to a newly proposed draft framework for PET Response Criteria in Solid Tumors (PERCIST).[155] The authors point out that, despite effective treatment, changes in tumor size can be minimal in tumors such as lymphomas, sarcomas, hepatomas, mesothelioma, and gastrointestinal stromal tumors. CT tumor density, contrast enhancement, or MRI characteristics appear more informative than size but are not yet routinely applied. In addition, RECIST criteria may show progression of tumor more slowly than may WHO criteria, and the revised RECIST 1.1 criteria (assessing a maximum of 5 tumor foci vs. 10 in RECIST) result in a higher complete response rate than the original RECIST criteria – at least in lymph nodes. [18F]FDG-PET response assessments, however, require a consistent PET methodology.[155] Statistically significant changes in tumor standardized uptake value (SUV) occur in studies of high-SUV tumors with a change of 20% in SUV of a region 1 cm or larger in diameter; however, medically relevant beneficial changes are often associated with a 30% or greater decline. Important components of the proposed PERCIST criteria include assessing normal reference tissue values in a 3-cm-diameter region of interest (ROI) in the liver using a consistent PET protocol; using a fixed, small ROI, approximately 1 cm^3 in volume, in the most active region of metabolically active tumors to minimize statistical variability; assessing tumor size; treating SUV lean measurements in the most metabolically active tumor focus as a continuous variable; requiring a 30% decline in SUV for "response"; and deferring to RECIST 1.1 in cases that do not have [18F]FDG avidity. In summary, the authors concluded that anatomic imaging alone using standard WHO, RECIST, and RECIST 1.1 criteria has limitations, particularly in assessing the activity of newer, noncytotoxic cancer therapies that stabilize disease, whereas [18F]FDG-PET appears particularly valuable in those instances.[155]

9.5.3. Imaging the Tumor Vasculature

Dynamic contrast-enhanced MRI (DCE-MRI) has evolved over the past 15 years and is now widely applied to the development of new antiangiogenic cancer therapies.[152,154,156–158] This development occurred as drugs targeting the angiogenesis process[159–161] were beginning to be developed and so found a natural role in the evaluation of drug effects on tumor vascular function. In its usual form, the DCE-MRI technique[162–166] involves the acquisition of a T_1-weighted image time series covering the tumor(s) of interest, during which a bolus of contrast agent is injected into a peripheral vein. Typically, the contrast agent comprises a gadolinium (Gd) chelate that increases the T_1 relaxation rate ($R_1 = 1/T_1$) of water protons local to the contrast agent and hence increases the signal intensity of T_1-weighted images in the time series. Thus, each pixel contains a signal intensity time course, the form of which reflects the perfusion and permeability characteristics of the tumor vasculature within that pixel. These time courses tend to differ qualitatively between tumor and normal tissue and between malignant and benign tumors.[166] Indeed, because the (in-plane) spatial resolution is typically on the order of millimeters, substantial heterogeneity in contrast agent uptake profiles within individual lesions is often observed. The form and heuristic parameterization of these contrast enhancement time courses can themselves be used as endpoints for tracking response to treatment.[167–169]

These changes in image intensity can be further processed to infer the local contrast agent concentration changes through time following injection, which are then amenable to compartmental PK modeling.[163] Most commonly, a two-compartment Tofts model is applied in which the compartments are the vasculature itself and the extravascular-extracellular space (EES). The model yields the intercompartmental transfer rate constants.[165] Indeed, reproducibility studies have shown that the vasculature-to-EES rate constant, K^{trans}, and the initial AUC (IAUC) are the most reliable summary measures from DCE-MRI analyses of this sort and so are generally recommended as primary endpoints in therapeutic trials.[170,171] DCE-MRI analyses are typically carried out pixel-wise (i.e., PK modeling for each pixel), generating parametric maps,[6,157,166] and histograms,[156,172] or both, of the DCE-MRI parameters to visualize heterogeneity within the tumor.[156] The application of DCE-MRI to drug development has been underpinned by a body of thorough analyses of the influence of acquisition parameters, modeling assumptions, and reproducibility of the technique[173–178] along with consensus recommendations for its use in this context.[170,171] Furthermore, for drug development applications, a single numeric primary endpoint is desirable. This endpoint is often calculated as the mean or median parameter value within the entire tumor or the strongest enhancing part thereof, or parameter values calculated from the average time course from pixels within a specified ROI. Nevertheless, substantial scope remains to extract alternative endpoints and additional information from the full – often heterogeneous – volume of tumor pixels and to leverage the fine spatial resolution of the data more fully. The stability of any such alternative endpoints to effects such as physiological motion and basic validation in terms of reproducibility needs to be evaluated.

Several clinical studies have demonstrated the application of DCE-MRI to the evaluation of novel therapeutics targeting vascular function.[152,168,179–181] Importantly, DCE-MRI can also be performed in rodent models, and a number of preclinical studies have also demonstrated the ability to detect drug effects on vascular parameters by using this technique.[182–186] Several reports have demonstrated fully translational DCE-MRI studies with both preclinical and clinical experiments performed with the same compound[187–189]: The vascular targeting agent combrestatin A4 phosphate (CA4P) was investigated in the P22 rat carcinosarcoma xenograft model using a DCE-MRI protocol designed to closely match that used in a subsequent Phase 1 clinical study.[187] The rat data showed a strong drug effect on vascular parameters at an early posttreatment time point (1 hour), informing the inclusion of an early posttreatment scan (4–6 hours) in the clinical study. The patient data, in turn, showed the strongest reduction in tumor DCE-MRI parameters at the 4- to 6-hour time point with reduced (but still significant) effects at 24 hours. The effects were selective to the tumor with minimal effects in normal tissues.

In another study,[188] the effects of the vascular targeting agent ZD6126, which acts by disrupting the tubulin cytoskeleton of tumor neoendothelial cells, were investigated in murine C38 colon adenocarcinoma models and in patients with liver metastases of mixed solid tumor origin. Both the mouse and the human data showed a dose-dependent reduction in IAUC in the tumors with no effects on skeletal muscle (Figure 9.4). In a third example,[189] the activity of the panvascular endothelial growth factor (VEGF) receptor tyrosine kinase inhibitor PTK787/ZK-222584 (vatalanib) in the orthotopic B16/BL6 mouse melanoma metastasis model[190] was compared with findings in Phase 1 DCE-MRI clinical trials.[191] Again, the preclinical measurements were designed to closely match the clinical situation and, despite potential interspecies differences, the mouse model yielded estimates of efficacious drug exposure (plasma AUC) levels that matched those corresponding to the antiangiogenic BED in humans. This study represents a good example of how a translational imaging approach can use preclinical data to inform and accelerate the selection of a BED in early clinical studies.

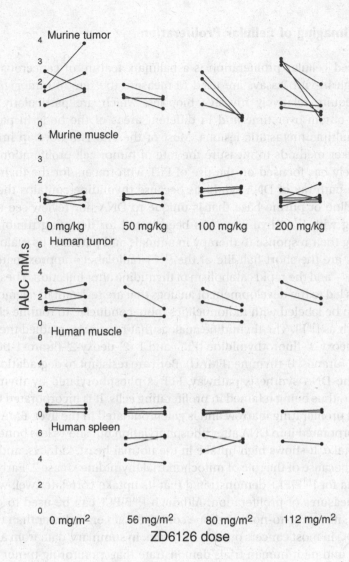

Fig. 9.4
Dose-dependent
reduction of the
DCE-MRI parameter
IAUC by the vascular
targeting agent
ZD6126 in both
murine and human
tumors with little
effect on other tissues.
[Reprinted from
ref. 188 with
permission of J.
Evelhoch and the
American Association
for Cancer Research.]

VEGF and its receptors are the most important regulators of angiogenesis. Lately, novel approaches were tested to probe the VEGF receptor with radiolabeled imaging probes. The uptake of the SPECT tracer [99mTc]-single-chain (sc)VEGF in turpentine-induced abscesses was specific and directly related to VEGF receptor-2 (R-2) expression in the neovasculature of the angiogenic rim.[192] In a different approach, VEGF(121) was conjugated with 1,4,7,10-tetra-azacylododecane *N,N′,N″,N‴*-tetraacetic acid (DOTA) and then labeled with [64Cu] for PET imaging in mice bearing different-sized human glioblastoma U87MG tumors.[193] The tumor uptake of [64Cu]DOTA-VEGF(121) measured by small-animal PET imaging reflected tumor VEGFR-2 expression level in vivo. It needs to be demonstrated whether such correlations translate to humans and are clinically useful for future treatment planning and treatment monitoring of cancer and potentially other angiogenesis-related diseases.

9.5.4. Imaging of Cellular Proliferation

Increased cellular proliferation is a hallmark feature of cancerous cells. Although in-vitro assays are used to measure the rate of tumor growth, they require relatively invasive biopsies, which are particularly difficult to obtain over time and in different areas of the body in patients with multiple metastatic lesions. Most of the effort to develop imaging biomarker methods to measure the rate of tumor cell proliferation noninvasively has focused on the use of PET with tracers for the thymidine salvage pathway of DNA synthesis because thymidine contains the only pyrimidine or purine base that is unique to DNA [for review see (194)]. Imaging with [^{11}C]thymidine has been tested for detecting tumors and tracking their response to therapy in animals and patients. Its major limitations are the short half-life of the [^{11}C]-radiolabel – approximately 20 minutes – and the rapid catabolism of thymidine after injection. These limitations led to the development of analogs that are resistant to degradation and can be labeled with radionuclides more conducive to routine clinical use such as [^{18}F]. The thymidine analogs that have been studied the most are 3′-deoxy-3′-fluorothymidine (FLT) and 1-(2′-deoxy-2′-fluoro-1-beta-D-arabinofuranosyl)-thymine (FMAU). Both are resistant to degradation and track the DNA synthesis pathway. FLT is phosphorylated by thymidine kinase 1, thus being retained in proliferating cells. It is incorporated by the normal proliferating marrow and is glucuronidated in the liver. FMAU can be incorporated into DNA after phosphorylation but shows less bone marrow uptake. It shows high uptake in the normal heart, kidneys, and liver, in part because of the role of mitochondrial thymidine kinase 2. Early clinical data for [^{18}F]FLT demonstrated that its uptake correlates well with in vitro measures of proliferation. Although [^{18}F]FLT can be used to detect tumors, its tumor-to-normal tissue contrast is generally lower than that of [^{18}F]FDG in most cancers outside the brain. In summary, data from animal studies and pilot human trials demonstrate that monitoring tumor treatment response appears to be the most promising use for thymidine and its analogs.[194] Although both FLT and FMAU appear to be promising candidates to eventually become surrogate markers for treatment response, it needs to be stressed that at present none of these imaging biomarkers has yet been adequately qualified to enable go/no-go decisions with novel cancer drug candidates.

An alternative probe on tumor metabolism is provided by proton magnetic resonance spectroscopy (^{1}H-MRS). This approach measures signals from mobile hydrogen nuclei within biochemical compounds in the tumor or other tissues. These compounds are present at much lower concentrations ($\sim 10^{-4}\times$) than water but can be distinguished from the much stronger water and lipid signals in spectroscopic measurements. The low concentrations of these metabolites result in a coarser temporal and spatial resolution of spectroscopic measurements relative to imaging sequences. Malignant lesions tend to be characterized by elevated levels of

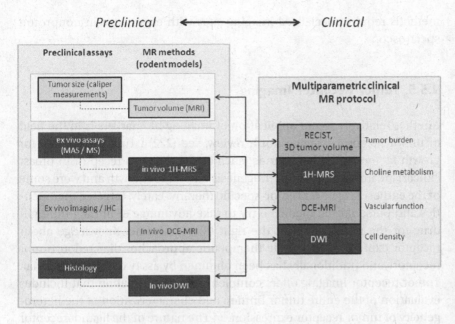

Preclinical ⟷ Clinical

Fig. 9.5
Schematic illustration of how the tumor microenvironment and its pharmacological modulation can be profiled by complementary imaging and experimental methods. Preclinically, ex-vivo assays and in-vivo MRI methods, or both, can provide a comprehensive picture of a compound's action at the level of the tumor phenotype. Many of these can translate into in-vivo clinical MRI measures that can be obtained within a single scan protocol. [IHC: immunohistochemistry; MAS: magic angle spinning; DWI = diffusion weighted imaging.]

choline-containing metabolites, which is a signal interpreted as reflecting increased cell membrane turnover in the proliferating tumor tissue. In brain and prostate cancer, this signature is superimposed on signals of native tissue metabolites,[195–200] whereas in other neoplasms (e.g., breast carcinoma, lymphoma) the choline signal is often the most reliably detectable metabolite.[150,151,201–206] Importantly, several studies have reported measurable decreases in the choline signal within a few days of initiating treatment that also correlate with subsequent clinical response.[150,151,207,208] Moreover, as with other MR-based methods, ^{1}H-MRS can also be implemented preclinically to probe tumor metabolism longitudinally in animal models[182,209,210] and thus provides a translatable, noninvasive biomarker of tumor choline metabolism.

The published clinical studies to date, however, are in relatively small cohorts with data acquired at single, specialized research sites; there remains a need for multicenter trials to develop standardized acquisition and analysis methodologies and to build a large body of comparable ^{1}H-MRS data linked to clinical outcome.[211] We also note that it is quite feasible to include ^{1}H-MRS within a multimethod MRI scanning session to provide a more complete in-vivo profile of tumor status, for example, alongside measurements of vascular parameters with DCE-MRI, cell density with diffusion-weighted imaging, as well as tumor volume and RECIST assessments (Figure 9.5).

MRS of other nuclei is also possible in – particular ^{31}P-MRS to examine phospholipid metabolism[212–214] and ^{19}F-MRS to study the PK, disposition, and metabolism of fluorine-containing compounds.[215–221] The latter is attractive as a means of determining drug concentration at the tumor site, for there is no background fluorine signal from native tissue, but it requires sufficient presence of drug to produce a detectable signal. These methods require specialized imaging sites with experience in nonproton spectroscopy.

9.5.5. Tumor Receptor Imaging

Another relatively recent application of imaging biomarkers is in the field of tumor receptor imaging [for a review, see (222)]. Tumor receptors for growth factors and other ligands (such as the estrogen receptor in breast cancer) are important for carcinogenesis and tumor growth and were some of the earliest targets for tumor-specific therapy. Lately, targeted therapeutics and personalized medicine try to take advantage of finding the right drug for the right patient at the right dose and time. Knowledge about receptor expression can guide therapeutic approaches directed at tumor receptors and traditionally has been obtained by assay of biopsy material. Tumor receptor imaging offers complementary information that includes evaluation of the entire tumor burden and characterization of the heterogeneity of tumor receptor expression.[222] The nature of the ligand–receptor interaction is challenging for imaging, however, for a low molecular concentration of the imaging probe is required to avoid saturating the receptor and increasing the background because of nonspecific uptake. Much of the work to date in tumor receptor imaging has been done with radionuclide probes. Examples of targets of tumor receptor imaging range are steroid receptors, such as the estrogen and progesterone receptors in breast cancer, and the androgen receptor in prostate cancer; somatostatin receptors (SSTRs) in neuroendocrine tumors and growth factor receptors, such as the epidermal growth factor receptor (EGFR).[222] Estrogen receptor imaging with [^{18}F]FES PET has given indications of promise as a tool to enhance breast cancer treatment.[223] Larger trials, however, are required to confirm the value of [^{18}F]FES PET as a prognostic assay and to determine an appropriate SUV cutoff for predicting a response to endocrine therapy.[222]

9.5.6. Imaging Apoptosis

The balance between proliferation and programmed cell death – apoptosis – is essential for organisms to regulate and maintain the number and type of their cells during embryogenesis, growth, and homeostasis. Increased cell proliferation or enhanced cell loss can be caused by dysregulated apoptosis and is observed in various diseases, including neurodegenerative disorders, myocardial infarction, and stroke, in which the rate of apoptosis is higher than normal. In cancer and autoimmune diseases, conditions with pathological proliferation, apoptosis is often downregulated. In addition, the mechanism of many newer targeted cancer drugs includes inhibition of the tumor's abnormal antiapoptosis-protective pathways. Therefore, noninvasive imaging of apoptosis is of clinical interest to diagnose cell loss postinfarction or to monitor apoptosis triggered by chemo- or radiation therapy of tumors.[224] Several biochemical transformations occur in apoptotic cells and present different biological targets for the development of specific molecular biomarkers of apoptosis: the externalization of phospholipid phosphatidylserine to the outer layer of the cell membrane, which can be visualized by labeled annexin V and the activation of caspases, especially effector caspase-3, which can be addressed by labeled enzyme substrates or synthetic caspase inhibitors. The field of apoptosis imaging is changing quite rapidly, but at the moment it appears that agents that bind to the surface of apoptotic cells, including annexin V and its derivatives, are superior to metabolically directed tracers, such as caspase-related radiopharmaceuticals, when sensitivity and specificity for apoptotic cells are probed.[225]

9.6. Imaging Cardiovascular Disease

A key biological target in atherosclerotic cardiovascular disease is the thickening of arterial walls due to the formation of atherosclerotic lesions or plaques.[226] This disease process involves inflammation, deposition of lipids (including cholesterol), and the formation of an extracellular matrix. Clinical symptoms are related to plaque instability, including a thinning of the fibrous cap and clot formation (thrombosis). Atherosclerotic plaques and the associated vessel walls are thus heterogeneous, and different lesions may comprise differing relative fractions of inflammatory cells, lipid-rich necrotic core (LRNC), and fibrous cap.[226]

In-vivo imaging of atherosclerotic disease in-situ has evolved rapidly over the past decade and has been demonstrated to be technically possible (despite the spatial resolution, signal-to-noise, and physiological confound challenges), reproducible, feasible in a multicenter clinical trial setting, and sensitive to drug effects.[226,227] Different imaging modalities offer complementary information on the status of the plaque(s). [^{18}F]FDG uptake measured via PET has been shown to correspond to macrophage-rich areas of the plaque[228,229] and thus provides a surrogate of inflammatory activity. Morphological imaging by MRI provides information on plaque composition with reproducible quantification of the vessel wall and lumen areas, as well as the LRNC and calcified areas.[227,230,231] A comprehensive MRI-based morphological characterization of plaque composition requires a multiparametric imaging protocol in which T_1-weighted, T_2-weighted, and proton density–weighted images are obtained alongside angiograms and, increasingly, gadolinium contrast-enhanced imaging[227,232,233] or full-fledged DCE-MRI as an alternative probe of inflammation.[234]

Multidetector CT provides another means of acquiring coronary angiograms and can also detect calcification – a strong risk factor in asymptomatic individuals.[226,235] These imaging techniques thus allow for the status of plaque pathology to be assayed alongside peripheral biomarkers such as high- and low-density lipoproteins or inflammatory markers.

9.6.1. Clinical Trials in Atherosclerosis Using Imaging Endpoints

Several clinical trials to date have demonstrated the use of imaging parameters as endpoints to assess drug effects on atherosclerosis.[227,236–239] The effect of simvastatin on plaque inflammation was evaluated by $[^{18}F]$FDG-PET in a trial of 43 completing subjects and showed that this drug decreased the FDG uptake by thoracic or carotid plaques over and above diet alone.[236] The treatment also decreased low-density lipoprotein (LDL) cholesterol and increased high-density lipoprotein (HDL) cholesterol, but only the latter was correlated with the attenuation in FDG uptake. Despite being a small trial (~20/arm) and having a relatively short treatment time of only 3 months, this study provided preliminary[240] in-vivo evidence that the statin treatment reduced plaque inflammation by the direct means of an imaging surrogate for this biological process in the pathological tissue.

Independent trials of the same drug using MRI endpoints have also been conducted. In a trial of 18 asymptomatic subjects with aortic or carotid plaques, simvastatin induced changes in vessel wall thickness (but not lumen area) that were significant after 12 months but not 6 months of treatment. This effect was interpreted as vascular remodeling.[237] Follow-up at later time points revealed increased reduction in vessel wall thickness at 18 and 24 months, at which times modest increases in lumen area also became apparent.[238] Another randomized trial compared conventional (20 mg/day) and aggressive (80 mg/day) doses of simvastatin in a similar population (total $N = 51$) with an ~18-month follow-up.[239] Vessel wall area was again reduced after 12 months in both dose cohorts, but the vessel wall parameters as measured by MRI were more associated with LDL cholesterol reduction than with treatment dose.

The prospective, randomized, double-blind ORION trial used high-resolution morphological MRI to assess the effects of 2 years of treatment with rosuvastatin (5 mg or 40/80 mg dose arms) on carotid plaque volume and composition in 33 patients with elevated LDL cholesterol (100 < LDL-C < 250 mg/dL) and carotid artery stenosis.[241] The total plaque volume did not change over the course of treatment; however, a 41% decrease in the LRNC fraction of the vessel wall was observed in the 18 patients with LRNC present at baseline. The ORION trial was the first prospective, long-term MRI study of statin effects on carotid plaque composition, and its results indicated an effect of the treatment on plaque stability by measuring parameters related to their composition, beyond total plaque size.

9.6.2. Practicality of Cardiovascular Imaging Trials and Application to Drug Development

Importantly, clinical trials such as those summarized earlier in the text have demonstrated the feasibility of multicenter cardiovascular imaging studies and have engendered the development of standardized acquisition protocols, QA/QC, data transfer logistics, and core analysis laboratories to provide a platform for robust clinical imaging trials.[233] Moreover, rigorous analyses of the reproducibility of these imaging endpoints have been undertaken, enabling informed power calculations of prospective trials.[227,230,231,233,242,243]

9.7. Conclusions

Imaging biomarkers are widely used in drug development. The maturity and degree of validation of different imaging biomarkers, however, vary not only by modality but also by therapeutic area. For instance, with CNS drug candidates aimed at brain targets, PET RO studies to determine brain penetration, target engagement, and, with an adequate PK/PD or PK/RO model, to subsequently inform dosing represent the current gold standard in the industry. This approach, however, requires substantial investment in developing novel tracers for new targets in parallel with the drug candidate. As there often is limited commercial value in the PET tracer, but substantial scientific interest in using those tools to probe basic biology of CNS conditions, that endeavor seems to be best addressed in public–private partnerships or industry consortia. A comprehensive review of the role of imaging biomarkers in POC trials for CNS drug development has been published recently.[244]

Moreover, although RO-PET represents a critical component of early CNS drug development, suitable PET ligands may not be available (or be able to be developed) for all CNS targets. Functional imaging, using methods such as fMRI, can provide additional insights into the downstream functional consequences of target engagement and can also be adapted to study direct mechanistic interactions between the drug and the brain by using phMRI designs. In the absence of a PET ligand, an fMRI approach might provide a suitable biomarker from which brain penetration and possibly target engagement could be inferred. Although there are many published studies on the effects of marketed drugs in fMRI paradigms, there are few compelling cases of fMRI's prospective use as a biomarker in early-phase drug development. This in part reflects a different set of exigencies associated with application to a novel compound (quite possibly with an unprecedented mechanism of action) for which the uncertainties and risks are much greater. Moreover, the extent and manner in which fMRI methods, for which the signal window will be lower than that expected for a good RO-PET ligand, can inform dose selection remain unknown. That said, several initiatives are under way to characterize specific fMRI methods systematically with a view to clinical trial and drug development applications. Moreover, if a functional imaging study can address key questions required for the progression of the drug candidate, the approach can provide additional data on how the compound is modulating brain function that can be linked to preclinical data to address mechanistic hypotheses about the compound's effect in humans.

As noted earlier, the public–private partnership around the ADNI focused on developing novel tools to improve drug development for AD. Besides the valuable insights into the usefulness of an imaging biomarker to establish the presence of β-amyloid in the living human brain, ADNI's goals were foremost to determine which, if any, imaging biomarker would be most sensitive to assay potentially disease-modifying interventions. As reviewed in this chapter, volumetric assessments of certain brain structures (in particular, the hippocampus) seem to have an edge over other modalities and may be useful not only to provide more objective information than can be obtained from clinical scales and interviews but may also help to minimize sample sizes as well as duration of clinical trials.

Most of the initial imaging biomarker research occurred in CNS-related applications. Oncology, however, is one of the most rapidly expanding areas in which novel imaging biomarkers are currently being tested. Imaging modalities span all the way from traditional anatomical assessments of tumor burden to more functional assays interrogating certain aspects of cancerous tumors such as metabolism, apoptosis, or tumor microenvironment (including angiogenesis). A robust link between the imaging endpoint and clinical outcome will need to be established for many of the emerging functional imaging methods. This endeavor will require large-scale clinical trials. Many methods are most suitable for use as biomarkers in early-phase studies to help establish confidence in the drug mechanism, particularly if the biological parameter measured can be tightly linked to target engagement but is not yet ready for large-scale application or to drive decisions regarding compound progression.

Cardiovascular imaging is one of the latest emerging fields for imaging biomarkers. For application to drug development, imaging methods have the possibility of relatively small ($N < 100$) trials in a Phase 2 setting to assess a drug candidate's action against relevant biological parameters of atherosclerotic plaque status, especially in terms of inflammatory activity and composition. Another likely role for cardiovascular imaging is as a screening tool at baseline for proof-of-concept studies to enrich the study population for one or more of these biological parameters with regard to the hypothesized effect of the compound to be studied or based on associated risk as data emerge on the association between imaging endpoints and subsequent clinical events.[245,246]

This chapter has highlighted examples of the utility of imaging biomarkers in the context of drug development ranging from (1) confirming the presence of a drug target in a population entering a clinical trial, to (2) assessing target engagement of a novel drug candidate, to (3) demonstrating pharmacology through a functional effect of a drug candidate, to (4) determining dosing for clinical trials, to (5) facilitating early go/no-go decisions, and, last but not least, to (6) serving as a surrogate for clinical response.

9.8. Conflict of Interest Statement

Both authors are employees and stockholders of Eli Lilly and Company in Indianapolis, Indiana.

9.9. References

1. Adams CP, & Brantner VV. (2006). Estimating the cost of new drug development: Is it really 802 million dollars? Health Aff. (Millwood). 25(2), 420–428.
2. Klunk WE, Engler H, Nordberg A, Wang Y, Blomqvist G, Holt DP, et al. (2004). Imaging brain amyloid in Alzheimer's disease with Pittsburgh Compound-B. Ann. Neurol. 55(3), 306–319.
3. Farde L, Hall H, Ehrin E, & Sedvall G. (1986). Quantitative analysis of D2 dopamine receptor binding in the living human brain by PET. Science. 231(4735), 258–261.
4. Deakin JF, Lees J, McKie S, Hallak JE, Williams SR, & Dursun SM. (2008). Glutamate and the neural basis of the subjective effects of ketamine: A pharmaco-magnetic resonance imaging study. Arch. Gen. Psychiatry. 65(2), 154–164.
5. Tauscher J, Kielbasa W, Iyengar S, Vandenhende F, Peng X, Mozley D, et al. (2009). Development of the 2nd generation neurokinin-1 receptor antagonist LY686017 for social anxiety disorder. Eur. Neuropsychopharmacol. 20, 80–87.
6. Galbraith SM. (2006). MR in oncology drug development. NMR Biomed. 19(6), 681–689.
7. Steiger P. (2009). Use of imaging biomarkers for regulatory studies. J. Bone Joint Surg. 91(Suppl 1), 132–136.
8. Eisenhauer EA, Therasse P, Bogaerts J, Schwartz LH, Sargent D, Ford R, et al. (2009). New response evaluation criteria in solid tumours: Revised RECIST guideline (version 1.1). Eur. J. Cancer. 45(2), 228–247.
9. Olson S, Robinson S, & Giffin R. (2009). Accelerating the Development of Biomarkers for Drug Safety: Workshop Summary. Washington, DC: The National Academies Press.
10. Woodcock J, & Woosley R. (2008). The FDA critical path initiative and its influence on new drug development. Ann. Rev. Med. 59, 1–12.
11. Kapur S, Remington G, Jones C, Wilson A, DaSilva J, Houle S, et al. (1996). High levels of dopamine D2 receptor occupancy with low-dose haloperidol treatment: A PET study. Am. J. Psychiatry. 153(7), 948–950.
12. Farde L, Nordstrom AL, Wiesel FA, Pauli S, Halldin C, & Sedvall G. (1992). Positron emission tomographic analysis of central D1 and D2 dopamine

receptor occupancy in patients treated with classical neuroleptics and clozapine. Relation to extrapyramidal side effects. Arch. Gen. Psychiatry. 49(7), 538–544.

13. Mintun MA, Raichle ME, Kilbourn MR, Wooten GF, & Welch MJ. (1984). A quantitative model for the in vivo assessment of drug binding sites with positron emission tomography. Ann. Neurol. 15(3), 217–227.

14. Kapur S, Zipursky R, Jones C, Remington G, & Houle S. (2000). Relationship between dopamine D(2) occupancy, clinical response, and side effects: A double-blind PET study of first-episode schizophrenia. Am. J. Psychiatry. 157(4), 514–520.

15. Tauscher J, & Kapur S. (2001). Choosing the right dose of antipsychotics in schizophrenia: Lessons from neuroimaging studies. CNS Drugs. 15(9), 671–678.

16. Grunder G, Yokoi F, Offord SJ, Ravert HT, Dannals RF, Salzmann JK, et al. (1997). Time course of 5-HT2A receptor occupancy in the human brain after a single oral dose of the putative antipsychotic drug MDL 100,907 measured by positron emission tomography. Neuropsychopharmacology. 17(3), 175–185.

17. Tauscher J, Jones C, Remington G, Zipursky RB, & Kapur S. (2002). Significant dissociation of brain and plasma kinetics with antipsychotics. Mol. Psychiatry. 7(3), 317–321.

18. Tauscher J, Pirker W, de Zwaan M, Asenbaum S, Brucke T, & Kasper S. (1999). In vivo visualization of serotonin transporters in the human brain during fluoxetine treatment. Eur. Neuropsychopharmacol. 9(1–2), 177–179.

19. Meyer JH. (2007). Imaging the serotonin transporter during major depressive disorder and antidepressant treatment. J. Psychiatry Neurosci. 32(2), 86–102.

20. Meyer JH, Wilson AA, Ginovart N, Goulding V, Hussey D, Hood K, et al. (2001). Occupancy of serotonin transporters by paroxetine and citalopram during treatment of depression: A [(11)C]DASB PET imaging study. Am. J. Psychiatry. 158(11), 1843–1849.

21. Meyer JH, Wilson AA, Sagrati S, Hussey D, Carella A, Potter WZ, et al. (2004). Serotonin transporter occupancy of five selective serotonin reuptake inhibitors at different doses: An [11C]DASB positron emission tomography study. Am. J. Psychiatry. 161(5), 826–835.

22. Suhara T, Takano A, Sudo Y, Ichimiya T, Inoue M, Yasuno F, et al. (2003). High levels of serotonin transporter occupancy with low-dose clomipramine in comparative occupancy study with fluvoxamine using positron emission tomography. Arch. Gen. Psychiatry. 60(4), 386–391.

23. Raichle ME. (1998). Imaging the mind. Semin. Nucl. Med. 28(4), 278–289.

24. Raichle ME. (2009). A brief history of human brain mapping. Trends Neurosci. 32(2), 118–126.

25. Ogawa S, Lee TM, Kay AR, & Tank DW. (1990). Brain magnetic resonance imaging with contrast dependent on blood oxygenation. Proc. Natl. Acad. Sci. U. S. A. 87(24), 9868–9872.

26. Bandettini PA, Wong EC, Hinks RS, Tikofsky RS, & Hyde JS. (1992). Time course EPI of human brain function during task activation. Magn. Reson. Med. 25(2), 390–397.

27. Blamire AM, Ogawa S, Ugurbil K, Rothman D, McCarthy G, Ellermann JM, et al. (1992). Dynamic mapping of the human visual cortex by high-speed magnetic resonance imaging. Proc. Natl. Acad. Sci. U. S. A. 89(22), 11069–11073.

28. Frahm J, Bruhn H, Merboldt KD, & Hanicke W. (1992). Dynamic MR imaging of human brain oxygenation during rest and photic stimulation. J. Magn. Reson. Imaging. 2(5), 501–505.

29. Kwong KK, Belliveau JW, Chesler DA, Goldberg IE, Weisskoff RM, Poncelet BP, et al. (1992). Dynamic magnetic resonance imaging of human brain activity

during primary sensory stimulation. Proc. Natl. Acad. Sci. U. S. A. 89(12), 5675–5679.

30. Honey G, & Bullmore E. (2004). Human pharmacological MRI. Trends. Pharmacol. Sci. 25(7), 366–374.

31. Schweinhardt P, Bountra C, & Tracey I. (2006). Pharmacological fMRI in the development of new analgesic compounds. NMR Biomed. 19(6), 702–711.

32. Abel KM, Allin MP, Kucharska-Pietura K, David A, Andrew C, Williams S, et al. (2003). Ketamine alters neural processing of facial emotion recognition in healthy men: An fMRI study. Neuroreport. 14(3), 387–391.

33. Anderson IM, Del-Ben CM, McKie S, Richardson P, Williams SR, Elliott R, et al. (2007). Citalopram modulation of neuronal responses to aversive face emotions: A functional MRI study. Neuroreport. 18(13), 1351–1355.

34. Anderson IM, McKie S, Elliott R, Williams SR, & Deakin JF. (2008). Assessing human 5-HT function in vivo with pharmaco MRI. Neuropharmacol. 55(6), 1029–1037.

35. Apud JA, Mattay V, Chen J, Kolachana BS, Callicott JH, Rasetti R, et al. (2007). Tolcapone improves cognition and cortical information processing in normal human subjects. Neuropsychopharmacol. 32(5), 1011–1020.

36. Becerra L, Harter K, Gonzalez RG, & Borsook D. (2006). Functional magnetic resonance imaging measures of the effects of morphine on central nervous system circuitry in opioid-naive healthy volunteers. Anesth. Analg. 103(1), 208–216.

37. Borsook D, Becerra L, & Hargreaves R. (2006). A role for fMRI in optimizing CNS drug development. Nat. Rev. Drug Discov. 5(5), 411–424.

38. Fu CH, Williams SC, Brammer MJ, Suckling J, Kim J, Cleare AJ, et al. (2007). Neural responses to happy facial expressions in major depression following antidepressant treatment. Am. J. Psychiatry. 164(4), 599–607.

39. Fu CH, Williams SC, Cleare AJ, Brammer MJ, Walsh ND, Kim J, et al. (2004). Attenuation of the neural response to sad faces in major depression by antidepressant treatment: A prospective, event-related functional magnetic resonance imaging study. Arch. Gen. Psychiatry. 61(9), 877–889.

40. Goekoop R, Barkhof F, Duschek EJ, Netelenbos C, Knol DL, Scheltens P, et al. (2006). Raloxifene treatment enhances brain activation during recognition of familiar items: A pharmacological fMRI study in healthy elderly males. Neuropsychopharmacol. 31(7), 1508–1518.

41. Honey GD, Suckling J, Zelaya F, Long C, Routledge C, Jackson S, et al. (2003). Dopaminergic drug effects on physiological connectivity in a human cortico-striato-thalamic system. Brain. 126(Pt 8), 1767–1781.

42. Honey RA, Honey GD, O'Loughlin C, Sharar SR, Kumaran D, Bullmore ET, et al. (2004). Acute ketamine administration alters the brain responses to executive demands in a verbal working memory task: An fMRI study. Neuropsychopharmacol. 29(6), 1203–1214.

43. Lorenz IH, Egger K, Schubert H, Schnurer C, Tiefenthaler W, Hohlrieder M, et al. (2008). Lornoxicam characteristically modulates cerebral pain-processing in human volunteers: A functional magnetic resonance imaging study. Br. J. Anaesth. 100(6), 827–833.

44. Sheline YI, Barch DM, Donnelly JM, Ollinger JM, Snyder AZ, & Mintun MA. (2001). Increased amygdala response to masked emotional faces in depressed subjects resolves with antidepressant treatment: An fMRI study. Biol. Psychiatry. 50(9), 651–658.

45. Stein EA, Pankiewicz J, Harsch HH, Cho JK, Fuller SA, Hoffmann RG, et al. (1998). Nicotine-induced limbic cortical activation in the human brain: A functional MRI study. Am. J. Psychiatry. 155(8), 1009–1015.

46. Thiel CM, Henson RN, & Dolan RJ. (2002). Scopolamine but not lorazepam modulates face repetition priming: A psychopharmacological fMRI study. Neuropsychopharmacol. 27(2), 282–292.

47. Wise RG, Rogers R, Painter D, Bantick S, Ploghaus A, Williams P, et al. (2002). Combining fMRI with a pharmacokinetic model to determine which brain areas activated by painful stimulation are specifically modulated by remifentanil. Neuroimage. 16(4), 999–1014.

48. Borsook D, Bleakman D, Hargreaves R, Upadhyay J, Schmidt KF, & Becerra L. (2008). A 'BOLD' experiment in defining the utility of fMRI in drug development. Neuroimage. 42(2), 461–466.

49. Logothetis NK. (2008). What we can do and what we cannot do with fMRI. Nature. 453(7197), 869–878.

50. Breiter HC, Gollub RL, Weisskoff RM, Kennedy DN, Makris N, Berke JD, et al. (1997). Acute effects of cocaine on human brain activity and emotion. Neuron. 19(3), 591–611.

51. Kufahl PR, Li Z, Risinger RC, Rainey CJ, Wu G, Bloom AS, et al. (2005). Neural responses to acute cocaine administration in the human brain detected by fMRI. Neuroimage. 28(4), 904–914.

52. Kufahl P, Li Z, Risinger R, Rainey C, Piacentine L, Wu G, et al. (2008). Expectation modulates human brain responses to acute cocaine: A functional magnetic resonance imaging study. Biol. Psychiatry. 63(2), 222–230.

53. Leppa M, Korvenoja A, Carlson S, Timonen P, Martinkauppi S, Ahonen J, et al. (2006). Acute opioid effects on human brain as revealed by functional magnetic resonance imaging. Neuroimage. 31(2), 661–669.

54. Chen YI, Choi JK, & Jenkins BG. (2005). Mapping interactions between dopamine and adenosine A2a receptors using pharmacologic MRI. Synapse. 55(2), 80–88.

55. Chen YC, Galpern WR, Brownell AL, Matthews RT, Bogdanov M, Isacson O, et al. (1997). Detection of dopaminergic neurotransmitter activity using pharmacologic MRI: Correlation with PET, microdialysis, and behavioral data. Magn. Reson. Med. 38(3), 389–398.

56. Chen YC, Choi JK, Andersen SL, Rosen BR, & Jenkins BG. (2005). Mapping dopamine D2/D3 receptor function using pharmacological magnetic resonance imaging. Psychopharmacol. (Berl). 180(4), 705–715.

57. Reese T, Bjelke B, Porszasz R, Baumann D, Bochelen D, Sauter A, et al. (2000). Regional brain activation by bicuculline visualized by functional magnetic resonance imaging. Time-resolved assessment of bicuculline-induced changes in local cerebral blood volume using an intravascular contrast agent. NMR Biomed. 13(1), 43–49.

58. Schwarz A, Gozzi A, Reese T, Bertani S, Crestan V, Hagan J, et al. (2004). Selective dopamine D(3) receptor antagonist SB-277011—A potentiates phMRI response to acute amphetamine challenge in the rat brain. Synapse. 54(1), 1–10.

59. Gozzi A, Schwarz A, Reese T, Bertani S, Crestan V, & Bifone A. (2006). Region-specific effects of nicotine on brain activity: A pharmacological MRI study in the drug-naive rat. Neuropsychopharmacol. 31(8), 1690–1703.

60. Gozzi A, Large CH, Schwarz A, Bertani S, Crestan V, & Bifone A. (2008). Differential effects of antipsychotic and glutamatergic agents on the phMRI response to phencyclidine. Neuropsychopharmacol. 33(7), 1690–1703.

61. Ireland MD, Lowe AS, Reavill C, James MF, Leslie RA, & Williams SC. (2005). Mapping the effects of the selective dopamine D2/D3 receptor agonist quinelorane using pharmacological magnetic resonance imaging. Neuroscience. 133(1), 315–326.

62. Skoubis PD, Hradil V, Chin CL, Luo Y, Fox GB, & McGaraughty S. (2006). Mapping brain activity following administration of a nicotinic acetylcholine receptor agonist, ABT-594, using functional magnetic resonance imaging in awake rats. Neuroscience. 137(2), 583–591.

63. Xu H, Li SJ, Bodurka J, Zhao X, Xi ZX, & Stein EA. (2000). Heroin-induced neuronal activation in rat brain assessed by functional MRI. Neuroreport. 11(5), 1085–1092.

64. Detre JA, & Wang J. (2002). Technical aspects and utility of fMRI using BOLD and ASL. Clin. Neurophysiol. 113(5), 621–634.

65. Williams DS. (2006). Quantitative perfusion imaging using arterial spin labeling. Methods Mol. Med. 124, 151–73.

66. O'Gorman RL, Mehta MA, Asherson P, Zelaya FO, Brookes KJ, Toone BK, et al. (2008). Increased cerebral perfusion in adult attention deficit hyperactivity disorder is normalised by stimulant treatment: A non-invasive MRI pilot study. Neuroimage. 42(1), 36–41.

67. Jenkins BG, Sanchez-Pernaute R, Brownell AL, Chen YC, & Isacson O. (2004). Mapping dopamine function in primates using pharmacologic magnetic resonance imaging. J. Neurosci. 24(43), 9553–9560.

68. Andersen AH, Zhang Z, Barber T, Rayens WS, Zhang J, Grondin R, et al. (2002). Functional MRI studies in awake rhesus monkeys: Methodological and analytical strategies. J. Neurosci. Methods. 118(2), 141–152.

69. Bingel U, Quante M, Knab R, Bromm B, Weiller C, & Buchel C. (2003). Single trial fMRI reveals significant contralateral bias in responses to laser pain within thalamus and somatosensory cortices. Neuroimage. 18(3), 740–748.

70. Borras MC, Becerra L, Ploghaus A, Gostic JM, DaSilva A, Gonzalez RG, et al. (2004). fMRI measurement of CNS responses to naloxone infusion and subsequent mild noxious thermal stimuli in healthy volunteers. J. Neurophysiol. 91(6), 2723–2733.

71. Wise RG, Williams P, & Tracey I. (2004). Using fMRI to quantify the time dependence of remifentanil analgesia in the human brain. Neuropsychopharmacol. 29(3), 626–635.

72. Borsook D, & Becerra LR. (2006). Breaking down the barriers: fMRI applications in pain, analgesia and analgesics. Mol. Pain. 2, 30.

73. Oertel BG, Preibisch C, Wallenhorst T, Hummel T, Geisslinger G, Lanfermann H, et al. (2008). Differential opioid action on sensory and affective cerebral pain processing. Clin. Pharmacol. Ther. 83(4), 577–588.

74. Iannetti GD, Zambreanu L, Wise RG, Buchanan TJ, Huggins JP, Smart TS, et al. (2005). Pharmacological modulation of pain-related brain activity during normal and central sensitization states in humans. Proc. Natl. Acad. Sci. U. S. A. 102(50), 18195–18200.

75. Nahas Z, George MS, Horner MD, Markowitz JS, Li X, Lorberbaum JP, et al. (2003). Augmenting atypical antipsychotics with a cognitive enhancer (donepezil) improves regional brain activity in schizophrenia patients: A pilot double-blind placebo controlled BOLD fMRI study. Neurocase. 9(3), 274–282.

76. Del-Ben CM, Deakin JF, McKie S, Delvai NA, Williams SR, Elliott R, et al. (2005). The effect of citalopram pretreatment on neuronal responses to neuropsychological tasks in normal volunteers: An FMRI study. Neuropsychopharmacol. 30(9), 1724–1734.

77. Muller U, Suckling J, Zelaya F, Honey G, Faessel H, Williams SC, et al. (2005). Plasma level-dependent effects of methylphenidate on task-related functional magnetic resonance imaging signal changes. Psychopharmacology (Berl). 180(4), 624–633.

78. Yahata N, Takahashi H, & Okubo Y. (2005). Pharmacological modulations in human cognitive processes: An fMRI study. J. Nippon Med. Sch. 72(1), 2–3.

79. Biswal B, Yetkin FZ, Haughton VM, & Hyde JS. (1995). Functional connectivity in the motor cortex of resting human brain using echo-planar MRI. Magn. Reson. Med. 34(4), 537–541.

80. Fox MD, Snyder AZ, Vincent JL, Corbetta M, Van Essen DC, & Raichle ME. (2005). The human brain is intrinsically organized into dynamic, anticorrelated functional networks. Proc. Natl. Acad. Sci. U. S. A. 102(27), 9673–9678.

81. Shehzad Z, Kelly AM, Reiss PT, Gee DG, Gotimer K, Uddin LQ, et al. (2009). The resting brain: Unconstrained yet reliable. Cereb. Cortex. 19(10), 2209–2229.

82. Damoiseaux JS, Rombouts SA, Barkhof F, Scheltens P, Stam CJ, Smith SM, et al. (2006). Consistent resting-state networks across healthy subjects. Proc. Natl. Acad. Sci. U. S. A. 103(37), 13848–13853.

83. Achard S, & Bullmore E. (2007). Efficiency and cost of economical brain functional networks. PloS Comput. Biol. 3(2), e17.

84. Anand A, Li Y, Wang Y, Wu J, Gao S, Bukhari L, et al. (2005). Antidepressant effect on connectivity of the mood-regulating circuit: An FMRI study. Neuropsychopharmacol. 30(7), 1334–1344.

85. Kelly C, de Zubicaray G, Di Martino A, Copland DA, Reiss PT, Klein DF, et al. (2009). L-dopa modulates functional connectivity in striatal cognitive and motor networks: A double-blind placebo-controlled study. J. Neurosci. 29(22), 7364–7378.

86. Greicius M. (2008). Resting-state functional connectivity in neuropsychiatric disorders. Curr. Opin. Neurol. 21(4), 424–430.

87. Verma A, Declercq R, Coimbra A, & Achten E. (2009). Incorporating functional MRI into clinical pharmacology trials. In: Imaging in CNS Drug Discovery and Development, edited by Borsook D. Springer, New York.

88. Large CH. (2007). Do NMDA receptor antagonist models of schizophrenia predict the clinical efficacy of antipsychotic drugs? J. Psychopharmacol. 21(3), 283–301.

89. Littlewood CL, Cash D, Dixon AL, Dix SL, White CT, O'Neill MJ, et al. (2006). Using the BOLD MR signal to differentiate the stereoisomers of ketamine in the rat. Neuroimage. 32(4), 1733–1746.

90. Littlewood CL, Jones N, O'Neill MJ, Mitchell SN, Tricklebank M, & Williams SC. (2006). Mapping the central effects of ketamine in the rat using pharmacological MRI. Psychopharmacol. (Berl). 186(1), 64–81.

91. Gozzi A, Schwarz A, Crestan V, & Bifone A. (2008). Drug-anaesthetic interaction in phMRI: The case of the psychotomimetic agent phencyclidine. Magn. Reson. Imaging. 26(7), 999–1006.

92. Gozzi A, Herdon H, Schwarz A, Bertani S, Crestan V, Turrini G, et al. (2008). Pharmacological stimulation of NMDA receptors via co-agonist site suppresses fMRI response to phencyclidine in the rat. Psychopharmacol. (Berl). 201(2), 273–284.

93. Duncan GE, Leipzig JN, Mailman RB, & Lieberman JA. (1998). Differential effects of clozapine and haloperidol on ketamine-induced brain metabolic activation. Brain Res. 812(1–2), 65–75.

94. Duncan GE, Miyamoto S, Leipzig JN, & Lieberman JA. (2000). Comparison of the effects of clozapine, risperidone, and olanzapine on ketamine-induced alterations in regional brain metabolism. J. Pharmacol. Exp. Ther. 293(1), 8–14.

95. Langsjo JW, Kaisti KK, Aalto S, Hinkka S, Aantaa R, Oikonen V, et al. (2003). Effects of subanesthetic doses of ketamine on regional cerebral blood flow, oxygen consumption, and blood volume in humans. Anesthesiology. 99(3), 614–623.

96. Langsjo JW, Maksimow A, Salmi E, Kaisti K, Aalto S, Oikonen V, et al. (2005). S-ketamine anesthesia increases cerebral blood flow in excess of the metabolic needs in humans. Anesthesiology. 103(2), 258–268.

97. Langsjo JW, Salmi E, Kaisti KK, Aalto S, Hinkka S, Aantaa R, et al. (2004). Effects of subanesthetic ketamine on regional cerebral glucose metabolism in humans. Anesthesiology. 100(5), 1065–1071.

98. Apkarian AV, Bushnell MC, Treede RD, & Zubieta JK. (2005). Human brain mechanisms of pain perception and regulation in health and disease. Eur. J. Pain. 9(4), 463–484.

99. Cole LJ, Farrell MJ, Duff EP, Barber JB, Egan GF, & Gibson SJ. (2006). Pain sensitivity and fMRI pain-related brain activity in Alzheimer's disease. Brain. 129(Pt 11), 2957–2965.

100. Davis KD, Kwan CL, Crawley AP, & Mikulis DJ. (1998). Event-related fMRI of pain: Entering a new era in imaging pain. Neuroreport. 9(13), 3019–3023.

101. Peyron R, Laurent B, & Garcia-Larrea L. (2000). Functional imaging of brain responses to pain. A review and meta-analysis. Neurophysiol. Clin. 30(5), 263–288.

102. Owen DG, Bureau Y, Thomas AW, Prato FS, & St. Lawrence KS. (2008). Quantification of pain-induced changes in cerebral blood flow by perfusion MRI. Pain. 136(1–2), 85–96.

103. Geha PY, & Apkarian AV. Brain imaging findings in neuropathic pain. (2005). Curr. Pain Headache Rep. 9(3), 184–188.

104. Moisset X, & Bouhassira D. (2007). Brain imaging of neuropathic pain. Neuroimage. 37(Suppl 1), S80–S88.

105. Meyer-Lindenberg A, & Weinberger DR. (2006). Intermediate phenotypes and genetic mechanisms of psychiatric disorders. Nat. Rev. Neurosci. 7(10), 818–827.

106. Meyer-Lindenberg A, & Zink CF. (2007). Imaging genetics for neuropsychiatric disorders. Child Adolesc. Psychiatr. Clin. N. Am. 16(3), 581–597.

107. Hariri AR, Drabant EM, Munoz KE, Kolachana BS, Mattay VS, Egan MF, et al. (2005). A susceptibility gene for affective disorders and the response of the human amygdala. Arch. Gen. Psychiatry. 62(2), 146–152.

108. Hariri AR, Mattay VS, Tessitore A, Kolachana B, Fera F, Goldman D, et al. (2002). Serotonin transporter genetic variation and the response of the human amygdala. Science. 297(5580), 400–403.

109. Hariri AR, & Weinberger DR. (2003). Functional neuroimaging of genetic variation in serotonergic neurotransmission. Genes Brain Behav. 2(6), 341–349.

110. Roiser JP, de Martino B, Tan GC, Kumaran D, Seymour B, Wood NW, et al. (2009). A genetically mediated bias in decision making driven by failure of amygdala control. J. Neurosci. 29(18), 5985–5991.

111. Dannlowski U, Ohrmann P, Bauer J, Kugel H, Baune BT, Hohoff C, et al. (2007). Serotonergic genes modulate amygdala activity in major depression. Genes Brain Behav. 6(7), 672–676.

112. Munafo MR, Brown SM, & Hariri AR. (2008). Serotonin transporter (5-HTTLPR) genotype and amygdala activation: A meta-analysis. Biol. Psychiatry. 63(9), 852–857.

113. Surguladze SA, Elkin A, Ecker C, Kalidindi S, Corsico A, Giampietro V, et al. (2008). Genetic variation in the serotonin transporter modulates neural system-wide response to fearful faces. Genes Brain Behav. 7(5), 543–551.

114. Meyer-Lindenberg A, Nichols T, Callicott JH, Ding J, Kolachana B, Buckholtz J, et al. (2006). Impact of complex genetic variation in COMT on human brain function. Mol. Psychiatry. 11(9), 867–877, 797.

115. Tan HY, Chen Q, Goldberg TE, Mattay VS, Meyer-Lindenberg A, Weinberger DR, et al. (2007). Catechol-O-methyltransferase Val158Met modulation of prefrontal-parietal-striatal brain systems during arithmetic and temporal transformations in working memory. J. Neurosci. 27(49), 13393–13401.

116. Egan MF, Goldberg TE, Kolachana BS, Callicott JH, Mazzanti CM, Straub RE, et al. (2001). Effect of COMT Val108/158 Met genotype on frontal lobe function and risk for schizophrenia. Proc. Natl. Acad. Sci. U. S. A. 98(12), 6917–6922.

117. Mattay VS, Goldberg TE, Fera F, Hariri AR, Tessitore A, Egan MF, et al. (2003). Catechol O-methyltransferase val158-met genotype and individual variation in the brain response to amphetamine. Proc. Natl. Acad. Sci. U. S. A. 100(10), 6186–6191.

118. Blasi G, Mattay VS, Bertolino A, Elvevag B, Callicott JH, Das S, et al. (2005). Effect of catechol-O-methyltransferase val158met genotype on attentional control. J. Neurosci. 25(20), 5038–5045.

119. Tan HY, Chen Q, Sust S, Buckholtz JW, Meyers JD, Egan MF, et al. (2007). Epistasis between catechol-O-methyltransferase and type II metabotropic glutamate receptor 3 genes on working memory brain function. Proc. Natl. Acad. Sci. U. S. A. 104(30), 12536–12541.

120. Buckholtz JW, Sust S, Tan HY, Mattay VS, Straub RE, Meyer-Lindenberg A, et al. (2007). fMRI evidence for functional epistasis between COMT and RGS4. Mol. Psychiatry. 12(10), 893–895, 885.

121. Tan HY, Nicodemus KK, Chen Q, Li Z, Brooke JK, Honea R, et al. (2008). Genetic variation in AKT1 is linked to dopamine-associated prefrontal cortical structure and function in humans. J. Clin. Invest. 118(6), 2200–2208.

122. Bertolino A, Caforio G, Blasi G, De Candia M, Latorre V, Petruzzella V, et al. (2004). Interaction of COMT (Val(108/158)Met) genotype and olanzapine treatment on prefrontal cortical function in patients with schizophrenia. Am. J. Psychiatry. 161(10), 1798–1805.

123. Glahn DC, Ragland JD, Abramoff A, Barrett J, Laird AR, Bearden CE, et al. (2005). Beyond hypofrontality: A quantitative meta-analysis of functional neuroimaging studies of working memory in schizophrenia. Hum. Brain Mapping. 25(1), 60–69.

124. Davidson RJ, Irwin W, Anderle MJ, & Kalin NH. (2003). The neural substrates of affective processing in depressed patients treated with venlafaxine. Am. J. Psychiatry. 160(1), 64–75.

125. Surguladze S, Brammer MJ, Keedwell P, Giampietro V, Young AW, Travis MJ, et al. (2005). A differential pattern of neural response toward sad versus happy facial expressions in major depressive disorder. Biol. Psychiatry. 57(3), 201–209.

126. Chen CH, Lennox B, Jacob R, Calder A, Lupson V, Bisbrown-Chippendale R, et al. (2006). Explicit and implicit facial affect recognition in manic and depressed states of bipolar disorder: A functional magnetic resonance imaging study. Biol. Psychiatry. 59(1), 31–39.

127. Ford JM, Roach BJ, Jorgensen KW, Turner JA, Brown GG, Notestine R, et al. (2009). Tuning in to the voices: A multisite fMRI study of auditory hallucinations. Schizophr. Bull. 35(1), 58–66.

128. Potkin SG, & Ford JM. (2009). Widespread cortical dysfunction in schizophrenia: The FBIRN imaging consortium. Schizophr. Bull. 35(1), 15–18.

129. Haller S, & Bartsch AJ. (2009). Pitfalls in fMRI. Eur. Radiol. 19(11), 2689–2706.

130. Iannetti GD, & Wise RG. (2007). BOLD functional MRI in disease and pharmacological studies: Room for improvement? Magn. Reson. Imaging. 25(6), 978–988.

131. Suckling J, Ohlssen D, Andrew C, Johnson G, Williams SC, Graves M, et al. (2008). Components of variance in a multicentre functional MRI study and implications for calculation of statistical power. Hum. Brain Mapping. 29(10), 1111–1122.

132. Desmond JE, & Glover GH. (2002). Estimating sample size in functional MRI (fMRI) neuroimaging studies: Statistical power analyses. J. Neurosci. Methods. 118(2), 115–128.

133. Mumford JA, & Nichols TE. (2008). Power calculation for group fMRI studies accounting for arbitrary design and temporal autocorrelation. Neuroimage. 39(1), 261–268.

134. Murphy K, & Garavan H. (2005). Deriving the optimal number of events for an event-related fMRI study based on the spatial extent of activation. Neuroimage. 27(4), 771–777.

135. Friedman L, & Glover GH. (2006). Report on a multicenter fMRI quality assurance protocol. J. Magn. Reson. Imaging. 23(6), 827–839.

136. Friedman L, Stern H, Brown GG, Mathalon DH, Turner J, Glover GH, et al. (2008). Test-retest and between-site reliability in a multicenter fMRI study. Hum. Brain Mapping. 29(8), 958–972.

137. Miller G. (2009). Alzheimer's biomarker initiative hits its stride. Science. 326(5951), 386–389.

138. Landau SM, Harvey D, Madison CM, Koeppe RA, Reiman EM, Foster NL, et al. (2009). Associations between cognitive, functional, and FDG-PET measures of decline in AD and MCI. Neurobiol. Aging. Aug. 4. E-pub ahead of print.

139. Hua X, Lee S, Yanovsky I, Leow AD, Chou YY, Ho AJ, et al. (2009). Optimizing power to track brain degeneration in Alzheimer's disease and mild cognitive impairment with tensor-based morphometry: An ADNI study of 515 subjects. Neuroimage. 48(4), 668–681.

140. Agdeppa ED, Kepe V, Liu J, Flores-Torres S, Satyamurthy N, Petric A, et al. (2001). Binding characteristics of radiofluorinated 6-dialkylamino-2-naphthylethylidene derivatives as positron emission tomography imaging probes for beta-amyloid plaques in Alzheimer's disease. J. Neurosci. 21(24), RC189.

141. Verhoeff NP, Wilson AA, Takeshita S, Trop L, Hussey D, Singh K, et al. (2004). In-vivo imaging of Alzheimer disease beta-amyloid with [11C]SB-13 PET. Am. J. Geriatr. Psychiatry. 12(6), 584–595.

142. Choi SR, Golding G, Zhuang Z, Zhang W, Lim N, Hefti F, et al. (2009). Preclinical properties of 18F-AV-45: A PET agent for Abeta plaques in the brain. J. Nucl. Med. 50(11), 1887–1894.

143. Okello A, Koivunen J, Edison P, Archer HA, Turkheimer FE, Nagren K, et al. (2009). Conversion of amyloid positive and negative MCI to AD over 3 years: An 11C-PIB PET study. Neurology. 73(10), 754–760.

144. Buyse M, Thirion P, Carlson RW, Burzykowski T, Molenberghs G, & Piedbois P. (2000). Relation between tumour response to first-line chemotherapy and survival in advanced colorectal cancer: A meta-analysis. Meta-Analysis Group in Cancer. Lancet. 356(9227), 373–378.

145. El-Maraghi RH, & Eisenhauer EA. (2008). Review of phase II trial designs used in studies of molecular targeted agents: Outcomes and predictors of success in phase III. J. Clin. Oncol. 26(8), 1346–1354.

146. Goffin J, Baral S, Tu D, Nomikos D, & Seymour L. (2005). Objective responses in patients with malignant melanoma or renal cell cancer in early clinical studies do not predict regulatory approval. Clin. Cancer Res. 11(16), 5928–5934.

147. Paesmans M, Sculier JP, Libert P, Bureau G, Dabouis G, Thiriaux J, et al. (1997). Response to chemotherapy has predictive value for further survival of patients with advanced non-small cell lung cancer: 10 years experience of the European Lung Cancer Working Party. Eur. J. Cancer. 33(14), 2326–2332.

148. Therasse P, Arbuck SG, Eisenhauer EA, Wanders J, Kaplan RS, Rubinstein L, et al. (2000). New guidelines to evaluate the response to treatment in solid tumors. European Organization for Research and Treatment of Cancer, National Cancer Institute of the United States, National Cancer Institute of Canada. J. Natl. Cancer Inst. 92(3), 205–216.

149. Workman P, Aboagye EO, Chung YL, Griffiths JR, Hart R, Leach MO, et al. (2006). Minimally invasive pharmacokinetic and pharmacodynamic technologies in hypothesis-testing clinical trials of innovative therapies. J. Natl. Cancer Inst. 98(9), 580–598.

150. Schwarz AJ, Maisey NR, Collins DJ, Cunningham D, Huddart R, & Leach MO. (2002). Early in vivo detection of metabolic response: A pilot study of 1H MR spectroscopy in extracranial lymphoma and germ cell tumours. Br. J. Radiol. 75(900), 959–966.

151. Meisamy S, Bolan PJ, Baker EH, Bliss RL, Gulbahce E, Everson LI, et al. (2004). Neoadjuvant chemotherapy of locally advanced breast cancer: Predicting response with in vivo (1)H MR spectroscopy – a pilot study at 4 T. Radiology. 233(2), 424–431.

152. O'Connor JP, Jackson A, Parker GJ, & Jayson GC. (2007). DCE-MRI biomarkers in the clinical evaluation of antiangiogenic and vascular disrupting agents. Br. J. Cancer. 96(2), 189–195.

153. Hamstra DA, Galban CJ, Meyer CR, Johnson TD, Sundgren PC, Tsien C, et al. (2008). Functional diffusion map as an early imaging biomarker for high-grade glioma: Correlation with conventional radiologic response and overall survival. J. Clin. Oncol. 26(20), 3387–3394.

154. Padhani AR, & Leach MO. (2005). Antivascular cancer treatments: Functional assessments by dynamic contrast-enhanced magnetic resonance imaging. Abdom. Imaging. 30(3), 324–341.

155. Wahl RL, Jacene H, Kasamon Y, & Lodge MA. (2009). From RECIST to PERCIST: Evolving considerations for PET response criteria in solid tumors. J. Nucl. Med. 50(Suppl 1), 122S–150S.

156. Hayes C, Padhani AR, & Leach MO. (2002). Assessing changes in tumour vascular function using dynamic contrast-enhanced magnetic resonance imaging. NMR Biomed. 15(2), 154–163.

157. Padhani AR. (2003). MRI for assessing antivascular cancer treatments. Br. J. Radiol. 76 Spec No 1, S60–S80.

158. Miller JC, Pien HH, Sahani D, Sorensen AG, & Thrall JH. (2005). Imaging angiogenesis: Applications and potential for drug development. J. Natl. Cancer Inst. 97(3), 172–187.

159. Folkman J. (1971). Tumor angiogenesis: Therapeutic implications. N. Engl. J. Med. 285(21), 1182–1186.

160. Folkman J. (1985). Tumor angiogenesis. Adv. Cancer Res. 43, 175–203.

161. Kerbel RS. (2008). Tumor angiogenesis. N. Engl. J. Med. 358(19), 2039–2049.

162. Jackson A, Buckley DL, & Parker GJM (eds.). (2005). Dynamic Contrast-Enhanced Magnetic Resonance Imaging in Oncology. Berlin: Springer-Verlag.

163. Tofts PS. (1997). Modeling tracer kinetics in dynamic Gd-DTPA MR imaging. J. Magn. Reson. Imaging. 7(1), 91–101.

164. Taylor JS, Tofts PS, Port R, Evelhoch JL, Knopp M, Reddick WE, et al. (1999). MR imaging of tumor microcirculation: Promise for the new millennium. J. Magn. Reson. Imaging. 10(6), 903–907.

165. Tofts PS, Brix G, Buckley DL, Evelhoch JL, Henderson E, Knopp MV, et al. (1999). Estimating kinetic parameters from dynamic contrast-enhanced T(1)-weighted MRI of a diffusible tracer: Standardized quantities and symbols. J. Magn. Reson. Imaging. 10(3), 223–232.

166. Parker GJ, Suckling J, Tanner SF, Padhani AR, Revell PB, Husband JE, et al. (1997). Probing tumor microvascularity by measurement, analysis and display of contrast agent uptake kinetics. J. Magn. Reson. Imaging. 7(3), 564–574.

167. Li KL, Henry RG, Wilmes LJ, Gibbs J, Zhu X, Lu Y, et al. (2007). Kinetic assessment of breast tumors using high spatial resolution signal enhancement ratio (SER) imaging. Magn. Reson. Med. 58(3), 572–581.

168. Wilmes LJ, Pallavicini MG, Fleming LM, Gibbs J, Wang D, Li KL, et al. (2007). AG-013736, a novel inhibitor of VEGF receptor tyrosine kinases, inhibits breast cancer growth and decreases vascular permeability as detected by dynamic contrast-enhanced magnetic resonance imaging. Magn. Reson. Imaging. 25(3), 319–327.

169. Hylton N. (2006). Dynamic contrast-enhanced magnetic resonance imaging as an imaging biomarker. J. Clin. Oncol. 24(20), 3293–3298.

170. Leach MO, Brindle KM, Evelhoch JL, Griffiths JR, Horsman MR, Jackson A, et al. (2003). Assessment of antiangiogenic and antivascular therapeutics using MRI: Recommendations for appropriate methodology for clinical trials. Br. J. Radiol. 76 Spec No. 1, S87–S91.

171. Leach MO, Brindle KM, Evelhoch JL, Griffiths JR, Horsman MR, Jackson A, et al. (2005). The assessment of antiangiogenic and antivascular therapies in early-stage clinical trials using magnetic resonance imaging: Issues and recommendations. Br. J. Cancer. 92(9), 1599–1610.

172. Robinson SP, McIntyre DJ, Checkley D, Tessier JJ, Howe FA, Griffiths JR, et al. (2003). Tumour dose response to the antivascular agent ZD6126 assessed by magnetic resonance imaging. Br. J. Cancer. 88(10), 1592–1597.

173. Roberts C, Issa B, Stone A, Jackson A, Waterton JC, & Parker GJ. (2006). Comparative study into the robustness of compartmental modeling and model-free analysis in DCE-MRI studies. J. Magn. Reson. Imaging. 23(4), 554–563.

174. Evelhoch JL. (1999). Key factors in the acquisition of contrast kinetic data for oncology. J. Magn. Reson. Imaging. 10(3), 254–259.

175. Padhani AR, & Husband JE. (2001). Dynamic contrast-enhanced MRI studies in oncology with an emphasis on quantification, validation and human studies. Clin. Radiol. 56(8), 607–620.

176. Galbraith SM, Lodge MA, Taylor NJ, Rustin GJ, Bentzen S, Stirling JJ, et al. (2002). Reproducibility of dynamic contrast-enhanced MRI in human muscle and tumours: Comparison of quantitative and semi-quantitative analysis. NMR Biomed. 15(2), 132–142.

177. Padhani AR, Hayes C, Landau S, & Leach MO. (2002). Reproducibility of quantitative dynamic MRI of normal human tissues. NMR Biomed. 15(2), 143–153.

178. Ashton E, Raunig D, Ng C, Kelcz F, McShane T, & Evelhoch J. (2008). Scan-rescan variability in perfusion assessment of tumors in MRI using both model and data-derived arterial input functions. J. Magn. Reson. Imaging. 28(3), 791–796.

179. Galbraith SM, Rustin GJ, Lodge MA, Taylor NJ, Stirling JJ, Jameson M, et al. (2002). Effects of 5,6-dimethylxanthenone-4-acetic acid on human tumor microcirculation assessed by dynamic contrast-enhanced magnetic resonance imaging. J. Clin. Oncol. 20(18), 3826–3840.

180. Lankester KJ, Taylor NJ, Stirling JJ, Boxall J, D'Arcy JA, Leach MO, et al. (2005). Effects of platinum/taxane based chemotherapy on acute perfusion in human pelvic tumours measured by dynamic MRI. Br. J. Cancer. 93(9), 979–985.

181. O'Donnell A, Padhani A, Hayes C, Kakkar AJ, Leach M, Trigo JM, et al. (2005). A phase I study of the angiogenesis inhibitor SU5416 (semaxanib) in solid tumours, incorporating dynamic contrast MR pharmacodynamic end points. Br. J. Cancer. 93(8), 876–883.

182. McPhail LD, Chung YL, Madhu B, Clark S, Griffiths JR, Kelland LR, et al. (2005). Tumor dose response to the vascular disrupting agent, 5,6-dimethylxanthenone-4-acetic acid, using in vivo magnetic resonance spectroscopy. Clin. Cancer Res. 11(10), 3705–3713.

183. McPhail LD, McIntyre DJ, Ludwig C, Kestell P, Griffiths JR, Kelland LR, et al. (2006). Rat tumor response to the vascular-disrupting agent

5,6-dimethylxanthenone-4-acetic acid as measured by dynamic contrast-enhanced magnetic resonance imaging, plasma 5-hydroxyindoleacetic acid levels, and tumor necrosis. Neoplasia. 8(3), 199–206.

184. Checkley D, Tessier JJ, Kendrew J, Waterton JC, & Wedge SR. (2003). Use of dynamic contrast-enhanced MRI to evaluate acute treatment with ZD6474, a VEGF signalling inhibitor, in PC-3 prostate tumours. Br. J. Cancer. 89(10), 1889–1895.

185. Marzola P, Degrassi A, Calderan L, Farace P, Crescimanno C, Nicolato E, et al. (2004). In vivo assessment of antiangiogenic activity of SU6668 in an experimental colon carcinoma model. Clin. Cancer Res. 10(2), 739–750.

186. Marzola P, Degrassi A, Calderan L, Farace P, Nicolato E, Crescimanno C, et al. (2005). Early antiangiogenic activity of SU11248 evaluated in vivo by dynamic contrast-enhanced magnetic resonance imaging in an experimental model of colon carcinoma. Clin. Cancer Res. 11(16), 5827–5832.

187. Galbraith SM, Maxwell RJ, Lodge MA, Tozer GM, Wilson J, Taylor NJ, et al. (2003). Combretastatin A4 phosphate has tumor antivascular activity in rat and man as demonstrated by dynamic magnetic resonance imaging. J. Clin. Oncol. 21(15), 2831–2842.

188. Evelhoch JL, LoRusso PM, He Z, DelProposto Z, Polin L, Corbett TH, et al. (2004). Magnetic resonance imaging measurements of the response of murine and human tumors to the vascular-targeting agent ZD6126. Clin. Cancer Res. 10(11), 3650–3657.

189. Lee L, Sharma S, Morgan B, Allegrini P, Schnell C, Brueggen J, et al. (2006). Biomarkers for assessment of pharmacologic activity for a vascular endothelial growth factor (VEGF) receptor inhibitor, PTK787/ZK 222584 (PTK/ZK): Translation of biological activity in a mouse melanoma metastasis model to phase I studies in patients with advanced colorectal cancer with liver metastases. Cancer Chemother. Pharmacol. 57(6), 761–771.

190. Rudin M, McSheehy PM, Allegrini PR, Rausch M, Baumann D, Becquet M, et al. (2005). PTK787/ZK222584, a tyrosine kinase inhibitor of vascular endothelial growth factor receptor, reduces uptake of the contrast agent GdDOTA by murine orthotopic B16/BL6 melanoma tumours and inhibits their growth in vivo. NMR Biomed. 18(5), 308–321.

191. Morgan B, Thomas AL, Drevs J, Hennig J, Buchert M, Jivan A, et al. (2003). Dynamic contrast-enhanced magnetic resonance imaging as a biomarker for the pharmacological response of PTK787/ZK 222584, an inhibitor of the vascular endothelial growth factor receptor tyrosine kinases, in patients with advanced colorectal cancer and liver metastases: Results from two phase I studies. J. Clin. Oncol. 21(21), 3955–3964.

192. Chen K, Cai W, Li ZB, Wang H, & Chen X. (2009). Quantitative PET imaging of VEGF receptor expression. Mol. Imaging Biol. 11(1), 15–22.

193. Levashova Z, Backer M, Backer JM, & Blankenberg FG. (2009). Imaging vascular endothelial growth factor (VEGF) receptors in turpentine-induced sterile thigh abscesses with radiolabeled single-chain VEGF. J. Nucl. Med. 50(12), 2058–2063.

194. Bading JR, & Shields AF. (2008). Imaging of cell proliferation: Status and prospects. J. Nucl. Med. 49(Suppl 2), 64S–80S.

195. Dowling C, Bollen AW, Noworolski SM, McDermott MW, Barbaro NM, Day MR, et al. (2001). Preoperative proton MR spectroscopic imaging of brain tumors: Correlation with histopathologic analysis of resection specimens. AJNR Am. J. Neuroradiol. 22(4), 604–612.

196. Nelson SJ, Graves E, Pirzkall A, Li X, Antiniw Chan A, Vigneron DB, et al. (2002). In vivo molecular imaging for planning radiation therapy of gliomas: An application of 1H MRSI. J. Magn. Reson. Imaging. 16(4), 464–476.

197. Vigneron D, Bollen A, McDermott M, Wald L, Day M, Moyher-Noworolski S, et al. (2001). Three-dimensional magnetic resonance spectroscopic imaging of histologically confirmed brain tumors. Magn. Reson. Imaging. 19(1), 89–101.

198. Kurhanewicz J, & Vigneron DB. (2008). Advances in MR spectroscopy of the prostate. Magn. Reson. Imaging Clin. N. Am. 16(4), 697–710, ix–x.

199. Scheenen TW, Klomp DW, Roll SA, Futterer JJ, Barentsz JO, & Heerschap A. (2004). Fast acquisition-weighted three-dimensional proton MR spectroscopic imaging of the human prostate. Magn. Reson. Med. 52(1), 80–88.

200. Jung JA, Coakley FV, Vigneron DB, Swanson MG, Qayyum A, Weinberg V, et al. (2004). Prostate depiction at endorectal MR spectroscopic imaging: Investigation of a standardized evaluation system. Radiology. 233(3), 701–708.

201. Bolan PJ, Meisamy S, Baker EH, Lin J, Emory T, Nelson M, et al. (2003). In vivo quantification of choline compounds in the breast with 1H MR spectroscopy. Magn. Reson. Med. 50(6), 1134–1143.

202. Baik HM, Su MY, Yu H, Mehta R, & Nalcioglu O. (2006). Quantification of choline-containing compounds in malignant breast tumors by 1H MR spectroscopy using water as an internal reference at 1.5 T. MAGMA. 19(2), 96–104.

203. Kim JK, Park SH, Lee HM, Lee YH, Sung NK, Chung DS, et al. (2003). In vivo 1H-MRS evaluation of malignant and benign breast diseases. Breast. 12(3), 179–182.

204. Booth SJ, Pickles MD, & Turnbull LW. (2009). In vivo magnetic resonance spectroscopy of gynaecological tumours at 3.0 Tesla. BJOG. 116(2), 300–303.

205. Wang CK, Li CW, Hsieh TJ, Chien SH, Liu GC, & Tsai KB. (2004). Characterization of bone and soft-tissue tumors with in vivo 1H MR spectroscopy: Initial results. Radiology. 232(2), 599–605.

206. Allen JR, Prost RW, Griffith OW, Erickson SJ, & Erickson BA. (2001). In vivo proton (H1) magnetic resonance spectroscopy for cervical carcinoma. Am. J. Clin. Oncol. 24(5), 522–529.

207. Baek HM, Chen JH, Nalcioglu O, & Su MY. (2008). Proton MR spectroscopy for monitoring early treatment response of breast cancer to neo-adjuvant chemotherapy. Ann. Oncol. 19(5), 1022–1024.

208. Hsieh TJ, Li CW, Chuang IIY, Liu GC, & Wang CK. (2008). Longitudinally monitoring chemotherapy effect of malignant musculoskeletal tumors with in vivo proton magnetic resonance spectroscopy: An initial experience. J. Comput. Assist. Tomogr. 32(6), 987–994.

209. Huang MQ, Nelson DS, Pickup S, Qiao H, Delikatny EJ, Poptani H, et al. (2007). In vivo monitoring response to chemotherapy of human diffuse large B-cell lymphoma xenografts in SCID mice by 1H and 31P MRS. Acad. Radiol. 14(12), 1531–1539.

210. Madhu B, Waterton JC, Griffiths JR, Ryan AJ, & Robinson SP. (2006). The response of RIF-1 fibrosarcomas to the vascular-disrupting agent ZD6126 assessed by in vivo and ex vivo 1H magnetic resonance spectroscopy. Neoplasia. 8(7), 560–567.

211. Evelhoch J, Garwood M, Vigneron D, Knopp M, Sullivan D, Menkens A, et al. (2005). Expanding the use of magnetic resonance in the assessment of tumor response to therapy: Workshop report. Cancer Res. 65(16), 7041–7044.

212. Negendank W, Li CW, Padavic-Shaller K, Murphy-Boesch J, & Brown TR. (1996). Phospholipid metabolites in 1H-decoupled 31P MRS in vivo in human cancer: Implications for experimental models and clinical studies. Anticancer Res. 16(3B), 1539–1544.

213. Arias-Mendoza F, Zakian K, Schwartz A, Howe FA, Koutcher JA, Leach MO, et al. (2004). Methodological standardization for a multi-institutional in vivo trial of

localized 31P MR spectroscopy in human cancer research. In vitro and normal volunteer studies. NMR Biomed. 17(6), 382–391.

214. Arias-Mendoza F, Payne GS, Zakian KL, Schwarz AJ, Stubbs M, Stoyanova R, et al. (2006). In vivo 31P MR spectral patterns and reproducibility in cancer patients studied in a multi-institutional trial. NMR Biomed. 19(4), 504–512.

215. Dzik-Jurasz AS, Collins DJ, Leach MO, & Rowland IJ. (2000). Gallbladder localization of (19)F MRS catabolite signals in patients receiving bolus and protracted venous infusional 5-fluorouracil. Magn. Reson. Med. 44(4), 516–520.

216. Wolf W, Presant CA, & Waluch V. (2000). 19F-MRS studies of fluorinated drugs in humans. Adv. Drug Deliv. Rev. 41(1), 55–74.

217. Klomp DW, Van Laarhoven HW, Kentgens AP, & Heerschap A. (2003). Optimization of localized 19F magnetic resonance spectroscopy for the detection of fluorinated drugs in the human liver. Magn. Reson. Med. 50(2), 303–308.

218. Kamm YJ, Heerschap A, Van Den Bergh EJ, & Wagener DJ. (2004). 19F-magnetic resonance spectroscopy in patients with liver metastases of colorectal cancer treated with 5-fluorouracil. Anticancer Drugs. 15(3), 229–233.

219. van Laarhoven HW, Punt CJ, Kamm YJ, & Heerschap A. (2005). Monitoring fluoropyrimidine metabolism in solid tumors with in vivo (19)F magnetic resonance spectroscopy. Crit. Rev. Oncol. Hematol. 56(3), 321–343.

220. Klomp D, van Laarhoven H, Scheenen T, Kamm Y, & Heerschap A. (2007). Quantitative 19F MR spectroscopy at 3 T to detect heterogeneous capecitabine metabolism in human liver. NMR Biomed. 20(5), 485–492.

221. Reid DG, & Murphy PS. (2008). Fluorine magnetic resonance in vivo: A powerful tool in the study of drug distribution and metabolism. Drug Discov. Today. 13(11–12), 473–480.

222. Mankoff DA, Link JM, Linden HM, Sundararajan L, & Krohn KA. (2008). Tumor receptor imaging. J. Nucl. Med. 49(Suppl 2), 149S–63S.

223. Linden HM, Stekhova SA, Link JM, Gralow JR, Livingston RB, Ellis GK, et al. (2006). Quantitative fluoroestradiol positron emission tomography imaging predicts response to endocrine treatment in breast cancer. J. Clin. Oncol. 24(18), 2793–2799.

224. Faust A, Hermann S, Wagner S, Haufe G, Schober O, Schafers M, et al. (2009). Molecular imaging of apoptosis in vivo with scintigraphic and optical biomarkers – a status report. Anticancer Agents Med. Chem. 9(9), 968–985.

225. Blankenberg FG. (2008). In vivo imaging of apoptosis. Cancer Biol. Ther. 7(10), 1525–1532.

226. Sanz J, & Fayad ZA. (2008). Imaging of atherosclerotic cardiovascular disease. Nature. 451(7181), 953–957.

227. Yuan C, Kerwin WS, Yarnykh VL, Cai J, Saam T, Chu B, et al. (2006). MRI of atherosclerosis in clinical trials. NMR Biomed. 19(6), 636–654.

228. Rudd JH, Warburton EA, Fryer TD, Jones HA, Clark JC, Antoun N, et al. (2002). Imaging atherosclerotic plaque inflammation with [18F]-fluorodeoxyglucose positron emission tomography. Circulation. 105(23), 2708–2711.

229. Tawakol A, Migrino RQ, Bashian GG, Bedri S, Vermylen D, Cury RC, et al. (2006). In vivo 18F-fluorodeoxyglucose positron emission tomography imaging provides a noninvasive measure of carotid plaque inflammation in patients. J. Am. Coll. Cardiol. 48(9), 1818–1824.

230. Takaya N, Cai J, Ferguson MS, Yarnykh VL, Chu B, Saam T, et al. (2006). Intra- and interreader reproducibility of magnetic resonance imaging for quantifying the lipid-rich necrotic core is improved with gadolinium contrast enhancement. J. Magn. Reson. Imaging. 24(1), 203–210.

231. Saam T, Hatsukami TS, Yarnykh VL, Hayes CE, Underhill H, Chu B, et al. (2007). Reader and platform reproducibility for quantitative assessment of carotid

atherosclerotic plaque using 1.5T Siemens, Philips, and General Electric scanners. J. Magn. Reson. Imaging. 26(2), 344–352.

232. Cai J, Hatsukami TS, Ferguson MS, Kerwin WS, Saam T, Chu B, et al. (2005). In vivo quantitative measurement of intact fibrous cap and lipid-rich necrotic core size in atherosclerotic carotid plaque: Comparison of high-resolution, contrast-enhanced magnetic resonance imaging and histology. Circulation. 112(22), 3437–3444.

233. Chu B, Zhao XQ, Saam T, Yarnykh VL, Kerwin WS, Flemming KD, et al. (2005). Feasibility of in vivo, multicontrast-weighted MR imaging of carotid atherosclerosis for multicenter studies. J. Magn. Reson. Imaging. 21(6), 809–817.

234. Kerwin WS, O'Brien KD, Ferguson MS, Polissar N, Hatsukami TS, & Yuan C. (2006). Inflammation in carotid atherosclerotic plaque: A dynamic contrast-enhanced MR imaging study. Radiology. 241(2), 459–468.

235. Rosen BD, Fernandes V, McClelland RL, Carr JJ, Detrano R, Bluemke DA, et al. (2009). Relationship between baseline coronary calcium score and demonstration of coronary artery stenoses during follow-up MESA (Multi-Ethnic Study of Atherosclerosis). JACC Cardiovasc. Imaging. 2(10), 1175–1183.

236. Tahara N, Kai H, Ishibashi M, Nakaura H, Kaida H, Baba K, et al. (2006). Simvastatin attenuates plaque inflammation: Evaluation by fluorodeoxyglucose positron emission tomography. J. Am. Coll. Cardiol. 48(9), 1825–1831.

237. Corti R, Fayad ZA, Fuster V, Worthley SG, Helft G, Chesebro J, et al. (2001). Effects of lipid-lowering by simvastatin on human atherosclerotic lesions: A longitudinal study by high-resolution, noninvasive magnetic resonance imaging. Circulation. 104(3), 249–252.

238. Corti R, Fuster V, Fayad ZA, Worthley SG, Helft G, Smith D, et al. (2002). Lipid lowering by simvastatin induces regression of human atherosclerotic lesions: Two years' follow-up by high-resolution noninvasive magnetic resonance imaging. Circulation. 106(23), 2884–2887.

239. Corti R, Fuster V, Fayad ZA, Worthley SG, Helft G, Chaplin WF, et al. (2005). Effects of aggressive versus conventional lipid-lowering therapy by simvastatin on human atherosclerotic lesions: A prospective, randomized, double-blind trial with high-resolution magnetic resonance imaging. J. Am. Coll. Cardiol. 46(1), 106–112.

240. Rudd JH, Machac J, & Fayad ZA. (2007). Simvastatin and plaque inflammation. J. Am. Coll. Cardiol. 49(19), 1991; author reply 1992.

241. Underhill HR, Yuan C, Zhao XQ, Kraiss LW, Parker DL, Saam T, et al. (2008). Effect of rosuvastatin therapy on carotid plaque morphology and composition in moderately hypercholesterolemic patients: A high-resolution magnetic resonance imaging trial. Am. Heart J. 155(3), 584.e1–e8.

242. Saam T, Kerwin WS, Chu B, Cai J, Kampschulte A, Hatsukami TS, et al. (2005). Sample size calculation for clinical trials using magnetic resonance imaging for the quantitative assessment of carotid atherosclerosis. J. Cardiovasc. Magn. Reson. 7(5), 799–808.

243. Rudd JH, Myers KS, Bansilal S, Machac J, Pinto CA, Tong C, et al. (2008). Atherosclerosis inflammation imaging with 18F-FDG PET: Carotid, iliac, and femoral uptake reproducibility, quantification methods, and recommendations. J Nucl. Med. 49(6), 871–878.

244. Wong DF, Tauscher J, & Grunder G. (2009). The role of imaging in proof of concept for CNS drug discovery and development. Neuropsychopharmacology. 34(1), 187–203.

245. Takaya N, Yuan C, Chu B, Saam T, Underhill H, Cai J, et al. (2006). Association between carotid plaque characteristics and subsequent ischemic

cerebrovascular events: A prospective assessment with MRI–initial results. Stroke. 37(3), 818–823.

246. Rominger A, Saam T, Wolpers S, Cyran CC, Schmidt M, Foerster S, et al. (2009). 18F-FDG PET/CT identifies patients at risk for future vascular events in an otherwise asymptomatic cohort with neoplastic disease. J. Nucl. Med. 50(10), 1611–1620.

European New Safe and Innovative Medicines Initiatives: History and Progress (through December 2009)

Ole J. Bjerrum and Hans H. Linden

10.1. Introduction

On April 30, 2008, the Innovative Medicines Initiative (IMI), worth 2 billion euros, was launched in Brussels, Belgium, as a joint undertaking (JU) by the European Union (EU) and the European Federation of Pharmaceutical Industries and Associations (EFPIA). The initiative is meant to boost the funding of research of the drug development process in Europe, by addressing the key bottlenecks in the drug development value chain.[1]

The IMI focuses on clinical safety concerns, and it is seeking to improve the efficacy of new pharmacological interventions in areas such as cancer and brain disorders, as well as inflammatory, metabolic, and infectious diseases. Projects to be funded through the IMI will also address current deficits in knowledge management and education and training for pharmaceutical research and development (R&D) in Europe. Strengthening these four pillars (efficacy, safety, information management, and education and training) is foreseen to lead to new discoveries and faster development of better therapies.

Such a program and its associated investment has a long history. In Section 10.2, we also report on the history of earlier initiatives with the involvement of many stakeholders over several years and how they have led to this successful outcome. The EU research funding system and the many European stakeholders of it should first be briefly described.

10.1.1. The EU Research Funding System

When the EU was established, there was also the intention to create a central funding system for research with the purpose of facilitating and supporting research collaboration between its member states. This funding system demands that researchers, based in at least three different countries, need to apply together to become eligible for available funding. The grant support was structured in European Framework Programmes for Research and Technological Development (FP's), each of 4 years' duration.

Over the years, the FP budgets have grown steadily. Today they account for nearly 5% of the all public research spending in the EU. For each 4-year funding period, certain research themes are typically selected. Through this, the EU gets a chance to focus on important new and emerging topics and issues for society. This funding system has encouraged an intense lobbying aimed at the European Commission (EC) to seek, obtain, and include a preferred research area into the FPs.

Both basic and applied research has been supported. For example, biotechnology was a theme in FP 5 (1998–2002). Here, the project support, among others, related to new targets, methodology, and tools for drug discovery. Drug development research, however, was neither included nor seen to be a funding consideration.

Each FP has received funds for identifying new and emergent themes to be incorporated in the next FPs. The European Federation for Pharmaceutical Sciences (EUFEPS) took advantage of this possibility for the New Safe Medicines Faster (NSMF) project, paving the way for today's IMI (see Section 10.2.3)

FP 7 opened up a new avenue of funding, the Joint Technology Initiatives, supporting public–private partnerships (PPPs). This initiative was a breakthrough for the establishment of current IMI funding.

10.1.2. Stakeholders

The European pharmaceutical sciences scene is fragmented both vertically (i.e., health care providers, universities, learned societies) and horizontally (i.e., between member states). The process-oriented thinking of the pharmaceutical industry is not always accepted by the discipline-oriented universities. Accordingly, translational and holistic approaches in drug development are less common in universities and schools of pharmacy or pharmaceutical sciences.

Until recently, competition – and even distrust – have hampered research collaboration among European pharmaceutical companies. The EFPIA seemed to focus on trade conditions and intellectual property rights rather than on research matters and precompetitive scientific or technological issues.

Professional societies, albeit including researchers from both the industry and universities, are organized by discipline. In addition, many European countries have one or more learned societies for each discipline, which have small membership numbers and thus obviously less than the "critical mass" needed, for example, for, larger-scale initiatives and cross-discipline collaborations. Influencing the EC in Brussels to support general funding of research dedicated to the drug development process required broad support by the scientific community.

In Europe, there is also a conflict between federative thinking (uniting forces) and national interests. This conflict also prevails in scientific and professional federations and associations. These scientific organizations should – or could be expected to – take on the tasks of joint or third-party interests. Keeping the interest balance among nations takes energy as do future-focused federative approaches.

10.2. Toward the IMI

In 1998–1999, there was only one European association that was aligned for approaching Brussels on the aforementioned matters and issues, namely, the EUFEPS. As the name indicates, EUFEPS is a multidisciplinary federation covering discovery, development, and use of drugs. Also, as a European Federation, the member societies represent 24 countries, including Israel and Turkey.[2]

Thus, the preconditions were the right substrate for a collaborative effort to influence and even change the funding conditions for research related to drug development in the EU. Moreover, EUFEPS had the foresight, leadership, capability, and capacity to drive and bring the new endeavor forward.

10.2.1. First Round: Establishment of the NSMF Project

In the EUFEPS, the Committee on Industrial Research Relations (CIRR), in 1998–1999, saw the emerging problems that the European pharmaceutical industry was facing regarding future productivity. The CIRR focused on the translational aspects – especially on how low-capacity techniques used in drug development could match the quickly emerging, high-throughput methods applied in drug discovery.

Massive funding in research aimed at drug development methodologies, procedures, and techniques was deemed necessary. Only one major potential funding body existed in Europe, namely the European Framework Programme for Research and Technological Development. On recommendation from the CIRR, the Executive Committee of the EUFEPS set up a EUFEPS task force to look at ways to support drug development in Europe. Ole J. Bjerrum became the chair of the task force and was supported by Hans H. Linden primarily in the EUFEPS Secretariat. Ambitions included presenting and drawing attention to research deficits in drug development and, it was hoped, convincing the EU Commission that (external) funding would be needed to cope with these deficits on a European scale.

A position paper on NSMF[3] was drafted and issued mimicking the structure of "Key Actions" known from the FP 5. It was proposed that the

Table 10.1. Improvement Recommendations Brought Forward at the NSMF Workshop in March 2000 for a Faster Drug Development Process[4,6]

- Improved quality of selected drug candidates through better prediction
- Full exploitation of simulation and modeling
- Enlarged databases
- Parallel tracks for the testing of new drug candidates
- Seamless processing
- Involvement of regulatory bodies early on
- Information technology (IT) integration and better management
- Faster access of test medicines into humans; e.g., through implementation of newer microdosing techniques
- Availability of researchers with appropriate education

effort include (1) a mission-oriented, problem-solving approach, integrating all necessary disciplines and sectors from basic research to development and demonstrations; (2) a strong networking element; and (3) design and implementation in consultation with all stakeholders, including the ultimate beneficiaries.

The position paper was then sent to the Directorate-General Research (DG Research) of the EC in September 1999. It was positively received by the Director of DG Research, Bruno Hansen, who suggested applying for a "Support Action" under FP 5 to arrange a workshop for further strengthening of the theme. Together with the EFPIA and the Danish Medicines Agency, the EUFEPS applied for 50,000 euros to arrange the workshop under the overarching theme New Safe Medicines Faster.

During March 15–16, 2000, the New Safe Medicine Faster Workshop gathered approximately 115 representatives from the pharmaceutical industry, academic institutions, and regulatory authorities and produced an outcomes report on research and technology required to bring safe new medicines to the market faster. The report was issued in July 2000. In addition to being presented to the EC, it was widely circulated in Europe.[4] Table 10.1 summarizes suggested improvements considered necessary for obtaining a faster drug development process. Table 10.2 lists the corresponding research topics. It is noteworthy that the listed items also appeared in the later published strategic research agenda (SRA) on Innovative Medicines.[5]

The NSMF initiative was followed by presentations in a series of conferences from 2000 through 2002 in Stockholm, Copenhagen, Budapest, Manchester, Helsinki, Madrid, Strasburg, and Basel.[6] The EUFEPS 2002

Table 10.2. Suggested Research Topics for a Faster Drug Development Process at the NSMF Workshop in March 2000[4,6]

- Functional gene analysis
- Pathophysiological understanding of diseases for target prioritization
- In-vivo and in-vitro disease models
- Expanded use of modeling tools for in-silico testing
- Miniaturized fast screens with a robotic base
- Use of the information technology (IT) solution throughout the development process
- Pharmacogenetic profiling and population genetics
- Predictive biomedical markers and surrogate endpoints
- Drug and gene delivery systems
- Toolboxes containing predictive methods and seamless scaling techniques
- Pharmacometrics, including noninvasive testing methods and sensor technologies
- Process measurement technologies to allow rational manufacturing
- Science-based regulatory guidelines reflecting the latest scientific developments

Congress in Stockholm was supported by the EU Commission and was dedicated to NSMF project.

10.2.2. Second Round: Incorporation of NSMF in FP 6

The NSMF initiative and recommendations fell on fertile ground at the DG Research in Brussels. Apparently, for some time there had been concerns about the growing gap between U.S. and European implementation of biotechnologies in the community and in the pharmaceutical industry.[7] Thus, the general FP 6 program published with the name "Life sciences, genomic and biotechnology for health" in 2002 had a section specifically dedicated to "Rational and accelerated development of new safer and more effective medicines."[8]

Subsequently, calls for proposals related to the NSMF project appeared in FP 6 with corresponding funding of approximately 200 million euros. Titles of the calls are listed in Table 10.3. The topics for the calls had been created by a concerted effort from national representatives, experts, and staff of the Commission. For this reason, the NSMF concept was spread all over Europe. Besides influencing DG Research, it also inspired national activities such as the DRUG 2000-biomedicines, drug development and

Table 10.3. New, Safer, and More Effective Medicine Calls in FP 6 (2002–2006)[8]

Individualized medicines

Optimization of test batteries for human acute toxicity

Nonanimal test methods for (bio)chemicals, medicines, and biomaterials

In-silico models as alternatives to animal experiments

Development of genetic tests allowing harmonization and validation

In-vivo molecular imaging: Identification of new markers

Modeling for drug discovery and testing; biopharmaceutical development platform; clinical testing of biopharmaceuticals; medicines for children

New approaches for accelerated development of new, safe medicines

Validations of in-vitro models for the study of absorption, distribution, metabolism, and elimination detoxification

Microdosing

Cell systems for toxicity testing

Risk assessment: Prediction for toxicity testing

Exploring the potential of stem cells and/or primary cells

Immunogenicity of biopharmaceuticals

pharmaceutical program in Finland and the Dutch Top Institute Pharma in The Netherlands. Furthermore, EUFEPS in 2001 founded an NSMF Award with support from Sanofi-aventis.[2]

Importantly, additional learned societies and groups, such as the Medicines Development Section of the European Biotechnology Federation (EFB), the European Federation for Medicinal Chemistry (EFMC), the Association of European Toxicologists and European Societies of Toxicology (Eurotox), and the European Clinical Research Infrastructure Network (ECRIN) became engaged in the NSMF initiative. The latter four associations, together with EUFEPS and EFPIA, arranged a workshop titled "How to Establish a European Technology Platform for Pharmaceutical Sciences" through a grant (250,000 euros) under FP 6. In the last phases, "Pharmaceutical Sciences" was changed to "Innovative Medicines." In any case, the workshop was held and organized by the EUFEPS-led consortium in April 2005 in Barcelona, Spain, significantly contributing to the work on the SRA of the IMI.[9] (see Section 10.2.3).

In the process of creating funding for and strengthening the NSMF project, EUREKA, the public-supported, market-oriented network on industrial R&D, was approached with little success.[10] In addition, the EFPIA did not seem to be receptive to the NSMF project recommendations. At least, there was little public follow-up on the outcomes of the first workshop in Brussels in 2000. Nevertheless, strong industry support was reflected by the large industry representation in the CIRR and EUFEPS conferences. In parallel, an EFPIA Research Directors' Group was formed to strengthen the EFPIA's role toward R&D perhaps by using a precompetitive approach.

A Brainstorm Workshop on Safety Sciences was held in April 2004 in Brussels and was preceded by a position paper in the EUFEPS newsletter in 2003.[11] The CIRR and EUFEPS addressed the foreseeable dramatic shortfall of safety scientists in Europe and made a series of recommendations for education and training initiatives, which later affected the IMI (see Section 10.3.4).[11]

It is also noteworthy that the U.S. Food and Drug Administration (FDA), on March 16, 2004, in parallel with the NSMF initiative, published a white paper titled "Innovation, Stagnation, Challenge and Opportunities on the Critical Path to New Medical Products," which covered essentially the same issues as the NSMF project by EUFEPS and partners.[12]

10.2.3. Third Round: The Rise of the IMI

In the autumn of 2003, the DG Research realized that the biopharmaceutical industry had shown limited interest in the calls relevant to NSMF in FP 6. For the industry, the application process was too complicated, and the chance for success was judged to be too small compared with the time and effort that would have to be invested. Thus, when preparing the FP 7, the Commission called industry representatives and other stakeholders to an informal, high-level meeting on research for NSMF. The meeting was held on November 20, 2003, in Brussels, and the attendees discussed what the Commission could do to assist the competitiveness of the European pharmaceutical industry in the global market and on their own terms.

The Commission had by then started fostering the idea of creating technology platforms that could become new tools in the funding system suitable for industrial partnerships.[7] The amount of funds that the Commission could make available for pharmaceutical research was set to 800 million to 1 billion euros. The message was conveyed to the EFPIA representatives present at the meeting, and the industry agreed to engage, including setting up a precursor project (under FP 6). As established, in 2005, it was named the InnoMed Integrated Project.[13,14]

It is fair to assume, we think, that the many NSMF activities and spin-offs of it in the European pharmaceutical community, the FP support and outcomes reports, together with the overall dissemination of information and many years of trustful collaboration with relevant officers of the DG Research paved the way for the successful launch of the IMI. It started with few resources and an identified urgent need, and it grew into a joint effort by many relevant stakeholders, including those on the European political scene (see Section 10.6).

The Commission's initiative to approach the European biopharmaceutical industry body officially with a generous offer was an ice-breaking moment. The intense EFPIA involvement that followed over the next 12 months resulted in a vision document that confirmed the need and listed key research bottlenecks hampering the drug development process. The vision document was ready in December 2004,[14] and the InnoMed Integrated Project was launched in October 2005.[1,13]

A series of workshops to refine and settle on plans for the European Technology Platform for Innovative Medicines and to liaise with other stakeholders was held in Spring 2005 and involved more than 200 researchers from biopharmaceutical companies, small and medium size enterprises (SMEs), universities, learned societies, regulatory authorities, health care providers, clinical centers, and patient organizations. The workshops focused on bottlenecked research issues that were brought together and categorized as the following four pillars: efficacy, safety, information management and education, and training.

The outcomes of these workshops were incorporated in an SRA made public in August 2005 with the latest revision in April 2008.[5] Discussions and negotiations with the Commission continued to identify common ground on which to build the IMI JU. In May 2007, a Commission proposal for an EU Council regulation was ready, and, in December 2007, there was final approval and a decision by the European Parliament and the EU Council. All had agreed to establish the IMI JU, under FP 7, as a PPP. The budget for it was set at 2 billion euros (1 billion public money and a 1 billion in-kind contribution by EFPIA IMI companies) to be spent in the period from 2008 through 2017.[1] The various steps toward this IMI JU are summarized in Table 10.4.

10.3. Organizational Structure of the IMI

Implementation of the IMI as a JU makes it more attractive for both partners. Companies are more actively involved in setting priorities and are able to access results from a large number of studies and participate in a larger network of partners with the EC acting as a representative of the public interest.

The IMI is structured with the following constituents:

1) An IMI governing board with equal participation of representatives from DG Research and the EFPIA to direct the operations of IMI and oversee the implementation;

2) An IMI Executive Director, together with the staff, to manage the operations required to support implementation of the IMI research agenda;

Table 10.4. History for the IMI JU

January 1998	EUFEPS CIRR meeting with officers of the EC in Brussels
January 1999	First version of the EUFEPS Task Force EU Position Paper on long-term actions for improving pharmaceutical research
September 1999	Publication of NSMF initiative by EUFEPS
March 2000	First EC-supported workshop on NSMF, Brussels
March 2002	Launch of the calls for "Rational and accelerated development of new, safer and more effective drugs" in the EU's FP 6
April 2003	Application under FP 6 by EUFEPS-organized consortium on creation of biopharmaceutical development platform filed and later transformed into the IMI under FP 6 by EUFEPS
November 2003	First informal, high-level contact between EC and EFPIA on large-scale support to NSMF
April 2004	Brainstorm Workshop on Safety Sciences in Brussels and Outcomes Report
May 2004	Start of official discussions between the EC and EFPIA
June 2004	Agreement of EFPIA to take leadership of the European Technology Platform for Innovative Medicines (IMI)
December 2004	Publication of IMI vision paper by EFPIA
April 2005	EUFEPS-organized workshop: "How to Establish a European Technology Platform for Innovative Medicines," Barcelona, Spain
August 2005	Publication of IMI SRA by EFPIA
October 2005	Start of pilot (precursor) project "InnoMed" funded under FP 6 (18 million euros)
September 2006	Publication of the IMI SRA version 2 (including draft governance and intellectual property IP Policy)
August 2007	Adoption of IMI Intellectual Property Policy
November 2007	Adoption of IMI legal package by the European Competitiveness Council
December 2007	Adoption of the European Parliament opinion
December 2007	Approval of the establishment of IMI JU by the European Council
December 2007	First (unofficial) drafts of calls for EoI available
March 2008	Establishment of IMI Government Board
April 2008	Announcement of first call for EoIs
July 2008	Establishment of IMI Scientific Committee
July 2008	Deadline for first call application of EoIs
November 2008	Deadline for first call submission of Project Proposals
January 2009	Start of Project Contract negotiations and first Research Activities
November 2009	Announcement of second call for EoIs

Fig. 10.1
Organizational
structure of IMI.

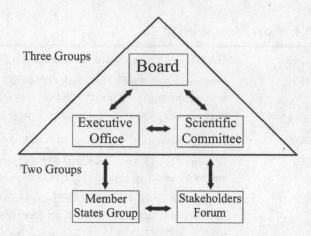

3) An IMI Scientific Committee, having an advisory role in future implementations (It is composed of 15 members representing public and private stakeholders from academia, patient groups, industry, and regulatory bodies. Its members combine expertise representing the entire
   medicine discovery and development process.);
4) An IMI States Representatives Group with an advisory role to facilitate
   coordination with member states; and
5) A stakeholder forum, acting as antennae for the IMI, to help disseminate information and to ensure openness and transparency for the
   stakeholders.

Figure 10.1 shows an organogram of the structure.[1]

10.4. How Does the SRA of the IMI Address Predictive Markers of Efficacy and Safety?

10.4.1. Predictive Markers of Efficacy

"Improved Predictability of Efficacy Evaluation" represents one of the four
pillars in the IMI. The main focus here is to bring together academic, clinical, and pharmaceutical expertise to identify the required biological tools
and to advance the use of emerging technologies, including "-omics" and
imaging.

The challenges to improving efficacy have these overarching goals:

■ Develop better understanding of disease mechanisms,
■ Develop in-vitro and in-vivo models that are predictive of clinical
  efficacy,
■ Develop in-silico simulations of disease pathology,

- Stimulate translational medicine in an integrated fashion across industry and academia,
- Create disease-specific European imaging networks to establish standards and validate imaging biomarkers,
- Create disease-specific European centers for validation of "-omics-" based biomarkers,
- Coordinate the development of national patient networks and databases to develop pan-European organizations, and
- Develop partnerships with regulators to devise innovative critical trial designs and analyses, to aid acceptance of biomarkers, and to promote data sharing and the joint consideration of ethical issues.

These needs are applicable to all diseases. In addition, better understanding of the individual disease pathophysiology will provide the basis for the predictive pharmacology that is essential to reducing attrition rates in clinical trials. The key output of this research will be the discovery and validation of biomarkers, which are of critical importance in modern drug development.

Because biomarkers are quantitative measures of biological responses that provide informative links between mechanism of action and clinical effectiveness, they can provide new insights into a drug's mechanism of action, metabolism, efficacy, and safety and into disease mechanisms as well as disease course. The application of biomarkers in the drug development process will translate into such benefits as increasing the probability of program success and, at the same time, reducing the cycle time by faster optimization of therapy for the right patients by a companion diagnostic test utilizing the identified biomarker.

The key issue is how to validate biomarkers as substitutes for clinical outcomes (surrogates). This exercise is lengthy and expensive, and it involves many patients and years. No real consensus exists among all the stakeholders. Proper validation is essential if biomarkers are to develop from being tools for internal use by the pharmaceutical industry to measures that can be used to drive approval decisions.

The successful development of biomarkers and their integration into the drug-discovery process require improvement and facilitated access to current technology. The -omics technologies are essential for the discovery of accessible biomarkers, for example, in blood, urine, or cerebrospinal fluid (CSF); for use as diagnostics, measures of disease progression, and prediction of treatment outcome; and as measurement of treatment effectiveness. Other essential technologies are bioimaging methods such as MRI or PET scanning. As with other biomarker methods, the development and validation of imaging biomarkers in animals are important precursors to the use of such techniques in humans. There is a need for further refinement in the technologies such as improvements in resolution, sensitivity, and comparability. For this refinement to happen, standards and registries of biomarker and clinical data will need to be developed and agreed on, and existing Europe-wide national networks will need to be coordinated to establish standards and validate imaging biomarkers. In addition, the use of genetic variables for patient stratification is in its infancy in many therapeutic areas.

It is beyond the scope of this chapter to summarize the specific recommendations for developing better biomarkers for predicting efficacy in the elected disease areas of the SRA: cancer, brain disorders, infections, and inflammatory and metabolic diseases. Instead we refer to the SRA for more detailed information.[5] Efficacy biomarkers to be studied in the first IMI proposals' descriptions are given in Section 10.7.2.

10.4.2. Predictive Markers of Safety

"Improved Predictability of Drug Safety Evaluation" represents the first pillar of the SRA. Regarding the predictive markers, the main focus is on development and validation but not the identification of biomarkers.

A proliferation of candidate biomarkers and surrogate endpoints is expected in the future "driven by -omics technology" and embracing proteins, metabolites, individual gene expression, and, perhaps, gene expression signature patterns. The major issues will be to clarify the utility and human relevance of these candidate biomarkers and their regulatory value.

The ideal (preclinical/clinical) biomarker for monitoring toxicity can be characterized as follows:

- Is specific for certain types of injury;
- Indicates injury in a variety of experimental species as well as in humans;
- Bridges nonclinical/preclinical studies to clinical and surveillance studies;
- Is more effective at indicating injury than any other biomarker currently used;
- Is used instead of classical biomarkers, not in addition to them;
- Is easily measured in real time, even at a later stage (not time critical);
- Is more reproducible, sensitive, and measurable than other toxicity endpoints; and
- Reduces the number of individuals tested, whether animals or humans.

Each new candidate biomarker requires validation in the preclinical and clinical arenas. To achieve general acceptance, in-house validation is not sufficient, as has been shown in the past for the development of in vitro tests. Therefore, collaboration between several stakeholders is essential to achieve proper validation. Because of this, validation it is a preeminent subject for the IMI proposed European Center of Drug Safety research (see Section 10.5).

The development of an individual biomarker (or a limited set of directly linked biomarkers) will be allocated to a project team under the leadership of a Biomarker Strategic Management Team.

Support to the following activities for biomarkers is expected: definition of transparent criteria for acceptance, kit development for different species, validation of acceptable criteria in preclinical species in a sufficient number of clinical studies, mechanistic understanding, and data analysis. These studies require extensive work that exceeds the resources of individual stakeholders. Furthermore, realizing these studies represents an excellent task for the IMI.

10.5. How Is Off-Target Toxicity Addressed in the SRA?

The SRA foresees that the IMI JU will finance the establishment of a small European Center of Drug Safety Research to coordinate research efforts in this area. The research foci within nonclinical safety will be (1) the issue of intractable toxicities, (2) relevance of nongenotoxic carcinogens, (3) development of in silico methods, and (4) biomarker development (see Section 10.4.2).

Intractable toxicities represent issues characterized by the fact that they occur in humans and that they are currently not well predicted by animal safety testing. Thus, many findings appear in nonclinical safety studies, the relevance of which in humans is unclear or questionable. Clinical observations, such as drug hypersensitivity, have to be worked backward to nonclinical models. The plan is that a safety data warehouse will play a key role in the research combining these two ends.

A few high-impact areas will be selected that are currently causing repetitive delays or compound terminations: testicular toxicity, biliary hyperplasia or hepatotoxicity, vasculitis phospholipidosis, and hypersensitivity. New areas will be included, such as new animal and cellular models, human tissues, imaging, and modeling.

Relevance of rodent nongenotoxic carcinogens will also be addressed. Although there are only approximately 20 known human carcinogens, substantial industry and regulatory resources are spent in unraveling (irrelevant) findings in rodent carcinogenicity assays. In contrast, approximately 50% of rodent carcinogenicity bioassays show a treatment-related increase in incidence of tumors. In most cases, these tumors occur through nongenotoxic mechanisms.

A carcinogenicity issue of high priority is receptor-mediated carcinogenesis as in the case of peroxisome proliferator-activated receptor (PPAR). In many cases, however, the possibility that the therapeutic and the rodent tumorigenic effects are driven by the same mechanism cannot be ruled out.

The scope of the research activities will be (1) application of mechanistic studies and -omics approaches to the development of predictive markers for nongenotoxic carcinogenicity, and (2) evaluation of alternative approaches, such as alternative carcinogenicity studies of shorter duration, subchronic studies in aged animals, or the use of transgenics with altered or deleted relevant receptors.

To better understand the relevance of rodent studies for the prediction of human carcinogens, several scientific approaches will be used. Mechanistic studies to evaluate the significance of receptor subtypes; differences in tissue distribution and other species differences; involvement in cell proliferation, nutritional interactions, cellular pathways, or cell–cell interactions; and secondary messengers will be performed.

New general assays will be developed (in vivo/in vitro/-omics), or existing ones will be refined for early identification of potential hazards through validation and standardization. Among others, these assays might include alternative carcinogenicity studies of shorter duration, subchronic studies in aged animals, or the use of transgenic models with altered or deleted relevant receptors.

In addition, there is an urgent need for development of in silico methods to (1) improve predictability for endpoints characterized in late, nonclinical safety studies (e.g., chronic target organ toxicity); (2) provide tools to screen and select the best chemical lead at the discovery stage; (3) identify and, if possible, avoid specific structural and activity characteristics linked to safety issues; and (4) help to tailor a specific toxicity testing program.

Safety biomarkers to be studied appear in the first proposal descriptions given in Section 10.7.1.

10.6. How Will the IMI Consortium Help in Transforming Current Science?

The formation of the IMI JU represents a promising change in the landscape for drug development research in Europe. On the industrial side, 24 research directors of the leading biopharmaceutical companies in Europe with their signatures have agreed that they will collaborate in a concerted effort to solve the key bottlenecks that exist in drug development today. To be eligible for funding, the involved industries (of which many are multinational) must all have research facilities in the EU.

On the academic side, it is also a requirement that the actual research take place in the member states or in the other research-associated countries of the EU: Iceland, Israel, Norway, Switzerland, and Turkey. The research collaboration is also open to participation from individual experts outside the EU. The collaboration takes place on a common technology platform created together with DG Research of the EC.[5] Industry and the EU will spend 1 billion euros each on the project in the next 10 years.[1] The reasons why this step is happening now are (1) the present falling productivity of industry and (2) the significant tasks necessary to validate new tools and methodologies, which will result in a faster and more efficient drug-development process. Such validation can no longer be performed in-house by a single company, for it requires collaboration between multiple stakeholders. It is noteworthy that the intellectual property rights (IPR) issues linked to this research already have been solved and adopted in a common paper (cf. Table 10.4).

That such collaboration on precompetitive issues of pharmaceutical research is more than intentions only is clear from the just-finished 18-million-euro InnoMed Integrated Project under FP 6 in which 13 companies worked together to find and validate biomarkers for neurodegenerative diseases as well as to validate the predictive value of -omics techniques for predictive liver and kidney safety biomarkers.[13]

This collaboration has shown that companies are ready to share best practices regarding analytical tools to be able to ensure that the analyses conducted have the same accuracy and predictability (during the collaboration many companies, proud of their technical performance, realized that they were not best in class). Furthermore, ways to share and exploit a common database have been found. A row of other stakeholders, also funded by the EU, participate in the project on equal terms.

If this culture of collaboration continues, and the right projects are wisely selected, it may revolutionize the drug development process, not the least because the European Medicines Agency (EMA) is also actively engaged in projects.

The education and training activities initiated will also change the current science. Placing the needed educational and training programs in universities or academic settings will introduce process-oriented thinking into the academic environment – which, in the long run, will influence the mindset of the graduates who aim for a career in the industry. It will also address recruitment to new areas such as safety science, for the students now can see a clear career path.[11]

The process-oriented and holistic view of the projects will favor translational medicine activities in general and facilitate the discovery of potential new therapies based on reported exciting new science that otherwise might never advance beyond the laboratory bench. A key to successful deployment of translational medicine research is to focus on comparative medicine, physiology, and pharmacology. Also, there is an imperfect understanding of the relevance of preclinical experiments and their relationship to clinical experience. A way forward is development of comprehensive disease lifestyle models and further refinement and validation of complex animal models.

Table 10.5. Topics Supported in First Call of the IMI JU[1]

Nongenotoxic carcinogenesis	9	M €*
Expert systems for in silico toxicity prediction	4	M €
Qualification of translational safety biomarkers	15	M €
Strengthening the monitoring of the risks and benefits	11	M €
Islet cell research	7	M €
Surrogate markers for vascular endpoints	14	M €
Pain research	5	M €
New tools for the development of novel therapies in psychiatric disorders	7	M €
Neurodegenerative disorders	5	M €
Understanding severe asthma	9	M €
COPD patient-reported outcomes	7	M €
European Medicines Research Training Network	4	M €
Safety sciences for medicines training program	2	M €
Pharmaceutical medicine training program	3	M €
Pharmacovigilance training program	3	M €
Total	105	M €

*M €: million euros.

10.7. The Topic Proposals in the First Call of the IMI

The IMI is developing the tools and methods to increase the efficiency of new molecule development. Accurately predicting the value of a molecule in terms of safety and efficacy for therapeutic application in humans will help in enhancing this process. By doing so, the resources can be focused on candidate medicines with a high probability of success. The following therapeutic areas or model diseases have been chosen as areas of focus to better define the research needs to develop the required tools and methods: metabolic diseases (e.g., diabetes, obesity); disorders of the central nervous system (e.g., Alzheimer's disease, stroke); inflammatory diseases (e.g., asthma, rheumatoid arthritis); cancer (e.g., breast cancer, leukemias, and lymphomas); and infectious diseases (e.g., antibiotic-resistant *Staphylococcus aureus* or methicillin-resistant *S. aureus*).

How are the challenges described in the SRA reflected in the call for proposals in first round of support? Table 10.5 lists the topics, and Section 10.7.1. provides a short description of the purpose of the calls. The full text can be found on the IMI Web site.[1]

10.7.1. Predictive Safety

The *immunogenicity* project encompasses finding ways to make immunogenicity analyses comparable between assays, compounds, and companies and to gain insight based on pooled relevant immunogenicity data. The predictive value of preclinical tools (in silico, in vitro, animal markers, and stratification markers) should be investigated and shared.

Because the observed in-vivo carcinogenesis rarely is genotoxic in nature given the early exclusion of genotoxic drugs identified by in vitro and in vivo assays, short-term assays to identify nongenotoxic carcinogens are in demand. Therefore, it would be valuable to establish the mechanisms by which early biomarkers are linked to tumor formation.

The project for in-silico toxicity prediction should collect pharmacology-related chemistry ("molecule war-heads") from known series of compounds to build predictive expert systems for secondary pharmacology ("off-target toxicity") prediction. The same approach should be used for pure chemistry-related toxicity.

For the *nonclinical* safety assessment, the goals will be to integrate new, validated methods into the safety assessment by combining results from -omics technologies with the results from conventional toxicology methods. In this context, identification and qualification of novel translational biomarkers of selected toxicities should be undertaken. The research program should consist of the performance of in-vivo animal studies based on standardized and optimized study protocols using well-characterized drug candidates selected on the basis of liver or kidney toxicity.

The predictability between nonclinical and early clinical studies of currently accepted biomarkers is poor. Furthermore, there is no clear scientific qualification process on how to generate enough clinical evidence to qualify new safety biomarkers for clinical regulatory decision making in certain contexts. The definition of such a generic scientific process needs to match the regulatory qualification processes. Critical drug-induced pathologies from the liver, kidney, and vascular bed should be identified from previous discoveries and/or other preclinical qualification exercises, and relevant assays should be developed.

The effort to improve the *predictability of safety evaluation* should address problems and bottlenecks related to safety evaluation and risk–benefit analyses. Research in this area will be a key to enhancing safety prediction and development of better and more applicable models of toxicity. The project of strengthening the monitoring of the risks and benefits should facilitate the application of existing data resources and/or expedite the generation of more reliable pharmacoepidemiological data for proactive pharmacovigilance. Work will have to be directed toward signal identification and detection, data mining based on large safety databases, integration of drug utilization information into pharmacovigilance, and/or postapproval risk–benefit optimization.

10.7.2. Predictive Efficacy

To improve the predictability of efficacy evaluations requires address-ing bottlenecks related to understanding disease mechanisms, predic-tive pharmacology, identification and validation of biomarkers for patient recruitment, and risk–benefit assessment.

In diabetes, significant β-*cell dysfunction* occurs prior to the diagnosis of insulin resistance. Current treatments are not able to prevent the contin-ued loss of β-cell mass and function in the progression to type 2 diabetes. Hyperglycemia results from the inability of β cells to adapt their functional mass to the prevailing insulin demand. The mechanisms leading to these alterations are poorly understood. A better understanding of β-cell prolif-eration, differentiation, and apoptosis will permit approaches to preserve β-cell function to be identified.

In diabetes, *micro- or macrovascular complications* are often seen after several years of disease. The factors that contribute to these complica-tions are not well understood. There is a need to develop ways to reduce the size of studies and timelines for evaluating therapeutic efficacy on the establishment and progression of micro- and macrovascular com-plications. The project aims to find validated and scientifically justified biomarkers and surrogate endpoints. It should also aim to develop and val-idate new in vivo animal models and in vitro or in silico tools to test novel therapies.

Existing treatments for *chronic pain* provide incomplete relief for some patients or carry a side-effect profile that is unacceptable. The project aims to improve our understanding of the pathways and mechanisms mediat-ing different kinds of pain; to develop translatable efficacy, pharmacody-namic and pharmacokinetic measures in animals and humans; to estab-lish and validate mechanism-based human pain models; and to develop robust markers for patient stratification and quantitative pain assessment so that potential novel analgesics can be tested efficiently and compared in relevant patient groups.

The pathophysiological processes and etiologic factors in *depression and schizophrenia* have so far proven elusive despite a growing under-standing of their genetic and biochemical determinants. The development of preclinical models with sensitive pharmacodynamic markers that are closely linked to the pathophysiology of the disease is essential to improve the validity of preclinical models. The project focuses on how to translate efficacy of therapeutic approaches into blood and/or CSF markers or imag-ing and/or electrophysiological measures suitable for clinical assessments.

To accelerate the successful development of molecules for the treat-ment of *neurodegenerative disorders*, it is essential to improve the predic-tive value of animal models, identify pharmacodynamic markers of drug response, and develop pharmacodynamic models that allow early predic-tion of efficacy and markers to aid stratification of the patient population. The project aims to ensure effective translation of efficacy from bench to bedside and vice versa by focusing on the development of translatable animal and human volunteer models predictive of clinical efficacy in patients in the areas of Alzheimer's disease, Parkinson's disease, and multiple sclerosis.

There is a high, unmet need for more effective, convenient, and safe therapies for patients with *severe asthma*. Development of new treatments for patients with severe asthma presents clear challenges. There is a need for effective use and further development of diagnostic criteria for mechanistic and therapeutic trials. Without better understanding of disease etiology and pathogenesis, relevant preclinical and clinical models cannot be developed to enable translational research strategies. The project aims at setting up a large, longitudinal patient cohort that will enable research to validate novel biomarkers and clinical measures and serve as a vehicle for developing translational models.

Demonstration of the efficacy for new therapies for *chronic obstructive pulmonary disease* (COPD) has relied on showing reduction of airflow obstruction. There is now a clear understanding that the measured reduction does not capture the potential benefits that the patient experiences. Capturing the COPD patients' experience of the disease and effects of treatment is an important aspect of evaluating treatments for COPD. The projects should develop a framework to understand the patients' experience of COPD that will inform strategies for measuring meaningful outcomes in clinical trials followed by development of a measurement tool for use in clinical trials to evaluate treatments.

10.7.3. Knowledge Management

There is no call directly related to knowledge management in the first round. This pillar is intended to close the existing gap by addressing bottlenecks related to information technology and by providing platforms to analyze large amounts of information in an integrated and predictive way. This area will be key to maximizing the potential of new technologies, such as genomics, and in analyzing data generated by IMI in a consistently integrated manner.

10.7.4. Education and Training

This pillar addresses existing gaps in expertise in biomedical R&D knowledge and skills needed for the biopharmaceutical industry. Current monitoring and prediction of gaps in knowledge and capabilities will be conducted. These funding possibilities represent a remarkable step forward, for it is the first time that real educational aspects are brought forward on a pan-European basis. Education and training used to be considered the responsibility of each country.

The pharmaceutical industry needs highly skilled professionals who understand cutting-edge technologies and life science disciplines. One of the five calls on education and training in this round establishes a *pan-European network of excellence for education and training in the biopharmaceutical field* covering the whole life cycle of a medicine from research to pharmacovigilance. The aim is to create a sustainable academia–industry cross-disciplinary approach to facilitate collaboration on education and training, to anticipate emerging needs, and to provide appropriate training solutions. In addition, the project should create a network to identify and explore options for responding to these needs through efficient organization of training courses on emerging sciences and technologies that can be made rapidly available across Europe.

Safety scientists with a much broader spectrum of knowledge than the traditional toxicologist are in demand.[11] The future safety scientist will have to integrate knowledge accumulated from many safety-relevant disciplines if he or she is to excel in modern risk assessment and risk management. The safety scientist should bridge classical pharmaceutical toxicology and human safety pharmacology. This project will establish a program to train scientists holding a postgraduate master's degree in life sciences to become knowledgeable in the fields necessary to perform a holistic evaluation of the safety of a new medicine by evaluating and linking animal and human and/or patient safety data.

Pharmaceutical medicine represents a medical–scientific interdisciplinary field. There is a need to improve the professional effectiveness of physicians but also other life science graduates in drug development. This improvement is to be accomplished by harmonizing existing and new courses and establishing a network of academic centers that will deliver advanced postgraduate training programs. External validity and appropriateness of the content will be ensured.

An *integrated overview of the medicine development process*, including ethics, scientific methodology, regulatory requirements, assessments of risk and benefit, intellectual property matters, business skills, and understanding of the business environment, is needed by many stakeholders involved to a greater or lesser extent in the process of medicine development. A modular course to provide an overview of the medicine development process, including regulatory, health economics, and ethics requirements, should be developed.

The science of *pharmacovigilance* is still developing from being traditionally reactive to having a more proactive focus on coordinating and analyzing the wealth of data on the use of medicines. This change of focus requires inclusion of disciplines such as advanced epidemiology, biostatistics, drug utilization, pharmacoepidemiology, and the use of large, automated, population-based exposure–outcome databases. There is thus a pressing need to expand the knowledge of pharmacovigilance professionals in both industry and at regulatory agencies. Furthermore, the development of better methodologies for risk communication is also needed. The project is expected to achieve these goals by customized educational and training programs.

10.8. The Call Procedures

The long-established procedure under the EU Framework Programmes has, on the recommendation of the biopharmaceutical industry, been radically changed for the IMI to make the application procedure easier. Thus, the IMI calls are conducted through a two-stage process: In the first stage of the call, "Applicants Consortia" (e.g., collaborations between academia, SMEs, patient organizations, non-EFPIA industries, etc.) are asked to submit an "Expression of Interest" (EoI) as a response to a call. In the second stage, following a peer review of the EoIs, the Applicant Consortium of the best EoI, together with the "EFPIA Consortium" that committed to engage in the topic, will be invited to form a joint/full "Project Consortium." The full project proposal to be developed in the next phase will also contain a draft "Project Agreement," which is to be concluded between all members of the consortium, governing their relationship, including detailed intellectual property rights. Full project proposals will then be evaluated based on consistency with the original EoI, on scientific excellence, the quality of the implementation plan, and on the potential impact. Favorably reviewed full project proposals will, after this evaluation, be invited to conclude a "Grant Agreement" governing the relationship between the selected Project Consortium and the IMI JU.

The first call for proposals, to a value of 128 million euros for nonindustrial applicants, was announced on April 30, 2008, with the EoI submission deadline set to July 15, 2008. The second stage was finalized in 2008, with projects starting in 2009. In Tables 10.5 and 10.6, the topics of the first and second calls are listed. The second call topics were made public in November 2009. All call texts can be found on the IMI Web site.[1]

10.9. Future Perspectives

With the IMI JU, Europe has developed a new model for public–private collaboration. Through the involvement of 23 large biopharmaceutical companies applying for a budget of 2 billion euros over 9 years, it will have a major impact on pharmaceutical research and drug development in Europe.

In fact, the IMI JU represents the closest collaboration that has ever been established on a large scale between competitors within the

Table 10.6. Topics Announced for the Second Call of the IMI JU

September 2009 with an estimated EU contribution of 76 M €*

Oncology: New tools for target validation to improve drug efficacy

Oncology: Molecular biomarkers – accelerating cancer-care therapy development and refining patient care

Oncology: Imaging biomarkers for anticancer drug development

Infectious disease: Identification and development of rapid point-of-care microbiologic diagnostic test to facilitate clinical practice and conduct of clinical trials

Inflammation: Understanding aberrant adaptive immunity mechanisms in human chronic immune-mediated diseases: Rheumatoid arthritis (RA), systemic lupus erythematosus, and inflammatory bowel disease

Inflammation: Translational research in RA and RA-like diseases: Bridging between animal models and humans

Knowledge Management: Drug/Disease modeling: Library & framework

Knowledge Management: Open pharmacological space

Knowledge Management: Using electronic health records and enhanced medical research

*M €: million euros.

biopharmaceutical industry. The InnoMed pilot project provided much inspiration for the IMI JU and also was successful in its own right. It was funded (as a precursor) under FP 6 (18 million euros). For the InnoMed Integrated Project, 16 large pharmaceutical companies, 14 universities, and 8 SMEs committed to collaborate effectively on precompetitive predictive safety and efficacy markers (see Table 10.3).[13] Moreover, the participation of academia, clinical centers, SMEs, patient organizations, and public authorities (including regulators) should ensure faster and more durable solutions. This increases transparency and provides a collaborative experience.

IMI has the potential to become a unique technological platform for future drug development in Europe. Through it, industrial and regulatory needs meet the public research system, with the EC acting as protector for public interest. The IMI allows the industry to share precompetitive data and the best analytical practice available. Wisely used, it can help Europe recover its former position as a world leader in pharmaceutical innovation.

The IMI will also activate more peripheral stakeholders in a bottom-up fashion and create a fruitful climate for drug development.[9] It has the potential of better direct links and strong collaboration between the two key European Directorates for medicines research, development, and use: DG Research and DG Enterprise. The latter has accountability to the EMA. For example, it should be possible to link the needs of the regulatory authorities to implement more efficient methods in the regulatory framework on the basis of scientifically validated results generated through funding by DG Research.

Finally, the impact of IMI as a vehicle for introducing and facilitating translational thinking in the academic environment will, undoubtedly, lead to more translational research and better medicines. The basic research needed in Europe to identify and validate new chemical, molecular, and biological therapy targets will most likely need more traditional funding options.

10.10. Acknowledgments

Thanks go to EUFEPS – its Constituency, the Executive Committee, other EUFEPS Committees, not the least the one on Industrial Research Relations (CIRR), but also the Committee on Education and Training (CTE) and the Committee on Academic Research Relations (CARR) as well as to EUFEPS Liaison Officers Ing-Marie Nilsson for EU and Larry Lesko for the FDA. Very fruitful collaboration with EUREKA, EFPIA, EFMC, ECRIN, Eurotox, and the Medicines Development Section of the EFB is also acknowledged. NovoNordisk A/S support of Ole J. Bjerrum in his early engagement in the NSMF project should also be gratefully acknowledged as should the Swedish Academy of Pharmaceutical Sciences, which was one of the key initiators of EUFEPS and made Hans H. Linden available for the EUFEPS Secretariat. Finally, without highly appreciated financial support from several NSMF and other initiatives by the EC, this progress would not have been possible.

10.11. References

1. Innovation Medicines Initiative (IMI), http://www.IMI.Europa.eu
2. European Federation of Pharmaceutical Sciences, http://www.EUFEPS.org
3. Bjerrum OJ. (2000). New safe medicines faster: A proposal for a key action within the European Union's 6th framework programme. Pharmacol. Toxicol. 86(Suppl 1), 23–26.
4. Alderborn G, Bjerrum OJ, Lehr CM, Linden H, Nilsson M-I, Reden J et al.(2000). New medicines faster: Proposals for research topics, methodologies, techniques and other means promoting the drug development process to the benefit of European citizens. March 15–16, Brussels. European Federation for Pharmaceutical Sciences (EUFEPS) workshop. Available at: http://www.eufeps.org/document/pdfs/nsmf.pdf
5. The Innovative Medicines Initiative (IMI) research agenda. (February 15, 2008). Creating biomedical R&D leadership for Europe to benefit patients and

society (version 2.0). Available at: http://imi.europa.eu/docs/imi-gb-006v2–15022008-research-agenda_en.pdf

6. Bjerrum OJ. (2002). New safe medicines faster: A proposition for a pan-European research effort. Nat. Rev. Drug Discovery. 1, 395–398.

7. Donnelly F, & Jehenson P. (2005). European technology platform on innovative medicines. Int. J. Pharm. Med. 19, 153–161.

8. FP6 Workprogramme. Integrating and strengthening the European Research Area in Life sciences, genomics and biotechnology for health Call 1–4, 2002–2006. January 2002. Available at: http://ec.europa/research/fp6/pdf/fp6-in-brief_en.pdf

9. Bjerrum OJ, Demotes J, Odysseos A, Sanz F, Seiler J, Strandgaard K (2005). New medicines faster: How to establish a European technology platform for innovative medicines. April 21–22, Barcelona. European Federation for Pharmaceutical Sciences (EUFEPS). Available at: http://www.eufeps.org/document/pdfs/nsmf_III_final_report.pdf

10. Ainsworth MA, Bjerrum OJ, Bühler FR, Dencker L, Dirach J, Hansen JG, et al. (2003). New medicines faster: How to rethink and accelerate the development and approval of innovative, new medicines for faster patient relief. April 28–29, Copenhagen. European Federation for Pharmaceutical Sciences (EUFEPS). Available at: http://www.eufeps.org/document/pdfs/nsmf_II_report.pdf

11. Bjerrum OJ, Caldwell J, Claude N, Linden H, Mulder GJ, Seiler, JP, et al. (2004). Report from European Federation for Pharmaceutical Sciences (EUFEPS) brainstorm workshop on safety sciences. April 2–3. Available at: http://www.eufeps.org/document/pdfs/safetysciences_report.pdf

12. U.S. Department of Health and Human Services, Food and Drug Administration. (March 2004). Innovation or stagnation: Challenge and opportunity on the critical path to new medical products. Available at: http://www.fda.gov/ScienceResearch/SpecialTopics/CriticalPathInitiative/CriticalPathOpportunitiesReports/ucm077262.htm

13. The European Federation of Pharmaceutical Industries and Associations (EFPIA). Vision paper. Innovative Medicines Initiative. October 2010. Available at: http://www.imi.europa.eu/sites/default/files/uploads/documents/vision-document_en.pdf14. Innovative Medicines Initiative. InnoMed project. 27 Sept. 2007. Available at: http://www.imi.europa.eu/innomed_en.html

Critical Path Institute and the Predictive Safety Testing Consortium

Elizabeth Gribble Walker

11.1. Introduction to the Critical Path in Medical Product Development

Critical Path Institute (C-Path) is an independent, nonprofit institute created in 2005 by the University of Arizona and the U.S. Food and Drug Administration (FDA). C-Path is dedicated to bringing scientists from the FDA, the European Medicines Agency (EMA), industry, and academia together in collaborative research, endeavoring to improve the path for innovative new drugs, diagnostics, and devices to reach patients in need. C-Path's programs are designed to address the scientific, safety, and educational aspects of medical product development in support of the FDA's Critical Path Initiative (http://www.fda.gov/oc/initiatives/criticalpath/initiative.html).[1-4] Released in 2004, the FDA's Critical Path Report analyzed input from FDA scientists and stakeholders on opportunities and challenges along the critical path of medical product development. Although not perfectly analogous, similar initiatives to improve drug safety or efficacy originating in Europe include the InnoMed PredTox collaboration (http://www.innomed-predtox.com) and, more recently, the Innovative Medicines Initiative (http://imi.europa.eu).[5,6] Although the operational model for governance and execution of research varies widely, the objectives of each endeavor include the regulator's stated priorities for improving drug development and have resulted in the creation of new pathways and processes at the FDA and the EMA for reviewing and applying novel data often independent of a particular drug application.

To serve as a neutral and trusted third party for collaborators, C-Path does not accept funding from organizations that develop products regulated by the FDA or that would create a real or perceived conflict of interest. C-Path's projects are established on the basis of industry's willingness to share precompetitive knowledge and work cooperatively in support of projects that are identified as high priority to the FDA in the interest of public health. All collaborative projects seek ongoing input from health authorities, and work toward results that will be submitted for formal regulatory review and opinion, thus enabling their incorporation into the drug development process and the overall evolution of regulatory science.

Current collaborative public–private endeavors at C-Path include the Predictive Safety Testing Consortium (PSTC), the Coalition against Major Disease (CAMD), and the Patient-Reported Outcomes (PRO) Consortium. The PSTC aims to improve safety assessment in drug development through the evaluation of novel safety biomarkers in animal models and humans and is thus the primary focus of this chapter. The CAMD, striking first at Alzheimer's and Parkinson's diseases, seeks to capitalize on clinical trial placebo data and patient registries to establish clinical models of the natural history of disease and qualify biomarkers to streamline clinical trial design and conduct in therapeutic areas with unmet medical need.

CAMD members, including pharmaceutical companies, patient research groups, and advisors from the FDA, the EMA, the National Institute of Neurological Disorders and Stroke (NINDS), and the National Institute on Aging (NIA), define clinical data standards and share clinical trial data for control groups to describe the natural history of these diseases and test biomarkers and endpoints that may more carefully identify potential drug responders and clearly detect therapeutic response.[7] Addressing another important aspect of clinical trials in many therapeutic areas, the PRO Consortium enables the harmonization and sharing of the costs involved in the development and testing of patient-reported outcome instruments aimed at measuring the patient's response and perspective regarding the outcomes of medical interventions (e.g., drug therapy in clinical trials). These instruments are increasingly recognized as critical in many therapeutic areas (e.g., irritable bowel syndrome [IBS], depression, asthma) in which the perceived impact of a drug on a patient's symptoms and functioning may provide the most relevant measure of efficacy – particularly in the absence of other validated response metrics.[8–10]

11.2. The Predictive Safety Testing Consortium

C-Path's flagship consortium, the PSTC, was established in 2006 and addresses several themes illustrated in the FDA's Critical Path Initiative Opportunities Report, a list of research endeavors that can help speed the development and approval of medical products (http://www.fda.gov/oc/initiatives/criticalpath/initiative.html). The PSTC has a singular objective: to compile data, generate scientific consensus, and submit for regulatory review data on new safety biomarkers to be used in drug development. In the PSTC, the term "biomarker" is used to describe any measurable physiological endpoint that may reflect injury to, or modulation of, function of a target organ or system of interest. Loss of potential therapeutics due to unmonitorable safety concerns is an all-too-familiar occurrence at pharmaceutical companies and is regularly cited to be a major factor contributing to high development costs and lengthy cycles from discovery to market.[11] Optimizing the predictivity of preclinical models and testing is a major effort in toxicology. In recognition, however, of the reality that animal toxicity models are unlikely to ever predict or reflect human susceptibility perfectly, an equally important endeavor is to use sensitive and specific tools to detect and monitor toxicity in both animal models and humans. The PSTC undertakes the evaluation of novel biomarkers that can detect drug toxicity in animal models and humans in a more specific and sensitive fashion than can endpoints currently used in regulated drug studies.

Many "new" safety biomarkers have been used for years at pharmaceutical companies, but their application has been limited to solely support internal decision making. Industry and academic publications on safety biomarkers in the scientific literature are plentiful. Several companies have amassed large databases of safety information on preclinical biomarkers (e.g., for liver and kidney toxicity); however, *because these biomarkers have never been formally evaluated by the health authorities*, reluctance to use them in regulated studies has prevailed due to uncertainty as to whether the regulatory body would interpret the data in the same way as the company. As opposed to chemical structure or identification of novel therapeutic targets, safety can reasonably be conceived as precompetitive information in drug development. The PSTC provides a framework for sharing internal data and experience with biomarkers and their assays. By capitalizing on existing studies and data, identifying gaps and needs, and prospectively filling those gaps, a rich and robust data set is generated that could not practically be achieved at any one member company alone. The intended deliverables – new biomarkers with formal regulatory evaluation and opinion as to their acceptability for specific uses in drug development – are motivating incentives for industry participation that can directly enable decision making and advance programs in a way not previously possible.

The PSTC is an established global, mostly virtual, effort with participation of more than 250 leading safety scientists and clinicians at 16 pharmaceutical member companies, the FDA, the EMA, and many academic institutions. The consortium is governed by a unique legal agreement that addresses confidentiality, intellectual property, antitrust, and materials and data sharing. The PSTC is organized into several working groups focused on biomarkers for a particular target organ toxicity determined and prioritized by the membership with input from the FDA. Currently, working groups are investigating biomarkers of nephrotoxicity, hepatotoxicity, vascular injury, skeletal muscle toxicity, cardiac hypertrophy, and a gene signature for nongenotoxic carcinogenicity in the rat. The consortium is overseen by an advisory committee with one voting representative for each member, and all working groups are advised by a translational team of clinical safety scientists who guide the design of translational studies to bridge from the animal models to patients. The C-Path provides scientific staffing, project management, and oversight of the Consortium's activities and infrastructure, and the working groups are chaired by volunteer expert scientists and clinicians from the membership.

The PSTC experienced quick success in early 2008 when, following the submission of data that showed how 7 urinary biomarkers of nephrotoxicity in the rat were more sensitive and specific for detecting tubular or glomerular injury than were standard endpoints (i.e., serum creatinine or blood urea nitrogen), the FDA and the EMA announced that the biomarkers were considered appropriate for voluntary use in nonclinical rat studies to support regulatory decision making.[12] The PSTC submitted the data for these 7 urinary proteins (kidney injury molecule-1 [Kim-1], albumin, total protein, β_2-microglobulin, cystatin C, clusterin, trefoil factor 3) to the FDA and the EMA in June 2007, enabling the health authorities to pilot a first-ever joint biomarker review under the Voluntary Exploratory Data Submissions (VXDS) process. In addition to the data set containing evidence from 23 studies during which rats were given a number of nephrotoxic and control compounds, the PSTC's biomarker submission contained a thorough summary of the clinical literature and proposed that 5 of the 7 biomarkers (Kim-1, albumin, total protein, β_2-microglobulin, and cystatin C) be considered qualified for use in clinical safety studies.[13] The FDA and the EMA determined that the evidence that was submitted supported the use of the biomarkers in clinical monitoring strategies but would need to be reviewed on a case-by-case basis.[12] In 2009–2010, the same data set were reviewed by the Japanese Pharmaceuticals and Manufacturing Devices Agency (PMDA) with subsequent approval for voluntary use of the 7 biomarkers for drug applications to this agency. Further dialogue with the FDA and the EMA has produced a prioritized body of clinical evidence and discrete studies to be conducted that should widen the context of regulatory clinical use of these biomarkers.[14] The next round of data submissions will be made in parallel with the FDA, the EMA, and the PMDA.

11.3. Regulatory and Public Health Impact of the PSTC

The success of this first submission has influenced how the health authorities consider and manage qualification of safety biomarkers. The EMA has since finalized a guidance for "Qualification of novel methodologies for use in drug development," the FDA has a draft biomarker qualification guidance expected in early 2011, and the PMDA has drafted a process for the review of biomarker data. Qualification by all agencies is conceived as a stepwise process whereby an initial specific context of use proposed for a biomarker may be expanded as further data are generated, submitted, and reviewed.[3] For example, the PSTC's Nephrotoxicity Working Group is currently striving to more carefully establish the kinetics with which the biomarkers rise and fall with rat kidney injury progression and recovery and to elaborate the specificity of the biomarkers for kidney (as opposed to other organ) injury by measuring the kidney biomarkers in animals treated with other target organ toxicants. To gather data to support applications for the biomarkers in early clinical trials, several clinical studies to determine human inter- and intrasubject variability and responsiveness of the biomarkers to nephrotoxic drug insult in acute kidney injury are actively enrolling subjects.

Through this unique partnership among health authorities, industry, academia, and C-Path, significant advances in not only drug development but in public health in general are being achieved. New tools that enhance safety assessment of potential therapeutics are now available for drug development use but ultimately should make their way into the standard of care for evaluating patient health. The PSTC also represents an encouraging example of industry's willingness to collaborate in precompetitive space and influence the field of safety assessment as a whole. Finally, the success of this first biomarker qualification and the opportunity provided in the process of scientific dialogue between regulatory and industry scientists undeniably demonstrate the value of directed communication, resources, and collaboration among these key stakeholders in drug development. Because of the PSTC's efforts and the new pathways created at the FDA, EMA, and PMDA, potential medicines with promising therapeutic potential will advance into clinical trials with the ability to carefully monitor and protect patient safety. Initiatives such as the FDA's Critical Path Initiative and C-Path's collaborative research endeavors fill critical gaps in regulatory science research with huge potential to improve drug development and positively affect patients' lives.

II.4. References

1. Woodcock J, & Woosley R. (2008). The FDA critical path initiative and its influence on new drug development. Ann. Rev. Med. 59, 1–12.
2. Coons SJ. (2009). The FDA's critical path initiative: A brief introduction. Clin. Ther. 31(11), 2572–2573.
3. Goodsaid FM, Frueh FW, & Mattes W. (2008). Strategic paths for biomarker qualification. Toxicol. 245(3), 219–223.
4. Goodsaid FM and Mendrick DL (2010). Translational Medicine and the Value of Biomarker Qualification. Sci. Transl. Med. 2, 47ps44.
5. Mattes WB. (2008). Public consortium efforts in toxicogenomics. Methods Mol. Biol. 460, 221–238.
6. Hunter AJ. (2008). The Innovative Medicines Initiative: A pre-competitive initiative to enhance the biomedical science base of Europe to expedite the development of new medicines for patients. Drug Discov. Today. 13(9–10), 371–373.

7. Romero K, de Mars M, Frank D, Anthony M, Neville J, Kirby L, et al. (2009). The coalition against major diseases: Developing tools for an integrated drug development process for Alzheimer's and Parkinson's diseases. Clin. Pharmacol. Ther. 86(4), 365–367.

8. Acquadro C, Berzon R, Dubois D, Leidy NK, Marquis P, Revicki D, et al. (2003). Incorporating the patient's perspective into drug development and communication: An ad hoc task force report of the patient-reported outcomes (PRO) harmonization group meeting at the Food and Drug Administration, February 16, 2001. Value in Health. 5, 521–533.

9. Willke RJ, Burke LB, & Erickson P. (2004). Measuring treatment impact: A review of patient-reported outcomes and other efficacy endpoints in approved product labels. Control. Clin. Trials. 25, 535–552.

10. U.S. Food and Drug Administration. (February 2006). Guidance for Industry: Patient-Reported Outcome Measures: Use in Medical Product Development to Support Labeling Claims (DRAFT). Available at: http://www.fda.gov/cder/guidance/5460dft.pdf

11. Kola I, & Landis J. (2004). Can the pharmaceutical industry reduce attrition rates? Nat. Rev. Drug Discov. 3, 711–715.

12. European Medicines Agency. (July 3, 2008). Final report on the pilot joint EMA/FDA VXDS experience on qualification of nephrotoxicity biomarkers. Available at: http://www.ema.europa.eu/pdfs/human/biomarkers/25088508en.pdf

13. Nature Biotechnology. May 2010, 28(5), 429–494 (multiple articles).

14. Mattes WB, & Walker EG. (2009). Translational toxicology and the work of the predictive safety testing consortium. Clin. Pharmacol. Ther. 85(3), 327–330.

The Biomarkers Consortium: Facilitating the Development and Qualification of Novel Biomarkers through a Precompetitive Public–Private Partnership

David Wholley and David B. Lee

The Biomarkers Consortium is a groundbreaking public–private biomedical research partnership managed by the Foundation for the National Institutes of Health (FNIH) (see Box 12.1) that endeavors to develop, validate, and qualify biomarkers to accelerate the development of new medicines and improve patient care.

The Consortium was founded in late 2006 by FNIH, the National Institutes of Health (NIH), the U.S. Food and Drug Administration (FDA), and the Pharmaceutical Research and Manufacturers of America (PhRMA). Other major stakeholders include the Centers for Medicare & Medicaid Services (CMS) and the Biotechnology Industry Organization (BIO). These stakeholders, and many others, are working together on an unprecedented scale to identify, develop, and qualify biomarkers that can be used to detect, prevent, diagnose, and treat disease. This integrated, cross-sector approach is helping to accelerate the use of biomarkers in research, development of treatments, and regulatory decision making.

The Consortium has more than 60 additional contributing members involved in helping to support its operations; these members represent the pharmaceutical and biotechnology industries, nonprofit organizations, and patient advocacy organizations. The biopharmaceutical members of the Consortium include Abbott Laboratories; Amgen; Amylin; AstraZeneca; Boehringer-Ingelheim; Bristol-Myers Squibb; Celgene Corporation; Daiichi Sanyko; Eisai, Inc.; GlaxoSmithKline; Johnson & Johnson; Eli Lilly and Company; Merck & Co., Inc.; Pfizer, Inc; F. Hoffman–La Roche, Ltd.; Sunovion; and Takeda Pharmaceuticals. Other industry members include Banyan Biomarkers; BG Medicine; Genstruct, Inc.; InfraReDx, Inc.; Meso Scale Discovery; Metabolon, Inc.; NextGen Sciences; Orasi Medical, Inc.; Scout Diagnostics, LLC; and XOMA, Ltd. The Consortium has more than 30 additional members representing nonprofit and advocacy organizations, including the Alzheimer's Association, the American Diabetes Association, the American Society for Clinical Oncology, the Arthritis

---

Box 12.1. FNIH Description

The FNIH was established by the U.S. Congress to support the NIH in its mission to improve public health by forming and facilitating public–private partnerships for biomedical research, education, and training. The foundation identifies and develops opportunities for innovative public–private partnerships involving industry, academia, and the philanthropic community. A nonprofit 501(c)(3) charitable corporation, the foundation raises private-sector funds for a broad portfolio of unique programs that complement and enhance NIH priorities and activities. To date, the foundation has raised over $500 million toward more than 100 projects. The FNIH's Web site is www.fnih.org.

Foundation, the Avon Foundation, the Immune Tolerance Institute, the Juvenile Diabetes Research Foundation, the Michael J. Fox Foundation for Parkinson's Research, the Osteoarthritis Research Society International, the PROOF Centre, and the Radiological Society of North America.

The Consortium is a unique platform able to identify, develop, fund, and execute multiple biomarker development and qualification projects in a variety of therapeutic areas. All projects must adhere to agreed-upon principles and policies regarding intellectual property and data sharing (available at www.biomarkersconsortium.org/index.php?option=com_content&task=section&id=6&Itemid=40).

Given the realization by these diverse stakeholders that the objectives of the Consortium to identify and qualify new biomarkers are beyond the capacity of any one sector, these groups are working together to combine their efforts and share the financial and scientific risk to execute these costly, scientifically challenging projects. Working in partnership will also help ensure the best chance of successfully identifying and qualifying new and existing biomarkers through the input of all sectors.

Projects are aimed at precompetitive research in translational areas that combine a significant public health benefit with a practical impact on drug development or clinical practice, and results are made available as broadly and quickly as possible. Projects are selected and developed within four disease/therapeutic area–oriented steering committees (SCs), which include representatives from all Consortium stakeholders in addition to prominent academic scientists.

The four SCs established to date are in cancer, inflammation and immunity, metabolic disorders (including cardiovascular disease), and neuroscience. Ideas can either come to an SC from external submitters or be dynamically developed within an SC into an approved "project concept." After a concept is approved, the SC forms a project team, which develops the concept into a detailed project plan that covers quantifiable objectives, qualification criteria, analysis plans, handling of intellectual property, data access, human subjects, and milestone-based project timelines and budgets. This project plan is approved by the relevant SC as well as by the Consortium's Executive Committee (which includes industry executives, senior FDA officials, and NIH Institute Directors) prior to project funding and launch.

The FNIH seeks formal funding for a project only after final approval, although it performs a feasibility scan for funding beginning at the concept stage. Projects are funded by private organizations on an à la carte basis (i.e., organizations can choose which projects they wish to fund). Funders are typically represented on the project team, which provides oversight of the project and review of results. Project management is provided by the FNIH – or in some cases, the NIH – on behalf of the Consortium. Although the NIH cannot directly contribute to a project budget for a project that is FNIH-managed, many approved projects to date have leveraged substantial in-kind or parallel investments by the NIH that in aggregate can represent 40% or more of total project cost. (See Box 12.1.)

The Consortium is open to receiving ideas from the scientific community for potential execution. Investigators need to complete a "Project Concept Submission Form," available at the Consortium's Web site (www.biomarkersconsortium.org) by clicking on the "Submit a Project Concept" tab.

The Consortium has launched 10 projects to date (1 of which is completed) and has developed and approved 4 additional projects that are in the process of being funded for launch.

A brief description of the projects launched to date can be found in Table 12.1. (See also Box 12.2.)

The Consortium announced its first completed project – to determine whether adiponectin has utility as a predictive biomarker of glycemic control – in June 2009. The project, which was conducted entirely via in-kind contributions, involved aggregating deidentified data from 8 trials of peroxisome proliferator-activated receptor (PPAR) agonists at GlaxoSmith-Kline; Eli Lilly and Company; Merck & Co., Inc.; and F. Hoffman–La Roche, Ltd. and subjecting the pooled data to analysis by statisticians at Quintiles Transnational Corporation and at the NIH NIDDK. These findings were published in *Clinical Pharmacology & Therapeutics* in June 2009.[1,2]

Among the projects currently approved and poised to be launched in early 2011 is the Clinical Studies to Evaluate and Qualify Kidney Safety Biomarkers Project. This project will compare performance, initiate clinical qualification, and advance regulatory acceptance of new urinary biomarkers of acute drug-induced kidney injury. This project will expand the work accomplished by the Critical Path Institute's Predictive Safety Testing Consortium, which successfully qualified a panel of 7 kidney safety biomarkers for regulatory use in preclinical studies. In addition, this project would expand these findings to the clinical setting.

Table 12.1. Launched/Completed Projects (as of October 2010)

Project	Brief Description	Status
Fluorodeoxyglucose (FDG)-PET Lung and Lymphoma Projects (2 projects – Cancer SC)	Build case for FDA incorporation of FDG-PET into outcome measures for lung cancer/lymphoma	Scheduled to complete in 2012
I-SPY 2 TRIAL (Investigation of Serial Studies to Predict Your Therapeutic Response with Imaging and molecular analysis) (Cancer SC)	A personalized medicine trial that promises to accelerate the pace of identifying effective novel agents for breast cancer; patients will be classified according to biomarker profiles and randomized to control therapy for up to 12 agents	Launched in March 2010 (5 year, $24 million project)
Adiponectin Project (Metabolic Disorders SC)	Determine whether adiponectin has utility as a predictive biomarker of glycemic control	**Completed**; results published in June 2009
Carotid MRI Reproducibility Project (Metabolic Disorders SC)	Establish a standardized carotid MRI protocol and impact of site/platform on reproducibility	Scheduled to complete by end of 2011
Sarcopenia Consensus Summit (Metabolic Disorders SC)	Generate a consensus definition of sarcopenia (age-related decrease in skeletal muscle mass) to provide specific guidelines for diagnosis and better enable regulatory decisions	Phase 1 launched in July 2009; anticipate completion by mid-2011
Alzheimer's Disease Targeted Plasma Proteomics Project (Neuroscience SC)	Qualify a multiplexed panel of known AD plasma-based biomarkers using plasma samples from the ADNI	Anticipate project completion and upload of data to ADNI Web site by end of 2010
Alzheimer's Disease Targeted Cerebrospinal Fluid (CSF) Proteomics Project (Neuroscience SC)	Qualify a multiplexed panel of known AD CSF-based biomarkers, examine Beta-Site APP Cleaving Enzyme (BACE) levels in CSF, and qualify a mass spectroscopy panel using the ADNI CSF samples	Launched in May 2010; anticipate completion in mid-2011
PET Radioligand Project (Neuroscience SC)	Develop improved, more sensitive radioligands with higher binding to the peripheral benzodiazepine receptor	On track for completion by end of 2011
Alzheimer's Disease/Mild Cognitive Impairment Placebo Data Analysis Project (Neuroscience SC)	Combine placebo data from large industry clinical trials and analyze them to provide better measures of cognition and disease progression for use in future Alzheimer's Disease/Mild Cognitive Impairment clinical trials	Launched in February 2010; 3-year project

Box 12.2. Alzheimer's Disease Neuroimaging Initiative

First described more than 100 years ago, Alzheimer's disease (AD) has no cure or lasting, effective treatment. Currently, more than 5 million people in the United States suffer from it, and its incidence is projected to increase dramatically over the next 20 years. The goal of the Alzheimer's Disease Neuroimaging Initiative (ADNI) is to alter that prognosis.

The NIH's largest public–private partnership on brain research, ADNI, tracks normal, mildly cognitively impaired (MCI), and AD brain changes to measure the progression of the condition. This study is cofunded by the NIH and the private sector through $27 million in support provided to the FNIH by 20 pharmaceutical companies and two nonprofit organizations.

The ADNI is using magnetic resonance imaging (MRI) and positron emission tomography (PET) imaging as well as laboratory and cognitive testing of 821 normal, MCI, and AD patients. Among the goals of the study is to provide better tools for carrying out effective clinical trials and to identify biomarkers that can predict clinical outcome.

The ADNI has, in fact, led to improved understanding of how to conduct such trials in a multicenter setting by using imaging technologies to analyze blood and cerebrospinal fluid biomarkers. As a result, pharmaceutical companies developing AD drugs have begun using ADNI methodologies in their clinical trials. The idea is that, by using drugs to treat validated biomarkers of AD instead of treating less precise cognitive measures, the cost and length of drug trials can be reduced.

Already, more than 1,700 investigators from across the globe have accessed ADNI data for their own analyses. The study has also fostered similar projects in Australia, Japan, Europe, and China. Additional projects are being discussed in Korea, India, and South America. The establishment of worldwide standards and a worldwide network for clinical trials has huge implications for the scientific community.

Growing data from ADNI's subjects at 57 sites across the United States and Canada are being published as well as findings and other materials on ADNI's two Web sites, www.loni.ucla.edu/ADNI and www.adni-info.org.

Launched in 2004, the ADNI concluded in late 2010. Study investigators were approved to continue the ADNI study for an additional 5 years (from late 2010 to late 2015), which will continue to track the current ADNI subjects and will enroll additional healthy, MCI, and AD patients as well as people with early or very mild cognitive impairment. Additional plans for ADNI II include PET imaging scans on every new patient enrolled. To date, FNIH has identified $22 million that will be provided through the private sector for ADNI II; NIH anticipates providing an additional $40 million. Among the important new supporters of ADNI II is the Canadian Institutes of Health Research, which will provide $1.5 million to the Canadian sites to help cover a portion of the ADNI II costs.

The most direct way for private organizations to get involved in the Consortium is to participate in the contributing membership program, which supports the Consortium's core operations and project development activities. Among the membership benefits is the ability to nominate members to one or more of the Consortium's SCs as well as to nominate candidates for Executive Committee and SC cochair elections as those seats become available (typically every 2 years). Members also receive regular progress reports on Consortium activities and project opportunities from the FNIH.

The Consortium's Web site is www.biomarkersconsortium.org.

12.1. References

1. Wagner JA, Wright EC, Ennis M, et al. (June 2009). Utility of adiponectin as a biomarker predictive of glycemic efficacy is demonstrated by collaborative pooling of data from clinical trials conducted by multiple sponsors. Clin. Pharmacol. Ther. 86(6), 619–625. http://www.nature.com/clpt/journal/v86/n6/full/clpt200988a.html
2. Eck SL and Paul SM (January 2010). Biomarker qualification via public-private partnerships, *Clin. Pharmacol. Ther.* 87(1), 21–23.

Future Directions

Improving the Quality and Productivity of Pharmacometric Modeling and Simulation Activities: The Foundation for Model-Based Drug Development

Thaddeus H. Grasela, Jill Fiedler-Kelly, and Robert Slusser

13.1. Introduction

There is little disagreement among the stakeholders in the pharmaceutical industry and other discovery and development establishments about the existence of a crisis in research and development (R&D) productivity. There are mounting concerns about the difficulty of securing regulatory approval, the recent spates of late-stage failures to lack of efficacy, the withdrawal of drugs after commercialization because of safety concerns, the threat of generic substitution, and complaints over the prices of new medicines.[1] Each of these concerns, and the corresponding societal, political, academic, and industrial responses, will have significant implications for the vitality and sustainability of the pharmaceutical industry and other similar establishments. These implications, in turn, will affect our ability to capitalize on new advances in biomedical knowledge and to develop innovations in diagnostic tools, therapeutic interventions, and preventive treatment.[2,3]

Although there is agreement on the challenges, reaching consensus on the solution is much more difficult. Each functional area in the drug development enterprise has engaged in a variety of initiatives to increase productivity and reduce costs, ranging from deploying new technology and enhancing the information technology (IT) infrastructure to outsourcing and relocating overseas. Although many of these initiatives have merit, it is becoming clearer that more radical changes are necessary. In particular, the central process of knowledge generation has come under scrutiny along with the strategic and governance aspects of the decision-making process.

The dominant paradigm for drug development and evaluation of the performance of new medicines is based on the conduct of empiric clinical trials and analysis of the data collected during these trials through hypothesis testing against the null hypothesis. One idea that has surfaced as an alternative is model-based drug development (MBDD). In MBDD, mathematical equations are used to create computer-based models representing links between drug treatments and observed effects. This application is generally referred to as "pharmacometric modeling and analysis." Pharmacometric modeling combines knowledge of a disease state, relevant biomarkers, and findings from preclinical and available clinical studies with knowledge of placebo responses and dropout rates to gain insights into the determinants of efficacy and safety outcomes. These models are then used in an attempt to improve the prediction of future events by simulating the outcomes of various alternative study designs and computing the probability of a successful trial given a characterized patient population and proposed treatment regimens.[2,4]

Over the past 10 years there has been a growing interest in performing modeling and simulation (M&S) of efficacy and safety endpoints to select and justify dosing regimens and to optimize trial designs in both preclinical and clinical venues.[5] Examples of the application of M&S can be found throughout the drug realization life cycle, and there has been growing regulatory demand for, and reliance on, M&S results to guide regulatory decision making.[6,7] Consequently, the effort to develop and implement of an efficient and effective process to support M&S activities is emerging as a critical enabling step in ensuring the timely availability of relevant results when they are needed.[8]

13.1.1. Chapter Overview

The goal of this chapter is to describe the steps that can be implemented to improve the quality and reliability of the pharmacometric analysis process. The focus is on the process and not on the technical details of performing M&S. We describe the subtasks that comprise the core process, outline strategies to improve the efficiency and effectiveness of M&S efforts, and describe initiatives to improve model-related data definitions and requirements to better inform the modeling process.

The major theme of this chapter is that the challenges currently encountered in providing M&S results to development teams are symptoms of larger enterprise-wide problems. Although pharmacometrics is just one input into the R&D decision-making process, our premise is that the study of the challenges encountered in providing M&S results is a valuable place to begin to address the larger issues that will be encountered as MBDD is more fully implemented.

13.2. The Pharmacometric Analysis Process

Pharmacometric analysis enables the synthesis of pharmacokinetic (PK) and pharmacodynamic (PD) information from preclinical and clinical studies into knowledge that can inform important decision-making milestones across the entire R&D life cycle. The principle outputs of pharmacometric analysis typically include characterizations of drug kinetics, drug dynamics, and predictions or extrapolations concerning any of these attributes. Thus, the primary mission of the pharmacometrics group performing the M&S activities is to identify and quantify the determinants of drug effects. Importantly, however, we maintain that to improve the productivity of pharmaceutical R&D enterprises significantly, the pharmacometrics group must embrace the organizational changes required to efficiently develop, effectively disseminate, and reliably maintain an accurate picture of the determinants of drug effects.[9]

The process for generating pharmacometric analyses typically consists of seven interrelated steps, namely, analysis planning, data assembly, exploratory analyses, model development, simulation, validation, and presentation of results. These tasks have been described in detail in a variety of publications and have been addressed in regulatory guidances.[10–13]

One of the key tasks of the pharmacometrics process is the development of PK and PD models that serve as a mathematical representation of physiologic or pharmacologic phenomena. The mathematical relationships are observationally based, but, with sufficient experiential history, the models are able to represent the drug–patient interaction in a scientifically and mathematically rigorous way across a wide range of drugs, patients, and interaction parameters (doses, frequency, patient history, genetic makeup, etc.). The simulations based on these models are used to predict the output of clinical testing long before such testing is feasible. These simulations are ideal for iterating across ranges of data inputs to determine output reaction sensitivity, and they function within a feedback loop to provide incremental cause–effect insight to researchers.[2] The models used for these simulations need to be revised when sufficient history has accumulated to prove that the previous relationships require change or when a new relationship accumulates enough data to be mathematically represented with scientific integrity. Whereas the mathematical relationships will vary across disease states and pharmacologic effects, the computational methods and supportive processes can be used unchanged across a wide range of drug development projects.

13.2.1. The M&S Process in Pharmacometrics – Current Practice

It is important to keep in mind that the current typical implementation of pharmacometrics and its role in drug development is more suggestive of model-supported drug development than of MBDD.[8] In many development programs, blood samples are obtained from subjects enrolled in trials and are used for the determination of drug concentration and biomarker data. The drug concentration–time data are subjected to a PK modeling effort to obtain estimates of the model parameters, including the magnitude of between- and within-subject variability in the population.

The data are investigated to identify sources of variability (e.g., age, gender, disease state), and individual estimates of drug exposure are generated. These exposure estimates are then used in a PD or exposure–response analysis of safety and efficacy endpoints, including the aforementioned biomarkers. The goal of these later assessments is to provide information on the determinants of subject outcomes, including characteristics associated with a higher (or lower) probability of desirable (or undesirable) outcomes. These exposure–response relationships, and the determinants of outcome, are then used in simulations to predict the outcomes of possible trial designs using different dosing schemes, enrollment criteria, and so forth. The goal at this stage is to explore strategies that will maximize the probability of success in future trials or to decide that continued development of a compound is unlikely to yield successful results.[4]

In the current implementation, the strategy for collecting the information for pharmacometric analysis is typically overlaid onto traditional study designs. Even with the current understanding and implementation of model-based clinical trial simulations, there is often little opportunity to adjust design characteristics prospectively to optimize the yield for pharmacometric modeling and analysis. The inability to shape experimental designs and data collection strategies prospectively has important implications with respect to the types of challenges experienced by pharmacometricians in the current operating milieu, and it also points to the significant changes that are needed if MBDD is to realize its potential to become an effective tool in the investigative process.[8]

13.2.2. The M&S Process in Pharmacometrics – Future Practice

The current implementation of pharmacometrics in model-supported development is mostly reactionary to the data collected and to the knowledge gaps manifested as the drug development team approaches a decision-making milestone. This ad hoc implementation of pharmacometrics and the "crisis" mode under which it frequently operates can obscure the important ways in which M&S can affect the entire life cycle of drug discovery, development, and commercialization. As the evolution to model-based development continues to unfold, the pharmacometric analysis process must make the important transition from a sidebar activity to a recognized critical path activity (i.e., a requisite step in the decision-making timeline).

In MBDD, quantitative models and the information bases on which they rest will play an increasingly dominant role.[4] The models will become the principal instruments for the design and evaluation of preclinical and clinical studies and will be considered to be among the major deliverables of drug development programs. Consequently, the models become (1) critical to drug development and regulatory decision making, and (2) the foundation for attempts to ensure the safe and effective use of medicines in clinical applications. Consequently, the pharmacometric process will become an integral part of the iterative drug discovery, development, and delivery enterprise, which will proceed via a design study – execute study – capture data – model – simulate – incorporate findings into new study design – run new study – capture new data – refine model – update simulations – and so forth paradigm. Moreover, the design of studies, data collection and management strategies, analysis plans, and all of the other entailments of MBDD will be consistent with the model.

In this future scenario it will be necessary to engage the M&S process early in the development program design process well before clinical trials have been implemented and data collected. The simulations will be performed regularly and iteratively with updated models as additional data are obtained. In this way, M&S becomes an integral part of the discovery and development process and guides the scientists as they evolve the development program design, thus reducing or eliminating work that will not produce the desired solutions before it is done by the project team. Furthermore, the development program design process will be organized first to produce the most important data for M&S and then to address important ancillary issues defined as having much less potential impact on the design – that can therefore be incorporated later at a relatively low cost in time and effort.

13.2.3. The Central Role of the Franchise Disease–Drug Model

Whereas most pharmacometric model–building efforts today begin with the availability of data from within the investigation itself, future development programs will be based on franchise disease–drug models. These models will be focused on specific therapeutic areas and will serve as the bridge between the systems biology models that describe the qualitative and quantitative relationships between relevant biological processes (and their genetic and environmental influences) and the empirical frequentist-based characterizations of safety and efficacy currently used as a basis for determining registrational trial success. Franchise disease–drug models will derive from specific components of the systems biology models (the relevant and related pathways of positive and negative effects) and will specifically address the relationship between one or more biomarkers and clinical outcomes (see Figure 13.1). These semimechanistic models will be developed to evaluate and characterize the time course of biomarker data in the presence of drug or placebo.[14] Recent examples of modeling efforts in diabetes mellitus illustrate the potential for successful bridging of information derived from other in-class compounds to exposure–response evaluations in support of decision making.[15,16]

In translational research, the development and application of mechanism-based PK/PD models are instrumental in informing activities such as candidate selection, lead optimization, and the optimization of early

Fig. 13.1
The pharmacometric
relations encoded in a
Franchise Disease–Drug
Model serve as the
interface between a
systems biology view
of disease and the
design and analysis of
informative trials.

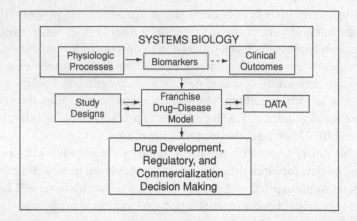

proof-of-concept trials based on knowledge gained in preclinical development.[17] Such mechanism-based models are specifically used to further elucidate and quantify characteristics of the processes linking exposure and response. When such models include estimation of both drug-specific properties and biological system parameters, they begin to demonstrate the benefits of franchise disease–drug models.

The diabetes literature is replete with examples of mechanism-based PK/PD models that characterize, to varying extents, both the mechanism of action of one or more drugs and the relevant physiological processes.[15] In this way, such models permit the distinction between drug-specific and system-specific parameters.[18] It is from this distinction that the true benefits of such models derive. Appropriately accounting for the homeostatic processes and interactions of various biomarkers in the presence and absence of drug allows for a more detailed and accurate description of drug effects in diabetes disease progression.

Beginning with the minimal model and the homeostatic model assessment (HOMA), both originally published in 1979,[19,20] numerous researchers have sought to extend and further characterize the description and understanding of the glucose–insulin system through modeling. In 2000, de Gaetano and Arino mathematically evaluated and described some of the limitations of the minimal model.[21] Silber et al. later built on the work of de Gaetano and Arino, developing an integrated model simultaneously fitting glucose and insulin and accounting for the control mechanisms between the two entities. Silber's model is based on several different kinds of intravenous glucose provocations in type 2 diabetic patients as well as healthy volunteers.[22]

In 2003, Frey et al. developed a disease progression model characterizing the long-term effect of gliclazide on fasting plasma glucose (FPG) in type 2 diabetic patients.[23] De Winter and coworkers sought to enhance the usefulness of this model by addressing the more fundamental level of the processes causing the disease. De Winter's model was developed using data comparing the long-term effects of pioglitazone, metformin, and gliclazide monotherapy on fasting serum insulin (FSI), FPG, and HbA1c in treatment-naive type 2 diabetic patients. DeWinter's model accounts for the differing physiological mechanisms by which each of these compounds achieves its antihyperglycemic effect and further differentiates between the immediate effects of each treatment and the long-term disease-modifying effects on the chronic β-cell function and insulin sensitivity.[18]

Hamren et al. (2008) added yet another feature to their mechanism-based PD model by incorporating red blood cell aging into their model for the interrelationships among plasma glucose, HbA1c, and hemoglobin in patients with type 2 diabetes receiving treatment with tesaglitazar, a dual peroxisome proliferator-activated receptor (PPAR) α/γ agonist.[24]

Nearly all of these models are described as having an immediate or future use beyond merely describing the data at hand. Model applications ranging from increasing understanding of the effects of different types of drugs with different mechanisms on the physiological system, to evaluating the disease-modifying properties of existing and newly developed antidiabetic agents, to supporting dose selection and optimizing trial design for subsequent development of current and future compounds are cited.[18,22]

Clearly, the development of drugs for metabolic disorders such as diabetes is situated in a complex physiological milieu, and yet, one in which decades of evolutionary model development efforts provide convincing evidence that franchise disease–drug models are not only the key to a more complete understanding of complex systems but also the promise of dramatic improvement in R&D productivity.

Importantly, the development of such disease–drug models can and should begin with the availability of data from in vitro and preclinical investigations. The continual refinement of these models with data from later phase trials will allow for the bridging of findings across animal data, healthy volunteers, and the intended patient population.[4] Furthermore, these franchise disease–drug models will be used, in the paradigm described earlier in this chapter, to provide initial feedback on the likelihood of desirable and undesirable pharmacologic effects based on the drug's mechanisms of action.[25] Given various development scenarios, including target population identification, disease severity considerations, and dosing schemas, such disease–drug models will be used to predict the probability of success with a proposed clinical trial and will serve as a basis for the analysis and presentation of results. Further expansion and elaboration of the underlying systems biology models via the introduction of pathological perturbations will then serve as a generator of hypotheses for subsequent model-based clinical trials.

Although this more proactive strategy of using pharmacometric models as critical constituents of development-related decision making is in place in a number of pharmaceutical establishments that have most effectively and aggressively implemented model-supported development, there is still a lack of formalization of the pharmacometric model building, analysis, and simulation process and a paucity of instances in which trial design and data collection strategies are truly dependent on, and therefore influenced by, the findings of pharmacometric modeling efforts.

13.2.4. Implications of the Future Scenario

As we continue to gain experience with M&S, we anticipate that considerable resources will be committed to the maintenance of the franchise disease–drug model because the demand for timely results will likely increase and the rigor required to justify regulatory decision making based on these pharmacometric models will become better appreciated. This aspect of the transition to model-based development will necessitate important changes that will affect the people, process, and technology currently invoked in performing an M&S project. In particular, the flow of information between disciplines is a significant but unrealized problem in the current data management environment in which data reside in functional area silos with minimal integration across studies or development programs. In particular, data definitions have been relatively discipline-specific. Integration of the data arising from different disciplines and functional areas requires that the definitions *between* disciplines be rationalized. Data definitions are the basic building blocks necessary for developing an interdisciplinary, synergistic process wherein team members are contributing to, and working with, a common franchise disease–drug model.[26]

Consistent data definitions will significantly improve productivity, substantially reduce errors and development missteps, and allow the effective integration of all primary stakeholders into the process. Inclusion of all primary stakeholders in M&S process design and execution will, in turn, help to ensure wider applicability of the results of the drug development process.

The pharmacometrics process, now often executed within the confines of the clinical pharmacology department structure, will develop much more intricate relationships with the larger drug R&D enterprise. A fully capable, efficient, and effective pharmacometric analysis process is a prerequisite for this comprehensive integration.[9] As companies deploy this fully capable process, a new view of the methodology and benefits of pharmacometrics will emerge with critical implications for the future of the pharmaceutical and biotechnology industries.

The strategic leveraging of M&S technology and results by a pharmaceutical company has the potential to provide a major increase in drug discovery and development competitiveness in the marketplace. With the fully capable process in place, the data analysis and simulation cycle time will be substantially reduced, and the application of model-based development will result in more formal definition and standardization of the drug development process, avoiding errors induced by faulty "one-of-a-kind" development plans. Last, data analysis process standardization will result in high-quality, consistent results across disciplines, allowing new discoveries through currently unrealized interdisciplinary synergy.

13.3. Challenges in the Delivery of M&S Results

The current processes for implementing a pharmacometric analysis have, for the most part, developed spontaneously from the ad hoc application of M&S activities. Historically, these applications have been selected based on the inclinations of individual drug development team leaders, and the result has been the lack of a formal connection to the larger drug development enterprise. The importance of M&S in a specific drug development program is often not clear at the beginning of a program when prospective planning can be implemented. The necessary data can be difficult to locate, and, often, the key data required for modeling are not available until the traditional efficacy and safety analyses have been completed.[27] The data assembly and scrubbing process is required to identify unusable data, often resulting in high discard rates, including the data that the development team so carefully generated. This process can be remarkably time-consuming, even delaying completion of M&S activities.[28] Furthermore, significant resistance to the use of M&S findings in decision making can be encountered because of unfamiliarity on the part of the development team with interpretation of the results and the urgent timelines of the development program.

These disconnects, generated when M&S activities are overlaid onto traditional development programs rather than being integrated into them, are an important source of the challenges to providing timely and relevant analysis results. Specifically, these challenges stem from the unmet process, informatics, and systematic needs of an MBDD program and represent critical obstacles to the delivery of timely results.[4]

13.3.1. Systematic Needs

There are three key sources of variability that affect the characteristics of a pharmacometric model and the nature of the results. The first source of variability relates to inherent characteristics of the drug and the extent to which they are known through previous experience with the compound itself or a class of similar compounds.

The second source of variability relates to the fact that the current implementation of M&S is executed more as art than science. This source of work product variability stems from M&S approaches that are driven by preference and experience rather than an objective analytic science based on industry- and regulatory agency–acceptable standards.

The third source of variability is the lack of sufficient data standards and data definitions, both within the individual projects and within the industry. Lack of such proper data definitions can result in the exclusion of much existing legacy data from analysis because of the time and expense associated with data normalization. It can also result in the exclusion of some of the data experimentally derived by the drug development program because of incompatibility of study conditions not easily addressed via modeling efforts.

These three sources of variability are commonly not differentiated, with the unfortunate effect of making each M&S project appear to be a unique creation of art rather than an instance of a systemic process. Although there is little that can be done about the inherent characteristics of a drug, minimizing the effects of unnecessary variability attributable to art versus science and establishing informatics standards specific to pharmacometric data are key to improving the efficiency, effectiveness, and acceptance of pharmacometric analyses. Pharmacometric models should appropriately reflect the unique drug absorption, distribution, metabolism, and excretion characteristics of a given compound, but the process for analyzing the data and using the modeling results should be the same across compounds.

This is why the application of M&S during the discovery phase is so important – it allows for the identification of the most productive lines of investigation so that the team can identify and understand the important sources of variability in outcome, thus reducing the chances of unexpected failed trials in later stages of development.

13.3.2. Informatics Needs

Informatics required for pharmacometric analysis encompasses a wide range of data types, including data from the franchise disease–drug model, information about the drug concentration–time data, covariates, preclinical and clinical biomarkers, clinical outcome data, and data from many other sources. Informatics in this regard includes, but is not limited to, metadata (e.g., specification of the structure and content of required data sets), prospectively defined data management and analysis plans, programming requirements and specifications, validation requirements, and the information to be used for guiding the content and format of the presentation of results.[26]

Informatics will eventually come to be recognized as a critical determinant of effectiveness and productivity, although it is not yet recognized as such by many of the stakeholders involved in the pharmacometrics process today. Each of the subtasks involved in the pharmacometrics process has special needs with respect to the informatics that must be explicitly defined to improve the performance of that task.

The lack of informatics to support the data management and programming tasks required for the preparation of analysis-ready data sets for pharmacometric analysis has emerged as a critical problem. Unlike traditional statistical analyses, pharmacometric analyses frequently use pooled data arising from multiple studies during various phases of drug development. It is not uncommon for data from multiple Phase 2 and 3 clinical trials to be combined for a pharmacometric analysis, particularly at the end of a large development program. These data-pooling efforts require heretofore unavailable definition data to specifically support this task.

In recent years, there has been considerable effort to improve the informatics available for the drug development process. One such effort is the Clinical Data Interchange Standards Consortium (CDISC), an open, multidisciplinary, nonprofit organization, the goal of which is to establish industry standards to support the electronic acquisition, exchange, submission, and archiving of clinical trial data and metadata for medical and biopharmaceutical product development.[29] In large measure, the initiatives that have been undertaken have focused on standardizing vocabulary, formats, and submission specifications of clinical trial data specifically from the perspective of traditional statistical analysis and database design. Although this effort has been significant, the initiative has not yet addressed the specialized needs of pharmacometric analyses. For example, current study data tabulation domain models do not cover the production of analysis data sets for population PK analysis.[29,30]

13.3.3. Process Needs

The performance of M&S activities and the appropriate interpretation of the results require the cooperation of a diverse group of scientists, statisticians, pharmacometricians, clinical pharmacologists, clinicians, and others. These groups have traditionally functioned independently, and the current operating milieu at most pharmaceutical companies is not geared for the synchronization of their activities in performing a pharmacometric analysis because the companies are typically organized by specialty discipline colocated with others of the same discipline working on different projects (functional departments) rather than by a colocated, multidisciplinary, integrated project team (IPT) all working on the same project. Many industries requiring complex development and design activities have now recognized that IPTs provide a much more focused and coordinated approach to the development process and produce higher quality, more timely results.[31]

As the demand for M&S techniques has continued to increase, there has been a growing urgency to expand and reorganize the role of pharmacometrics in the drug development project team. Some companies have already embraced this change, but it needs to become a widespread practice. Formation of a colocated drug development project team, which includes pharmacometricians, will improve the working environment by addressing obvious operational obstacles, such as early specification of the franchise disease–drug model and the corresponding data requirements. These challenges highlight the need for a formalization of the pharmacometrics process and its critical tasks. Full integration of the pharmacometrician into the drug development team and formalization of processes with defined accountabilities, responsibilities, and lines of communication are required to achieve desired levels of productivity and impact.

13.4. Next Steps

The foregoing discussion of the needs of an MBDD paradigm highlights the ongoing operational challenges that must be addressed if M&S results can be applied reliably in decision making. No improvement can be expected if we simply increase demands on the existing ad hoc process. Importantly, these needs also indicate that simple solutions, such as the hiring of additional scientists and support staff, are unlikely to yield successful and sustainable results. Successfully addressing these issues will require a rigorous effort to transform pharmacometrics from an ad hoc activity to one that is formally integrated into the R&D life cycle.[9]

The high degree of complexity of the interactions between the stakeholders involved in generating, interpreting, and applying M&S results creates a challenge for the successful design of a functional operational process and its requisite informatics infrastructure. Other scientific and development-based industries have used the disciplines encompassed by enterprise engineering, namely systems engineering,[32] strategic management,[33] informatics,[26] systematics,[34] and ontology,[35] to improve their enterprise processes, and therefore, their competitiveness significantly.

In the two sections that follow, we describe a series of initiatives, based on the disciplines encompassed by enterprise engineering, to improve the quality and productivity of the pharmacometrics process. The first set of initiatives speaks to changes in the way drug development teams and the pharmacometrics group are constituted, governed, and improved. The second set of initiatives provides an approach to overcoming the informatics deficiencies of the current process. The overarching goals of these initiatives are as follows:

- To significantly reduce the flow times associated with provisioning and performing M&S activities for MBDD;
- To increase the quality and consistency of M&S results and work products;

- To improve the effectiveness of M&S results as a basis for recommendations for selecting drug development targets and improving the probability of successful drug development and regulatory and commercialization decision making; and
- To provide the foundation for developing a suite of analytic, communications, and publishing tools to enhance pharmacometrics productivity.

The implementation of these initiatives will result in a pharmacometric process that functions more effectively in the short term while laying the groundwork for future initiatives to further the transition to model-based development. Perhaps the most important aspect of this transition is the idea that the model will drive the development program design and decision making rather than follow along as a supportive function.

13.4.1. Strategies for Improving the Quality and Productivity of the Pharmacometrics Process

13.4.1.1. Implement IPTs

In the proposed organizational structure for MBDD, the core operational unit is the colocated IPT, which includes pharmacometricians as a key team participant in all phases of the project. Ideally, the IPT would be organized around a long-term, problem-centered drug development program. Each team would be responsible for all work in the therapeutic area and could expand (or contract) as necessary to handle the workload.

Proper integration of the benefits of M&S activities into the drug development IPT and appropriate interpretation of the M&S results require the cooperation of a diverse group of scientists, including statisticians, pharmacometricians, clinical pharmacologists, and clinicians, as well as IT specialists, medical writers, and other support personnel, as required by the scope of the development program.

13.4.1.2. Perform Design Reviews at Critical Milestones

Design reviews (DRs) represent a comprehensive, structured, and disciplined approach to evaluating project progress and the efforts conducted to resolve issues that arise during all phases of a drug development program (discovery, development, approval, and production).[36] As a control system for project execution, DRs provide for the assessment and review of project progress; traceability of technical, strategic, and scientific inputs and changes; integration of data and new knowledge; configuration management (the task of identifying, organizing, and controlling modifications to the project design baseline); and risk management (the process of making decisions under uncertainty, while meeting cost, schedule, and quality requirements during the completion of a project). DRs are used during either small- or large-scale projects to demonstrate that required decision points have been carefully considered before proceeding beyond critical events and key program milestones. Implementation of the DR process will also serve to highlight gaps requiring continued core competency development and to define core curriculum elements to provide additional training. In addition to the relevant team members, senior management and senior nonproject scientific staff should also attend such DRs to provide feedback, assist in decision making, and further ensure consistency of scientific approach and data definitions for franchise disease–drug models between programs.

Examples of two types of DRs include the Preliminary Design Review (PDR) and the Base Model Design Review (MDR). The PDR, conducted at the conclusion of the exploratory analysis phase, is intended to determine whether the initial analysis plan is executable, based on the presentation of evidence that key assumptions are met, with acceptable risk in terms of the agreed-upon cost, quality, and scheduling requirements. The MDR is conducted to verify that the base structural model meets the requirements of the analysis. It ensures that technical problems and design anomalies have been resolved, checks the technical performance measures of the base model, and ensures that the early results justify the decision to complete the remainder of the analysis plan.

13.4.1.3. Implement a Lean Six-Sigma Approach to Process Improvement

During the development of the analysis plan and specification of analysis and data assembly requirements, the pharmacometrician and other members of the IPT should focus on three questions: (1) What are the requirements of the analysis? (2) What data are needed to perform an analysis that will meet these requirements? (3) What data are actually available for inclusion in the analysis? It is important to recognize that the process of answering these questions must for several reasons be iterative because the requirements for an analysis will likely change over time, the development team or regulatory agency may raise new questions, new findings and understandings may emerge, and new data may become available as the development program matures.

In the process of developing answers to these questions, a series of more specific questions are formulated as the pharmacometrician and members of the IPT go back and forth to clarify issues and resolve uncertainties. This cycle of questioning, assessment, and discussion inherent in the current manual – and largely experiential – process is a valuable source of information about the fundamental entities and relationships invoked by pharmacometric analysis.

Figure 13.2 illustrates how a broad-based initiative to perform a systematic analysis of pharmacometric processes and work products can be

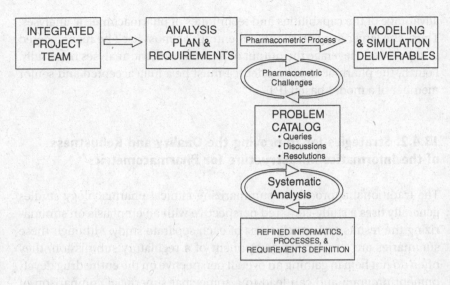

Fig. 13.2 Strategy for systematic analysis of pharmacometric challenges to continuously improve pharmacometric processes and work products. Reprinted with permission from Grasela TH, Fiedler-Kelly J, Cirincione BB, Hitchcock D, Reitz KE, Sardella S, et al. (2007). Informatics: the fuel for pharmacometric analysis. AAPS J. 9(1), E84–E91.

superimposed on existing pharmacometrics processes in such a way as to improve the delivery of M&S results. The challenges in performing these M&S activities, including data set assembly, can yield a rich catalogue of the problems currently faced by an MBDD IPT. Coupled with a critical consideration of CDISC and other standards, these data would provide a basis on which to improve the performance of subtasks, such as data assembly; provide needed insight into future CDISC improvements for pharmacometrics; and create functional specifications for future software development to facilitate pharmacometric analysis.

13.4.1.4. Implement Training Programs for Scientists and Support Staff

The pharmacometrics analysis process is growing increasingly sophisticated, and stakeholders are placing an increased emphasis on the results as a basis for decision making. The ability to perform these analyses with the requisite level of timeliness, quality, and sophistication creates the need for identifying personnel who have appropriate levels of scientific, technical, and business skills.

Training for such scientists and their support staff must encompass not only the technical and scientific aspects of pharmacometric analysis but also begin to develop the skills required for assessing and balancing risk, performance, schedule, and cost considerations in developing innovative study designs and contributing to the future redesign of the upstream and downstream processes.[37]

Properly trained scientists will be key to the successful implementation of model-based development for four reasons. First, there is a need to design the operating environment based on the comparative performance and capabilities of various strategies for performing M&S activities. Second, specific drug development programs must be designed to take full advantage of the capabilities and techniques of pharmacometric analyses. Third, the larger drug development enterprise must itself be reengineered to support and leverage the output of pharmacometric analyses more fully. Fourth, the pharmacometric scientist must be a fully accepted and senior member of a model-based IPT.

13.4.2. Strategies for Improving the Quality and Robustness of the Informatics Infrastructure for Pharmacometrics

The traditional approach to summarizing clinical pharmacology studies generally uses a study-centered perspective with an emphasis on summarizing the results and conclusions of each separate study. Although these summaries are a necessary component of a regulatory submission, they often do not help in gaining an overall perspective on the entire drug development program and can lead to a somewhat superficial comparison of study results. For example, a table of mean PK parameter estimates across studies can result in multiple estimates of drug half-life that may not be comparable because of study conditions or targeted patient populations, thus precluding an appropriate estimate of an overall population mean value or an understanding of the sources of variability. Moreover, a knowledge base derived from this study-centered approach necessarily relies on the key findings of specific studies to define key results. For example, the estimate of drug half-life in an elderly population may be obtained from a single age–gender study. Consequently, PK data collected in other studies that might contribute to a more representative estimate of the half-life, as well as the magnitude of interindividual variability across an elderly patient population, are underutilized or wasted.

We can anticipate that regulatory submissions and regulatory review will continue to require deeper levels of summarization and synthesis of outcomes across studies.[38] This synthesis will likely involve M&S techniques to perform pooled analyses and extrapolate and interpolate, as appropriate, for various decision-making purposes. Importantly, the all-or-none approach to risk–benefit assessments will give way to more granular risk–benefit assessments and the design of risk mitigation strategies that take into consideration the risk profile of individual patients or subpopulations of patients.[39]

At the same time, the mostly empirical PK and PD models currently used for these analyses are likely to become even more complicated and mechanistic. These models will evolve into the previously described franchise disease–drug models and incorporate the details of intermediary effects of the drugs into various aspects of the disease process. This trend is spurred on by both the proliferation of biomarker data, improvements in study design, data collection strategies, and bioassay technologies and the desire among the development teams to move beyond empirical and superficial descriptions of exposure–response relationships to gain insight into the various factors that influence a disease process or its severity.[25]

There are emerging concerns about the time and effort required to build complex models and about the subsequent costs of maintaining the models so that they can be leveraged for future purposes. Clearly the advantages of these complex models and the value realized across the life cycle of drug development and commercialization must outweigh these costs to justify the effort to senior management. Consequently, it is important to develop an efficient and systematic process that can determine the scope, resource requirements, and probability of success for the franchise disease–drug model.[40]

13.4.3. A Systematic Process for Assessing Franchise Disease–Drug Model Feasibility

An assessment of the feasibility of a complex model development or refinement effort, such as a model for neurohormonal control of blood glucose in diabetes, has three components. First, the mathematical equations required to describe the posited interrelationships adequately must be understood. Second, the extent of knowledge in the published literature on the various aspects of the model and the attendant data requirements must be defined. Finally, the quality and quantity of data available for the M&S effort for a particular development program must be ascertained. This latter component must take into consideration completed studies as well as those in progress and expected to be completed by decision-making milestones. A systematic assessment of each of these components entails the following steps:

1. Perform a literature review to identify published variants, if any, of a franchise disease–drug model for the targeted disease or drug effect.

    To develop a disease model, we need to consider the underlying physiologic relationships, the pathophysiologic alterations due to disease process, and the influence of drug therapy. We also need to consider the types of models that have been previously reported and develop an understanding of the differences and gaps between these previous models and the current development scenario for which a model is sought. It is important to recognize that various authors of published models handle components of the model differently – in part because of the varied quality and quantity of available data, which undoubtedly has an impact on the results and their interpretation. Consequently, parameter estimates of specific model components may not be informative in future model-building efforts due to differences in the extant knowledge and data behind the estimates.

2. Perform an inventory of available preclinical and clinical studies and create and populate a study index database to guide data selection for the model-building effort.

    The study index provides a listing of the studies available to contribute data to a modeling effort as well as pertinent information about the study designs. This latter content entails the development of a taxonomy to characterize the study conditions, subject characteristics, interventions, and comparators used in each study. For example, the taxonomy might differentiate the use of single or multiple dosing, intensive or sparse PK sampling strategy, and the types of endpoints measured (e.g., postprandial glucose measurements, insulin secretion rates). An important piece of information that is often underappreciated is the nature of study-specific investigations such as the type of test meal administered for investigations of postprandial glucose response. The timing and nature of these interventions is a critical determinant of the value of these data in a modeling effort. The study index database is useful in sorting out inconsistencies in the interventions that might render the data incompatible with the modeling goals.

3. Create and populate cross-study database(s) for each physiologic endpoint for an exploratory graphical analysis.

    A database consisting of the pooled data for the endpoints of interest must be assembled. Typically, data are stored in separate data files associated with a specific study. The metadata available for these data typically presume that an analysis will focus on the study-specific data as a separate entity. Consequently, considerable effort is required to find the information necessary to assess the poolability of such data. In addition, the data must be conditioned for use in a modeling effort, which generally involves creating a time-ordered sequence of events of interest.

4. Perform a gap analysis on the desired model versus the available data to guide future studies and formalization efforts.

    This step consists of a series of exploratory graphical analyses and simulations with a core model to assess model feasibility and define the conditions of use for the model. These graphical displays also play an important role in the development of the mathematical equations used in programming the model, including guiding the functional form of the equations and setting initial parameter estimates.

    A model for blood glucose control posits certain relationships that should exist if the model is a reasonable representation of diabetes. A review of composite data can provide evidence that the posited relationships do or do not exist. After the information in the study index and comparative assessment databases has been assembled, a series of exploratory graphical displays can be created to provide cross-study assessment of key relationships. Figure 13.3 illustrates the relationships among the components of the model feasibility assessment process.

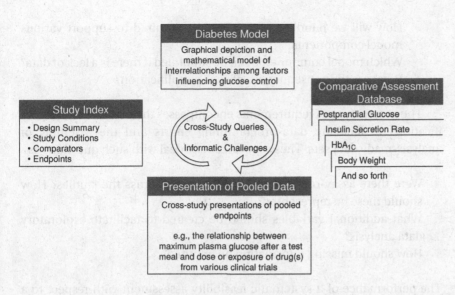

Fig. 13.3
The role of cross-study queries in helping to define informatic elements required to support complex model-building efforts.

There is an intricate relationship that arises when we consider the disease–drug model, the study index, and the pooled databases of the endpoints. This relationship is complex because there are many relationships of interest, all interacting with one another in complex and perhaps poorly understood ways. Because studies are currently not designed to specifically inform disease–drug models, the range of interventions in any one study, such as dose, may not cover the necessary range to support the modeling efforts. This is one of the key reasons for the need to pool data. The relationship is perplexingly detailed because the information required to pool data for a particular modeling effort may not be manifest until efforts are made at combining data and the modeling effort commences. For example, the need for a strategy to normalize nutritional intake across different studies becomes apparent when you recognize that one study used an oral glucose tolerance test, another used a test meal of a specific composition, and yet another used Similac (Abbott Laboratories. Abbott Park, IL) for the test meal.

5. Develop the analysis requirements and accompanying programming specifications for the data-assembly efforts.

    Analysis requirements are one of the critical pieces of information often misunderstood and undervalued in the process of summarizing and synthesizing information across the studies performed for a drug development program. Analysis requirements actually consist of at least two types. The first type encompasses the scientific requirements that drive the pharmacometric modeling efforts and deal with questions such as

    ■ What issues are to be addressed with the model?
    ■ What level of detail in the model structure is required?

- How will we handle gaps in the data required to support various model components?
- Which model components can be simplified if there is a lack of data?
- What are the consequences of such simplification?

The second type of requirements encompasses the programming specifications to facilitate data-programming efforts and the assembly of analysis-ready data sets. These specifications deal with such questions as

- Were there assay or formulation differences across the studies? How should these be represented?
- What additional variables should be created to facilitate exploratory data analysis?
- How should missing information be imputed?

The performance of a systematic feasibility assessment with respect to a specific franchise disease–drug model is illustrative of the gaps in informatics and the data generated from the development programs. It provides information that is valuable to

- Define the elements required for the modeling process,
- Identify sources of variability in critical measurements and interventions,
- Develop standards or limits to allowable variation, and
- Identify information important to future queries of composite data drawn from multiple studies.

This work can reduce the time and effort required to deliver results of the current modeling effort and can serve as a basis for formalizing future development program activities in terms of data collection, database design, study design, and technology deployment. The disciplined capture of this level of information would facilitate future assessments of the data. Perhaps more importantly, it would also help to ensure that unnecessary variability in study design or data collection has not crept into the studies that could have a negative impact on the compatibility of combining data for future M&S efforts.

13.4.4. Systematizing the Requirements Definition Management Process

The requirements of the drug development process encompass a wide range of inputs and a multitude of uses.[41] Properly defined requirements are critical to the workings of the many processes invoked in a drug development program and include the requirements for the M&S activities to ensure that the results are relevant to decision making, the programmer instructions for the assembly of analysis-ready data sets, and the necessary knowledge base required to secure regulatory approval and commercial success. Often, these processes are handicapped by a lack of systematically developed and clearly defined requirements, particularly in the early stages. Nowhere is this lack so obvious as in the initial selection of data for the franchise disease–drug model.

The process of specifying implies that the IPT must outline the goals of the modeling effort and define the information required to support decision making. The team must specify the data needed, drawing from the information provided in clinical study protocols or reports for the studies to be included in the analysis. These modeling requirements are then used to develop the modeling plans specifying the study conditions, key analysis variables, instructions for the preparation of analysis-ready data sets, and specifications for graphical and tabular outputs.

If the IPT can define project requirements in a way that allows some or all of the existing data from other investigations to be used, then the costs to the project in time and resources may be positively affected. This is why it is important to have all of the participants in the drug development program jointly develop the requirements. If the initial requirements definition effort shows that the prior data structures or analysis methodology of the existing franchise disease–drug model will not be sufficient for a clinical development program, the various IPT members can then define how the model should be updated and modified. This assessment of the need for model revision or modification, in turn, provides the scientist investigators with the ability to understand what additional data they must produce to allow such revision to take place and to include these requirements in their investigation plans and budgets.

As one example, to develop data for the franchise disease–drug model, the IPT must decide how to match its current data requirements with pre-existing data, such as drug concentrations, drug dosing histories, patient demography, laboratory data, use of concomitant medicines, and measures of efficacy and safety. These determinations will guide preclinical or clinical investigations in the near term through use of the outputs of the model, and they will also strongly influence downstream activities, such as the specification of the time-ordered sequence of events for each patient from the time of enrollment in a trial until its conclusion. Currently this information is often assembled by the pharmacometrician after the completion of clinical trials and therefore cannot affect the early design of the project's investigations.

Planning, forethought, and the benefit of experience are necessary to specify the requirements of the content and structure of the data sets to be consistent with the franchise disease–drug model. The investigating scientists must structure their experiments to produce necessary model data inputs. Minimally, requirements are based on content (variables to be included, definitions, and calculations) and structure (number of dosing history records, other physiological events).

Currently, requirements are often missing, incomplete, poorly communicated, ambiguous, and misinterpreted. These shortcomings in the requirements can lead to time-consuming rework to produce the desired data set. Regardless of the level of pharmacometric understanding of the person performing the investigation, an accurate and appropriate set of requirements is critical to achieving efficient, high-quality, and timely results for the development program.

The overall efficiency and quality of an M&S effort can be improved by systematizing the requirements definition process based on an understanding of the information required for unambiguous communications between IPT members. First, the common sources of miscommunication must be identified. Second, formalized model output specifications that meet the needs of scientists and programmers must be developed. Finally, a strategy for continually refining and expanding the comprehensiveness of the franchise disease–drug model must be implemented.

In our experience, the most common sources of confusion and error are ambiguities in the upstream clinical trial designs and the resulting laboratory investigations and database structure and content. These ambiguities can produce inconsistent requirements for the downstream programming efforts to work with dosing records, uncertainty regarding the composition of the analysis population, and confusion in the handling of concentration records and concomitant medication information.

By developing an understanding of the root causes of these ambiguities for franchise disease–drug models, new strategies can be implemented to improve the quality and robustness of the requirements specification process. This implementation process might include the development of dynamically linked databases that query the scientist and programmer to clarify ambiguities and address contingencies. The ongoing assessment of questions not yet addressed by the requirements specifications can serve as a continuous process improvement effort for further refinement of the requirements specification process.

13.5. Summary

The pharmaceutical industry is undergoing major structural change in several dimensions simultaneously, and these changes will completely transform the industry's fundamental business models, core processes, and socio-techno-logistical infrastructures. The accelerating shift from empirical to model-based methods and the growing reliance on M&S in decision making is forcing important and urgent changes to occur in the nature of the work of the drug discovery and development process. Effectively meeting the challenges of model-based drug discovery and development mandates the use of systematic and rigorous methods to consciously and deliberately engineer the process to ensure that it is fully capable of the timely delivery of effective results for decision-making purposes. Accordingly, requirements to establish or strengthen the pharmacometrics processes are also changing significantly.

Pharmacometrics is faced with a significant, but ephemeral, opportunity. The tools of pharmacometric analysis are sufficiently understood at the same time that the limitations of empirically based development are becoming more widely appreciated. Ad hoc implementations of the pharmacometrics process, however, incur a high risk of failure in the face of cost, quality, and schedule constraints. Only by envisioning and engineering a complete pharmacometrics process can the full promise of model-based development be realized.

13.6. References

1. U.S. Department of Health and Human Services, Food and Drug Administration. (2004). Innovation or stagnation: challenge and opportunity on the critical path to new medical products. Available at: http://www.fda.gov/Science Research/SpecialTopics/CriticalPathInitiative/CriticalPathOpportunities Reports/ucm077262.htm#intro

2. Lesko LJ. (2007). Paving the critical path: How can clinical pharmacology help achieve the vision? Clin. Pharmacol. Ther. 81(2), 170–177.

3. Critical path opportunity list. Available at: http://www.fda.gov/oc/initiatives/criticalpath/reports/opp_list.pdf

4. Sheiner LB. (1997). Learning versus confirming in clinical drug development. Clin. Pharmacol. Ther. 61(3), 275–291.

5. Grasela TH, Dement CW, Kolterman OG, Fineman MS, Grasela DM, Honig P, et al. (2007). Pharmacometrics and the transition to model-based development. Clin. Pharmacol. Ther. 82(2), 137–142.

6. Bhattaram VA, Bonapace C, Chilukuri DM, Duan JZ, Garnett C, Gobburu JV, et al. (2007). Impact of pharmacometric reviews on new drug approval and labeling decisions – a survey of 31 new drug applications submitted between 2005 and 2006. Clin. Pharmacol. Ther. 81(2), 213–221.

7. Bhattaram VA, Booth BP, Ramchandani RP, Beasley BN, Wang Y, Tandon V, et al. (2005). Impact of pharmacometrics on drug approval and labeling decisions: A survey of 42 new drug applications. AAPS J. 7(3), E503–E512.

8. Grasela TH, Fiedler-Kelly J, Walawander CA, Owen JS, Cirincione BB, Reitz KE, et al. (2005). Challenges in the transition to model-based development. Special Issue: Population Pharmacokinetics-A memorial tribute to Lewis Sheiner, M.D. 7(2), E488–E495. Available at: http://www.aapsj.org/default.asp

9. Grasela TH, & Dement CW. (2007). Engineering a pharmacometrics enterprise (pp. 903–924). In: The Science of Quantitative Pharmacology, edited by Ette EI, & Williams P. Hoboken, NJ: John Wiley & Sons, Inc.

10. Sheiner LB, & Steimer JL. (2000). Pharmacokinetic/pharmacodynamic modeling in drug development. Ann. Rev. Pharmacol. Toxicol. 40, 67–95.

11. Holford NH, Kimko HC, Monteleone JP, & Peck CC. (2000). Simulation of clinical trials. Ann. Rev. Pharmacol. Toxicol. 40, 209–234.

12. Wade JR, Edholm M, & Salmonson ST. (2005). A guide for reporting the results of population pharmacokinetic analyses: A Swedish perspective. AAPS J. 7(2), E456–E460.

13. U.S. Department of Health and Human Services, Food and Drug Administration. (1999). Guidance for industry: Population pharmacokinetics. Available at: www.fda.gov/downloads/Drugs/GuidanceComplianceRegulatory Information/Guidances/ucm072137.pdf

14. Gobburu JVS, & Lesko LJ. (2009). Quantitative disease, drug, and trial models. Ann. Rev. Pharmacol. Toxicol. 49, 291–301.

15. Landersdorfer CB, & Jusko WJ. (2008). Pharmacokinetic/pharmacodynamic modelling in diabetes mellitus. Clin. Pharmacokinet. 47(7), 417–448.

16. Rohatagi S, Carrothers TJ, Jin J, Jusko WJ, Khariton T, Walker J, et al. (2008). Model-based development of a PPARgamma agonist, rivoglitazone, to aid dose selection and optimize clinical trial designs. J. Clin. Pharmacol. 48(12), 1420–1429.

17. Danhof M, de Lange EC, Della Pasqua OE, Ploeger BA, & Voskuyl RA. (2008). Mechanism-based pharmacokinetic-pharmacodynamic (PK-PD) modeling in translational drug research. Trends Pharmacol. Sci. 29, 186–191.

18. de Winter W, DeJongh J, Post T, Ploeger B, Urquhart R, Moules I, et al. (2006). A mechanism-based disease progression model for comparison of long-term effects of pioglitazone, metformin and gliclazide on disease processes underlying type 2 diabetes mellitus. J. Pharmacokinet. Pharmacodyn. 33, 313–343.

19. Bergman RN, Ider YZ, Bowden CR, & Cobelli C. (1979). Quantitative estimation of insulin sensitivity. Am. J. Physiol. 236(6), E667–E677.

20. Turner RC, Holman RR, Matthews D, Hockaday TD, & Peto J. (1979). Insulin deficiency and insulin resistance interaction in diabetes: Estimation of their relative contribution of feedback analysis from basal plasma insulin and glucose concentrations. Metabolism. 28(11), 1086–1096.

21. de Gaetano A, & Arino O. (2000). Mathematical modelling of the intravenous glucose tolerance test. J. Math. Biol. 40, 136–168.

22. Silber HE, Jauslin PM, Frey N, Gieschke R, Simonsson US, & Karlsson MO. (2007). An integrated model for glucose and insulin regulation in healthy volunteers and type 2 diabetic patients following intravenous glucose provocations. J. Clin. Pharmacol. 47, 1159–1171.

23. Frey N, Laveille C, Paraire M, Francillard M, Holford NH, & Jochemsen R. (2003). Population PKPD modelling of the long-term hypoglycaemic effect of gliclazide given as a once-a-day modified release (MR) formulation. Br. J. Clin. Pharmacol. 55, 147–157.

24. Hamren B, Bjork E, Sunzel M, & Karlsson M. (2008). Models for plasma glucose, HbA1c, and hemoglobin interrelationships in patients with type 2 diabetes following tesaglitazar treatment. Clin. Pharmacol. Ther. 84, 228–235.

25. Krishna R, Schaefer HG, & Bjeffum OJ. (2007). Effective integration of systems biology, biomarkers, biosimulation, and modeling in streamlining drug development. J. Clin. Pharmacol. 47, 738–743.

26. Grasela TH, Fiedler-Kelly J, Cirincione B, Hitchcock D, Reitz K, Sardella S, et al. (2007). Informatics: The fuel for pharmacometric analysis. AAPS J. 9(1), E84–E91.

27. Antal EJ, Grasela TH Jr, & Smith RB. (1989). An evaluation of population pharmacokinetics in therapeutic trials. Part III. Prospective data collection versus retrospective data assembly. Clin. Pharmacol. Ther. 46(5), 552–559.

28. Grasela TH, Antal EJ, Fiedler-Kelly J, Foit D, & Barth B. (1999). An automated drug concentration screening and quality assurance program for clinical trials. Drug Inf. J. 33, 273–279.

29. Clinical Data Interchange Standards Consortium (CDISC), http://www.cdisc .org/about/index.html

30. CDISC SDTM pharmacokinetic domains: Individual subject drug concentrations (PC) and parameters (PP). Available at: http://www.cdisc.org/models/ sdtm/v1.1/Pharmacokinetic_Domains.zip

31. Gryna FM. (1988). Quality improvement (pp. 22.1–22.74). In: Juran's Quality Control Handbook, Fourth ed. edited by Juran JM. New York: McGraw-Hill, Inc.

32. Blanchard BS, & Fabrycky WJ. (1998). Systems Engineering and Analysis. Upper Saddle River, NJ: Prentice-Hall, Inc.

33. David FR. (1999). Strategic Management Concepts. Upper Saddle River, NJ: Prentice-Hall, Inc.

34. Mayr E. (1982). The Growth of Biological Thought: Diversity, Evolution, and Inheritance. Cambridge, MA: The Belknap Press of Harvard University Press.

35. Smith B. (2003). Ontology (pp. 155–166). In: Blackwell Guide to the Philosophy of Computing and Information, edited by Floridi L. Oxford, UK: Oxford Blackwell.

36. Gryna FM. (1988). Product Development (pp. 13.1–13.78). In: Juran's Quality Control Handbook, Fourth ed. edited by Juran JM. New York: McGraw-Hill, Inc.

37. Rechtin E, & Maier M. (1997). Social Systems (pp. 75–86). In: The Art of Systems Architecting, edited by Bahill T. Boca Raton, FL: CRC Press.

38. Lesko L, & Williams RL. (1999). The question-based review: A conceptual framework for good review practices. Appl. Clin. Trials. 8, 56–62.

39. Woodcock J. (2007). The prospects for "personalized medicine" in drug development and drug therapy. Clin. Pharmacol. Ther. 81, 164–169.

40. Cirincione B, Blasé E, Cummings M, Fineman MSD, & Grasela TH. (2008). Model feasibility assessment as a driver for model-based drug development. Presented at the American Society of Clinical Pharmacology and Therapeutics 109th Annual Meeting, April, Orlando, FL. Clin. Pharmacol. Ther. 83(Suppl 1), S588.

41. Bahill T, & Dean FF. (1999). Discovering system requirements (pp. 175–219). In: Handbook of Systems Engineering and Management, edited by Sage AP, & Rouse WB. New York: John Wiley & Sons, Inc.

Embracing Change: A Pharmaceutical Industry Guide to the 21st Century

Mervyn Turner

14.1. Introduction

> The art of progress is to preserve order amid change and to preserve change amid order.
> – Alfred North Whitehead, 1861–1947

With its focus on applying the latest in medical science to deliver products to address unmet medical need, change in the modern pharmaceutical industry is fueled by the need to drive innovation in search of the next therapeutic product. Historically, pharmaceutical companies have themselves led the way in medical research by using knowledge generated through internal basic research programs or licensed from academic institutions to develop products that would in turn fuel the next generation of drugs. This leadership position was solidified by the substantial capital and infrastructure requirements of the drug development process that created significant barriers to entry for others. Academic institutions and small companies generally lacked the expertise, infrastructure, and financial resources to engage in drug discovery and development. As a result, these groups had few options for advancing or realizing the value of their own scientific breakthroughs beyond licensing to a company that had the capabilities to transform scientific discoveries into therapeutic products. Consequently, the pharmaceutical industry was the primary innovator of biomedical science for most of the second half of the 20th century.

The advent of molecular biology, the Bayh–Dole act, and increasing recognition by entrepreneurs of the potential upside of innovative drugs spawned the biotechnology revolution. Suddenly, individuals from academic backgrounds empowered with new technologies were able to make important scientific breakthroughs using tools that were more widely accessible – it was "the democratization of drug discovery." There were new sources of competition, both for innovative discoveries and for licensing cutting-edge technologies. The early days of the biotechnology revolution provided fledgling companies with an edge over established pharmaceutical companies in the area of biologic and large-molecule therapies. More recently, the expansion of targeted therapies to include small molecule compounds has played to the established strength of big pharma, further democratizing the drug development process.

In addition, competition from generic drug companies began to accelerate following passage of the Hatch–Waxman act in 1984.[1] At the same time, increasing health care costs led managed care organizations to use their formularies as both an economic tool for excluding newer and more costly drugs and as a negotiating tool for demanding price concessions from manufacturers. Concurrently, the pharmaceutical industry entered a period of declining productivity, driven in large part by its own success in innovating therapies for diseases with clear-cut etiologies and treatment paradigms that essentially made differentiated new drugs more difficult to discover and develop. In the ongoing search for new blockbusters, pharmaceutical companies turned to more complex, high-risk diseases, which necessitated greater investment in research, extended the development timeline, and increased development and commercialization risk. Not only did these extended development times increase the cost of bringing new products to market, they also had the effect of shortening their patent life and therefore their revenue-generating period of exclusivity. Thus, even as development costs, time, and risk increased, replenishing research and development (R&D) investments became more challenging.

To address slowing productivity, pharmaceutical companies initially sought the most rapid path to accessing new technologies and novel drug candidates, leading to a wave of industry mergers (see Figure 14.1). These mergers failed to ignite productivity, which remains down even as sales and R&D spending dollars have increased. Moreover, the number of new molecular entities (NMEs) approved today is down slightly over the same period.[2] Only 19 new drugs or vaccines were approved in 2007, the lowest numbers since 1983. On average, it continues to take 10 to 15 years and more than $800 million to develop a single new medicine.[3] On the basis of our observations, we estimate that the top of the spending range is approaching $2 billion. This large increase is also compounded by an increase in regulatory requirements, particularly the need for pre- and postregistration studies designed to assess patient outcomes over the longer term. As an example, in July 2008, the U.S. Food and Drug Administration's (FDA's) Endocrinologic and Metabolic Drugs Advisory Committee recommended that new diabetes drugs should be evaluated in cardiovascular outcomes studies.[4] The panel voted in favor of a requirement to conduct a long-term trial or provide equivalent evidence to rule out an unacceptable cardiovascular risk for diabetes drugs that show no cardiovascular safety signals in Phase 2 or 3 studies.

In summary, a confluence of internal and external factors is now transforming the landscape for discovering, developing, commercializing, and

Large Pharma Consolidation – from 23 to 8

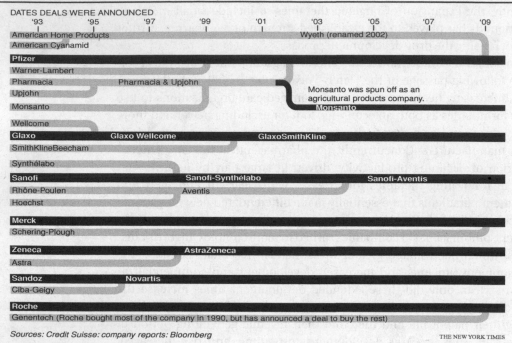

Fig. 14.1
Overview of industry mergers since 1993.

marketing pharmaceuticals, and the old rules simply no longer apply to an industry now facing (1) pressure to increase sales, (2) pressure to decrease development time and cost, (3) competition from smaller companies, (4) looming patent expirations, (5) increased regulatory scrutiny, and (6) unparalleled pricing pressures. Companies now need to embrace two critical realities.

14.1.1. Toward a New Paradigm of Drug Development

As yet, there is no evidence that increasing the number of programs entering clinical development drives a corresponding increase in late-stage trials or drug approvals. In fact, the number of product candidates in Phase 3 trials is largely unchanged since 1997.[5] The bottleneck is driven by the failure of many investigational therapies to demonstrate efficacy in Phase 2 trials. The high rate of failures in Phase 2 is a direct consequence of having an increasingly large number of candidate targets and a decreased capacity to fully validate the properties and clinical potential of any individual target. Failures in Phase 2 are mostly the result of an inherent flaw in the strategy of taking as many candidates forward as possible with minimal upfront investment in clinical validation. Rather than diversifying risk across multiple programs, this strategy has increased costs and the risk that an individual program will fail.

The high rate of candidate failures in Phase 2 appears to be a direct outcome of the 20th-century drug development paradigms. If the pharmaceutical industry is to regain its prominence in advancing human health, companies need to take a leadership position in establishing a wholly new, agile, and pragmatic approach to delivering differentiated drugs to the market. Critically, this process must incorporate effective decision making to identify candidates with a high probability of success earlier in the development process to relieve the burden of late-stage failure.

14.1.2. Embracing Democratization: Partner or Perish

The democratization of drug discovery has lowered the barrier to initiating Phase 1 trials, as evidenced by a two- to threefold increase in the number of compounds in Phase 1 trials and a similar increase in Phase 2 trials.[5]

14.2. Toward a New Paradigm of Drug Development: It's a State of Mind

As defined largely by regulatory agencies, the pharmaceutical process has routinely moved methodically from bench to bedside, identifying pharmacological activity and evaluating it in animal models before marching in orderly fashion through Phase 1 safety trials, Phase 2 trials designed to evaluate efficacy in small populations, and ultimately to pivotal Phase 3 trials. Drug candidates that failed along the way, for the most part, were placed on the shelf with little follow-up devoted to understanding the basis for failure.

Today's translational medicine approaches highlight the limitations of the old linear process, which was designed to reinforce existing hypotheses rather than to generate insight into clinically relevant interactions among drugs, targets, pathways, and disease. What we learn in the clinic now can – and must – inform our efforts in the laboratory. The path from bench to bedside has become a two-way street.

Translational medicine uses innovative, short-term clinical trials of small groups of human subjects to gain a preliminary assessment of pharmacological activity, efficacy, and safety of new chemical entities. Data from such trials should enable more rapid decision making earlier in the development process and make it possible to guide activities at the bench toward endpoints that truly matter at the bedside. Furthermore, such trials enable early identification of populations more likely to benefit from a specific compound, allowing stratification of downstream clinical trials in the hope of tailoring therapies effectively to improve the probability of success.

14.3. Fail Fast, Fail Cheap

Today's genomic technologies have made it relatively easy to identify disease-related targets and pathways that can be mapped and characterized. Critically assessing the clinical relevance of a target or drug candidate remains the industry's biggest bottleneck. For many years, the prevailing wisdom was to allocate the majority of development dollars to mid- and late-stage trials. After all, why make a significant investment in a program that might not advance beyond Phase 2? It made sense to ask this question a decade ago, when companies had only a handful of targets or lead candidates to consider. In today's environment, we need to ask different questions. Rather than considering the cost per program, companies need to evaluate their early-stage investments in the context of an entire product portfolio. Failing early is substantially less expensive than failing late, and investing in more intelligent early-stage evaluation will produce substantial returns if it increases the quality of the programs that advance, which will subsequently improve their probability of later stage success.

Moreover, it is time to reassess how the industry defines success or failure at the earliest stages of development. Can a preclinical or Phase 1 study be deemed a failure if it yields knowledge that informs the understanding of a target, compound, off-target interactions, disease biology, or clinical need? If such studies provide insight of important relevance to other programs within the portfolio and reduce the risk of failures in Phase 2 and Phase 3, do they not contribute to success?

Merck has embraced the concept of failing quickly and cheaply because it shortens the timeline and substantially reduces the risk for those programs that do move forward. This approach has helped the company to reduce its Phase 1 and 2 development timeline from the industry average of 3.7 years to 2.5 years.[6] Our early-stage R&D process uses technology and outsourcing to generate as much data as quickly and cost effectively as possible. Elements of the company's fail fast, fail cheap strategy are as follows:

1. Employing biomarkers and translational medicine to look at changes in gene expression, protein activity, or metabolites that may be indicative of efficacy, off-target interactions, or toxicity. Biomarker analyses provide additional insight into the activity of a target or compound, and oftentimes these data may be informative before clear evidence of clinical benefit or side effects can be determined. Small, short-term studies designed by Merck's experimental medicine team provide rapid feedback as to whether the data generated in preclinical

pharmacologic assays and efficacy models are consistent with clinical observations. This translational medicine approach has also been called proof of mechanism (POM) at some companies and represents an important decision point for the target, mechanism, and drug candidate (see Chapter 1). Although it may sound obvious that humans are not rodents, innumerable dollars have been spent pursuing programs that cure disease in animals but have limited benefit or demonstrate significant safety issues in humans. By using experimental medicine studies to get an early read on a drug candidate's pharmacologic profile and interactions with its target in humans, Merck is able to better guide its decision-making and investment process.

2. Incorporating more animal and human genetic studies early in the drug development process to better understand the role that potential targets play in the disease process and how they interact with other targets and pathways. These studies speak to target validation, can provide critical insight into interactions that might lead to unacceptable side effects or toxicities, and can help kill a program before it even enters the clinic. At Merck, we have pioneered the effective incorporation of integrative genomics into diverse development programs. Integrative genomics is a multistep procedure for identifying potential key drivers of complex traits that integrates DNA variation and gene-expression data with other complex trait data in defined populations. Ordering gene-expression traits relative to one another and with respect to other complex traits is achieved by systematically testing whether variations in DNA that lead to variations in relative transcript abundances statistically support an independent, causative, or reactive function in relation to the complex traits under consideration. This approach goes beyond the traditional whole genome-wide association studies that focus only on attempting to find the role of a single gene as a driver of disease traits. The end result is a much more complete and comprehensive view of the biology of the disease itself.

3. Conducting more extensive preclinical pharmacology and toxicology studies. Setting strict selection criteria at this stage of development may help to identify – and remove from the pipeline – those candidates that might be associated with clinically or commercially unacceptable dosing requirements, toxicities, or side effects.

4. Tapping into medicinal chemistry capabilities in emerging economies such as Asia to screen a greater number of candidates at a lower cost than could be achieved using internal resources. Asia – particularly China and India – has a large and expanding pool of scientists with strong chemistry and biology expertise, and many of them originally received training in the United States and Europe. Governments and entre-preneurs in Asia are dedicated to the growth of bioindustry, which has resulted in state-of-the art chemistry facilities and an R&D infrastructure that can be accessed for a fraction of the cost that U.S. and European companies would incur to build these resources.

14.4. Philosophy in Action: Merck's Clinical Pharmacology and Experimental Medicine Strategies

In both of the examples mentioned earlier in the text, the unifying principle between the subsidiary and Merck is the focus on the end goal of helping patients. Pursuing a portfolio mindset allows each employee to contribute to Merck's raison d'être in a manner that is both meaningful to the individual and beneficial to the company as a whole. In this context, it is less difficult to implement change and pursue new strategies because individuals retain a clear view of how their own work relates to and supports the company's overall success. Merck's transition to making experimental medicine a pillar of its research decision-making process demonstrates how a portfolio mindset can facilitate implementation and acceptance of wholly new processes and strategies.

In pursuing a philosophy of fail cheap, fail early, Merck was looking for technologies and processes that would allow it to kill compounds off faster and to be able to make go/no go decisions as early in development as possible. Merck established the Experimental Medicine department alongside our Clinical Pharmacology department to create tools that permit good choices earlier in the R&D process. Both teams can now use small, short-term clinical studies to provide early answers to important questions regarding pharmacological activity, efficacy, and safety of candidate drugs, including the following:

- Target engagement: How hard and how long is the target being hit?
- Proof-of-pharmacology: Does hitting the target elicit the intended biological effect?
- Biomarker (linkage to clinical outcomes) qualification: Are the resulting changes meaningful in the context of the disease?
- Disease mechanism: How do the clinical data enhance the understanding of disease pathways and development and use of disease models?

Drug candidates that failed to meet strict selection criteria in early experimental medicine studies would not advance.

Recently, U.S. and European regulators announced that they will accept data from seven new biomarker tests designed to assess kidney damage in animal studies of investigational therapies. Merck scientists worked collaboratively with colleagues at other companies to identify the markers and demonstrate their utility in detecting renal toxicity within hours of exposure to investigational drugs. These biomarkers are a significant advance over the standard assays for renal toxicity, which detect kidney damage at least 1 week after it has started.[7] The difference between hours and weeks can dramatically enhance early-stage development timelines and enable rapid elimination of compounds likely to cause renal toxicity, which is a common factor in late drug candidate failure.

Experimental medicine allows Merck to evaluate the efficacy and safety of drug candidates in Phase 0/1 using proof-of-concept platforms that provide reasonable certainty rather than absolute proof. Given the low probability of success of new mechanisms, experimental medicine enables Merck to interrogate as many mechanisms as possible while controlling R&D costs, for the savings associated with early decision making can be invested in more novel compounds. This translational medicine approach increases the chance that Merck will fulfill its vision of delivering innovative new medicines and vaccines that benefit patients. Merck has implemented translational medicine approaches in its oncology, neuroscience, cardiovascular disease, diabetes, obesity, bone, respiratory, immunology, and endocrinology programs. The benefits of the approach include the following:

- Increased capability to identify compound failures more quickly and cheaply earlier in development;
- Increased capability for better, faster, and more efficient assessment of proof of concept for new chemical entities;
- Increased probability of success;
- Reduced cycle times (i.e., ability to move more quickly between phases of clinical development); and
- Reduced costs.

In implementing a translational medicine approach to our R&D process, we have established a process that allows key decisions to be made in days or weeks instead of months or years without compromising commitment to patient safety. The portfolio mindset helped to create an environment in which finding a compelling rationale for taking something out of development is considered as valuable to the organization as demonstrating why it should move forward. In such an environment, the philosophy of failing fast and failing cheap can be embraced throughout Merck without fear that individuals or teams associated with failed products will be stigmatized. This change in mindset was essential to Merck's transition to establishing an environment in which translational medicine is incorporated across its development portfolio.

The cultural shift also facilitated the reallocation of financial and personnel resources from drug discovery to biomarkers and experimental medicine practices because the discovery teams recognized the value that these trials would bring to the portfolio as a whole. It also helped Merck's scientists transition from a decision-making process predicated on gathering data on every aspect of a compound or target to one based on more limited (but more clinically relevant) data. Rather than aiming for 100% analysis, decision makers now follow the "80/20 rule" in determining if a program merits continued investment. The power of translational medicine makes that 80% confidence level nearly as informative as 100% confidence based on less clinically relevant data. That 20% reduction can significantly decrease development time and costs because it enables the company to get into and out of Phase 1 and 2 development more rapidly. The uncommonly rapid development and tremendous market uptake of Merck's Januvia (sitagliptin) diabetes therapy demonstrates the benefits of this approach – particularly because the rapid timeline did not compromise the rigorous safety testing that is a critical component of all of Merck's development programs.

14.4.1. Embrace Democratization – Partner or Perish

Biology has become "open source," and pharmaceutical companies no longer control the resources and infrastructure for generating insight into disease and therapeutic strategies and advancing discoveries through the clinic. The emergence of a service industry that provides quality drug development resources outside of the pharmaceutical industry (including large compound libraries; state-of-the-art, high-throughput screening for both on- and off-target activities; standard absorption, distribution, metabolism, and elimination (ADME) testing capabilities; clinical research organizations; and pilot manufacturing facilities) has empowered individuals and institutions with innovative ideas, intellectual property, and financial backing to develop their own drug candidates rather than license technology to the pharmaceutical industry at an early stage. The ability to outsource most early-stage research functions has spurred an increase in the number of virtual companies, allowing inventors to remain engaged in advancing their own innovations at minimal cost. This democratization simultaneously expands competition at the early stages of drug development while reducing the pool of intellectual property that big pharma can license for its own development initiatives.

Rather than posing a competitive threat, democratization has created numerous and diverse opportunities for companies to tap into the entrepreneurial drive of these organizations while sharing both risk and reward. A growing number of companies and entrepreneurs have the resources to enter the development process, but few if any of these companies have the capital resources, physical infrastructure, or development expertise to undertake late-stage development and commercialization activities. Pharmaceutical companies still retain the vast amount of expertise and manufacturing capacity necessary for successful drug commercialization. The industry's ability to maintain its leadership in these areas rests on its ability to continue to convince earlier-stage companies and academic institutions that collaboration is a more compelling strategic option than pursuing commercial activities on their own. At Merck we say, "We know YOU do great science, so we want to partner with you!" Our mantra is "Combining our Strengths, Sharing our Successes."

Since the earliest days of the biotechnology industry, there was a need to establish pharmaceutical partnerships. Increasingly, business development strategies have become more sophisticated, and intellectual property continues to spawn biotechnology companies. Collaborations provide a biotechnology company with money and resources while providing the pharmaceutical company access to cutting-edge technologies. In addition, by collaborating with multiple partners, pharmaceutical companies today decentralize parts of their R&D activities. This decentralization provides a mechanism by which companies can (1) evaluate multiple new platform or product opportunities without increasing the size and cost of their own operations and (2) effectively increase the bandwidth of their operations.

Although collaborations at later product development stages may reduce the risk of product failure, such deals are usually characterized by less favorable economics. In the new era of fail fast, fail cheap, collaborations around early-stage products provide improved economics and an enhanced ability to rapidly evaluate and prioritize new technologies and products in the context of a company's overall asset portfolio. The success of any collaboration, however, is as dependent on a culture of accepting externally generated knowledge as it is on the performance of the technology or therapy itself.

14.4.2. Adapt Culture to Recognize the Benefits and Necessities of Diversifying Pathways to Knowledge

For most of its history, the pharmaceutical industry has had a severe case of "not invented here" syndrome, a reluctance to accept that external knowledge could be as or more valuable than internal research. Overcoming this philosophy was essential in an era during which the research contributions of any single company comprise less than 1/10 of 1% of collective biomedical research. Companies that devalue knowledge generated beyond their own walls do so at the peril of losing access to the vast majority of biomedical advances.

Recognizing the need to build and expand its connections to the greater research community, Merck made the strategic decision in 2000 to place greater emphasis on external research collaborations to supplement internal efforts.

14.4.2.1. Defining Areas of Internal and External Focus

Although Merck may have direct control of less than 1/10 of 1% of total biomedical research, the company has a track record of high standards and scientific excellence in broadly applied technologies. For example, Merck scientists have received worldwide recognition in the scientific community for the development and application of critical drug discovery and development tools in the areas of imaging and molecular profiling.

Structuring collaborations in a manner that empowers company scientists to focus on what they do best while enhancing their data-generating capabilities with external resources creates productive – rather than competitive – working environments. Celebrating the diversity of drug discovery opportunities while appreciating the company's unique resources has allowed us to be both an employer and a partner of choice for today's top scientists.

14.4.2.2. Identifying and Implementing Incentives That Encourage Scientists to Collaborate Effectively

Merck scientists have been charged with building a "virtual lab" by mounting the best scientific program in their area, whether it comes from internal research, external collaborations, or both. Several critical factors have enabled the successful execution of this strategy:

- Ensuring that Merck scientists receive equal incentives for work on internal and external programs;
- Creating an environment at the highest levels of the organizations that recognizes in-licensing proposals as a sign of innovation rather than internal deficits;
- Helping Merck scientists understand the needs, capabilities, and limitations facing scientists at our partner organizations; and
- Encouraging Merck scientists to recognize their scientific collaborators as equals with shared commitments to achieving mutual goals and objectives.

14.4.2.3. Building Expertise in Managing External Resources for Long-Term Productivity and Success (or, Put More Plainly, Play Well with Others So That They Will Want to Stay in Your Sandbox)

Recognize that any collaboration that interests you is likely to interest your competitors, and manage collaborations as you would any other competitive asset. Establish clear goals, objectives, and responsibilities for each team and the program as a whole and ensure that everyone has – or feels empowered to ask for – the resources needed to succeed.

In 2008, more than 65% of Merck's revenue was attributable to alliance products and patents (including 50% of all joint venture revenue; see Figure 14.2). In the past 8 years, Merck has established in excess of 300 collaborations with leading academic centers and biotechnology companies

Merck licensing strategy results in high-value alliances

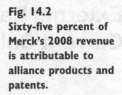

Fig. 14.2
Sixty-five percent of Merck's 2008 revenue is attributable to alliance products and patents.

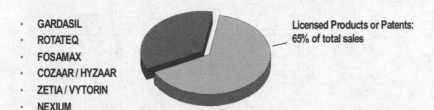

65% of Merck's 2008 revenue is attributable to alliance products and patents

- GARDASIL
- ROTATEQ
- FOSAMAX
- COZAAR / HYZAAR
- ZETIA / VYTORIN
- NEXIUM
- VARIVAX

Licensed Products or Patents: 65% of total sales

Revenue includes 50% of all JV revenue (Merck/Schering-Plough, Merial, Sanofi-Pasteur MSD, Johnson&Johnson °Merck)

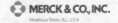

MERCK & CO., INC.
Whitehouse Station, N.J., USA

(see Figure 14.3). These collaborations have allowed the company to participate in breakthrough discoveries in important therapeutic areas, including Alzheimer's disease, ophthalmology, cancer, bone disease, and psychiatric disorders.

14.4.3. Advance Experimental Medicine through Acquisition and Partnering

In 2001, recognizing the potential power of applying molecular profiling technology across all of its research initiatives, Merck acquired Rosetta Inpharmatics. As with collaborations, successful management of acquisitions requires a culture that can accommodate new people, ideas, and processes. An acquiring company may own the physical and intellectual property assets of its latest purchase, but employees are free agents who can take critical institutional and technical knowledge with them if they are not provided appropriate incentives. Rosetta's genomics-focused technology platform has transformed our process of drug discovery from asking specific questions about a single target or disease state to evaluating diseases and therapies in the context of a complete biological system. The incorporation and continuing investment in this technology at our Boston location, as a critical component of Merck's fail fast, fail cheap approach to early-stage development, is a testament to the success of the acquisition. Moreover, today this technology forms a platform for ongoing collaborations with key scientific institutions such as the H. Lee Moffitt Cancer Center and

External Basic Research
Current Collaborations

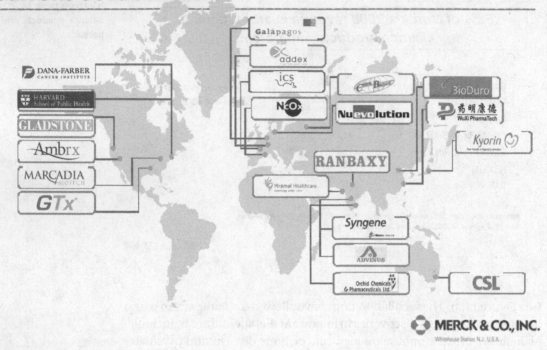

Fig. 14.3
A sampling of Merck's current External Basic Research collaborations.

the Dana–Farber Cancer Center, to apply the latest translational medicine approaches to drive cancer drug development.

Moffitt provides tumor samples excised from patients to Merck. We are then able to evaluate the biology of tumor samples in the context of clinical outcomes through the application of molecular profiling. Upon analysis of the samples, a detailed readout of the data is shared with Moffitt, where it is used internally for clinical research. In turn, Merck is able to use the clinical data associated with each sample. This collaboration is a pioneering approach to integrating medical data. The clinical data flow securely between Moffitt and Merck's clinical data repository on a customized network. Joint project teams made up of Merck and Moffitt clinical and basic researchers are together mining the shared data, designing experiments and trials, and identifying new mechanisms of action. This collaboration demonstrates how strong internal technologies can be used by leading internal and external researchers to enable leading edge science. The company is continuing its strong relationship with Moffitt and other external institutions to better integrate information and resources.

Merck's acquisition of GlycoFi exemplifies the benefits of partnership and acquisition. In December 2005, Merck established a broad strategic alliance and multiyear research collaboration with GlycoFi, a venture-backed platform technology company. The alliance provided Merck with access to GlycoFi's yeast-based glycoprotein optimization platform to develop novel biologic and vaccine drug candidates. Less than 6 months later, in May 2006, Merck acquired 100% of GlycoFi's equity, and the company became a wholly owned subsidiary. The strategic value of GlycoFi's patent estate and robust technology platform to Merck's long-term objective of discovering, optimizing, and developing novel biologic drugs to serve the needs of patients worldwide was self-evident and had been a driver for the initial collaboration. Yet, the positive and productive relationship that had been established in just a few short months was also a critical factor in the decision to make GlycoFi a part of Merck. The companies' complementary technologies have the potential to leapfrog Merck's vaccine and therapeutic protein development capabilities, but the relationships between Merck and GlycoFi scientists are the drivers for realizing that potential. Such excellent relationships were made possible by Merck's culture of valuing good science wherever it is done.

14.5. A Blueprint for Change

Charles Darwin observed that it is not necessarily the strongest or most intelligent that survive but those most responsive to change. The pharmaceutical industry stands at an important juncture facing patent expirations, increased generic competition, increasing regulatory standards, and decreasing profit margins. Those companies that embrace change by seizing the opportunity for innovation are more likely to thrive and evolve over the long term. Fundamentally, the ability to adapt to a new environment is as much a matter of state of the art as it is state of mind for the pharmaceutical industry. At Merck, we have established four pillars that support an environment for change:

1. Having a portfolio mindset that unifies all aspects of the organization because it creates a shared mark of success. Motivating individuals and teams to focus on the success of the portfolio rather than on that of a particular compound greatly facilitates continued prioritization and rationalization of the early-stage pipeline.
2. Redefining failure. A failed trial or program is really a success if it happens early enough to allow advancement of better programs and provides insight that can improve future development efforts.
3. Valuing quality science, regardless of its source.
4. Recognizing that owning part of a great product is ultimately more valuable than owning 100% of a failure.

These four pillars are applicable across diverse R&D models. With the advent of molecular biology as a critical component in the drug discovery and development process, pharmaceutical companies have generally pursued one of two divergent paths to commercial success. Some have opted to focus on specialty medicines for acute or serious diseases that have a clear molecular etiology, offer greater risk–benefit ratios, and have the potential to be used with a companion diagnostic test. Others continue to drive toward the challenge of the large, primary care markets in areas of major unmet medical need such as metabolic disease and the neurosciences.

A key driver in choosing the path of specialization is a belief in the power of personalized medicine. This belief derives from the simple but elegant logic of understanding the molecular basis for an individual's disease and matching treatment to a specific disease mechanism. Nowhere is this philosophy more apparent than in oncology, in which targeted therapies addressing cancer-related signaling pathways are transforming both the understanding and the treatment of disease. Cancer is, by any definition, a genetic disease that results from an accumulation of mutations in affected tissue. Consequently, if personalized medicine is likely to succeed anywhere, it will likely be in oncology.

Despite the logic on which personalized medicine is founded, and the expanding base of knowledge focused on how specific genes and pathways contribute to the development and progression of disease and response to therapy, success with this approach in major, primary care diseases has been frustratingly elusive. Although a small number of examples give hope that personalized medicine will play a transformative role in these widespread diseases, the path to achieving that transformation remains unclear. For example, diabetes patients are still segmented by the temporal stage of their disease and degree of insulin resistance even though these are symptoms of the disease rather than the underlying cause.

Another challenge is that, in many cases of primary care disease, the additional economic cost of molecular diagnostics may not be consistent with the approach to making treatment decisions. For example, the general agreement that selecting the right drug the first time is critical in treating cancer leads to a willingness to take on additional cost to make that possible. A different mindset, however, prevails in many primary care diseases. Decisions about hypertensive therapies are typically handled by trial and error without a sense of urgency to get it right the first time.

Thus, realizing the potential of personalized medicine in the treatment of primary care diseases will require not only scientific innovation but a transformation in mindset and a rejection of the trial-and-error approach to patient care. Critical to making this transformation is the adoption of a strategic developmental path informed by an ascending ladder of information on pharmacodynamic response, early indicators of how a drug affects pathophysiological mediators of disease, and true disease readouts. This data-driven, pragmatic readiness to kill all but the most clearly effective medicines stands as a new paradigm for those companies with the fortitude and the pockets to pursue it.

The industry-wide need for improved efficiency coupled with a growing demand among payers and physicians for demonstrable value will demand improved tools and strategies for matching patients with therapies. Although the industry continues to work hard to adapt to this new environment, a few early success stories have established new and better paths to success. Several products have provided a strong indication of how development times may be condensed. Using clinically relevant biomarkers early in development can dramatically shorten the timeline for late-stage trials, reduce the risk of clinical failures, and enable the development of new therapies. Early successes are at the leading edge of what must be a fundamental transformation.

14.6. References

1. Gilbert C, & Sarkar RG. (2005) Merck: Conflict and change. Harvard Business Review, May 2005.
2. Global pipelines quantified (2007). Merrill Lynch Research Report. August 23, 2007.
3. DiMasi JA, Hansen RW, & Grabowski HG. (2003). The price of innovation: New estimates of drug development costs. J. Health Econ. 22, 151–185.
4. Hughes S. (2008). FDA advisory committee recommends cardiovascular safety studies for diabetes drugs. The Heart.org, July 3, 2008.
5. Parexel International. (2007). Pharmaceutical R&D Statistical Source Book 2007/2008, edited by Mathieu MP. Waltham, MA: Parexel International.
6. CMR International, 2001–2005 (Major Company Median Comparison). June 2006.
7. FDA. (2008). European Medicines Agency to consider additional test results when assessing new drug safety. FDA News, June 12, 2008.

Printed in the United States
By Bookmasters